COMPANION HANDBOOK to

THE
CHEMOTHERAPY
SOURCE BOOK

COMPANION HANDBOOK to

THE
CHEMOTHERAPY
SOURCE BOOK

Michael C. Perry, MD, FACP
Professor of Medicine
Nellie B. Smith Chair of Oncology
Director, Division of Hematology/Medical Oncology
University of Missouri/Ellis Fischel Cancer Center
Columbia, Missouri

Clay M. Anderson, MD
Assistant Professor
Division of Hematology/Medical Oncology
University of Missouri/Ellis Fischel Cancer Center
Columbia, Missouri

Victoria J. Dorr, MD
Assistant Professor
Division of Hematology/Medical Oncology
University of Missouri/Ellis Fischel Cancer Center
Columbia, Missouri

John D. Wilkes, MD
Assistant Professor
Division of Hematology/Medical Oncology
University of Missouri/Ellis Fischel Cancer Center
Columbia, Missouri

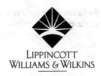

LIPPINCOTT
WILLIAMS & WILKINS

Editor: Jonathan W. Pine, Jr
Managing Editor: Molly L. Mullen
Project Editor: Ulita Lushnycky

351 West Camden Street
Baltimore, Maryland 21201-2436 USA

Rose Tree Corporate Center
1400 North Providence Road
Building II, Suite 5025
Media, Pennsylvania 19063-2043 USA

Printed in the United States of America

Library of Congress Cataloging-in-Publication Data

Companion handbook to the chemotherapy source book / Michael C. Perry . . . [et al.].
    p. cm.
    Companion v. to: The chemotherapy source book. 2nd ed. c1996.
    Includes bibliographical references and index.
    ISBN 0-683-30248-5
    1. Cancer—Chemotherapy—Handbooks, manuals, etc. I. Perry,
Michael C. (Michael Clinton), 1945– II. Chemotherapy source book.
    RC271.C5 C63 1998
    616.99'4061—ddc21

        98-42010
        CIP

The publishers have made every effort to trace the copyright holders for borrowed material. If they have inadvertently overlooked any, they will be pleased to make the necessary arrangements at the first opportunity.

To purchase additional copies of this book, call our customer service department at **(800) 638-0672** or fax orders to **(800) 447-8438.** For other book services, including chapter reprints and large quantity sales, ask for the Special Sales department.

Canadian customers should call **(800) 665-1148,** or fax **(800) 665-0103.** For all other calls originating outside of the United States, please call **(410) 528-4223** or fax us at **(410) 528-8550.**

Visit Williams & Wilkins on the Internet: http://www.wwilkins.com or contact our customer service department at **custserv@wwilkins.com.** Williams & Wilkins customer service representatives are available from 8:30 am to 6:00 pm, EST, Monday through Friday, for telephone access.

99 00 01 02 03
2 3 4 5 6 7 8 9 10

Preface

We have designed this handbook to accompany *The Chemotherapy Source Book*, with the idea that this volume may reside in the oncologist's pocket.

The book is divided into three sections. Section I deals with staging and treatment recommendations for hematologic malignancies and solid tumors, along with a separate list of chemotherapy programs, toxicity grading, and dose modifications.

Section II includes descriptions of currently used chemotherapeutic agents, listed alphabetically by generic name, altretamine through vinorelbine.

Section III includes our version of symptom control measures, presenting chapters on gastrointestinal complaints (e.g., anorexia, diarrhea, constipation, nausea, and vomiting), pain control, and miscellaneous other problems.

We would appreciate your comments and suggestions.

Michael C. Perry
Clay M. Anderson
Victoria J. Dorr
John D. Wilkes

Contributors

Clay M. Anderson, MD
Assistant Professor
Division of Hematology/Medical
　Oncology
University of Missouri
Ellis Fischel Cancer Center
Columbia, Missouri

Somasekhara Bandi, MD
Post-Doctoral Fellow
Division of Hematology/Medical
　Oncology
University of Missouri
Ellis Fischel Cancer Center
Columbia, Missouri

Victoria J. Dorr, MD
Assistant Professor
Division of Hematology/Medical
　Oncology
University of Missouri
Ellis Fischel Cancer Center
Columbia, Missouri

**Mary Johnson, MS, RN, CS, GNP,
　AOCN**
Nurse Practitioner
Division of Hematology/Medical
　Oncology
University of Missouri
Ellis Fischel Cancer Center
Columbia, Missouri

Irfan Maghfoor, MD
Post-Doctoral Fellow
Division of Hematology/Medical
　Oncology
University of Missouri
Ellis Fischel Cancer Center
Columbia, Missouri

**Deborah Morris, RN, MN, CS,
　GNP, AOCN**
Division of Hematology/Medical
　Oncology
University of Missouri
Ellis Fischel Cancer Center
Columbia, Missouri

**Michael C. Perry, MD,
　FACP**
Professor of Medicine
Nellie B. Smith Chair of
　Oncology
Director, Division of
　Hematology/Medical
　Oncology
University of Missouri
Ellis Fischel Cancer Center
Columbia, Missouri

Mohammed A. Raheem, MD
Post-Doctoral Fellow
Division of Hematology/Medical
　Oncology
University of Missouri
Ellis Fischel Cancer Center
Columbia, Missouri

Haleem J. Rasool, MD
Post-Doctoral Fellow
Division of Hematology/Medical
　Oncology
University of Missouri
Ellis Fischel Cancer Center
Columbia, Missouri

Nasir Shahab, MD
Post-Doctoral Fellow
Division of Hematology/Medical
　Oncology
University of Missouri
Ellis Fischel Cancer Center
Columbia, Missouri

John D. Wilkes, MD
Assistant Professor
Division of Hematology/Medical
　Oncology
University of Missouri
Ellis Fischel Cancer Center
Columbia, Missouri

Contents

Preface v
Contributors vii

Section One / **Therapy**
1/Staging Tables and Treatment Recommendations 3

A/HEMATOLOGIC MALIGNANCIES

Acute Lymphocytic Leukemia 3
Irfan Maghfoor and Victoria J. Dorr

Acute Myelogenous Leukemia 11
Irfan Maghfoor and Victoria J. Dorr

Chronic Lymphocytic Leukemia 16
Nasir Shahab and Victoria J. Dorr

Hairy Cell Leukemia 20
Nasir Shahab and Victoria J. Dorr

Chronic Myelogenous Leukemia 23
Nasir Shahab and Victoria J. Dorr

Myelodysplastic Syndromes 26
Irfan Maghfoor and Victoria J. Dorr

Plasma Cell Dyscrasias 32
Somasekhara Bandi and John D. Wilkes

Hodgkin's Disease 40
Irfan Maghfoor and John D. Wilkes

Non-Hodgkin's Lymphoma 47
Haleem J. Rasool and John D. Wilkes

B/SOLID TUMORS

Malignant Melanoma 57
Clay M. Anderson and John D. Wilkes

Adult Central Nervous System Tumors 65
John D. Wilkes

Head and Neck Cancer 70
John D. Wilkes

Thyroid Cancer 77
Victoria J. Dorr

Breast Cancer 84
Victoria J. Dorr

Lung Cancer   104
Mohammed A. Raheem and Victoria J. Dorr

Esophageal Cancer   113
John D. Wilkes

Gastric Cancer   118
John D. Wilkes

Pancreatic Cancer   122
John D. Wilkes

Neuroendocrine Tumors of the Gastrointestinal Tract   128
John D. Wilkes

Hepatobiliary Cancer   133
John D. Wilkes

Colorectal Cancer   143
John D. Wilkes

Anal Cancer   151
John D. Wilkes

Adrenal Gland Cancer   156
Victoria J. Dorr

Bladder Cancer   164
Victoria J. Dorr

Renal Cancer   170
Victoria J. Dorr

Prostate Cancer   175
Victoria J. Dorr

Penile Cancer   186
Victoria J. Dorr

Testicular Cancer   190
Victoria J. Dorr

Cervical Cancer   198
Victoria J. Dorr

Endometrial Cancer   205
Victoria J. Dorr

Gestational Trophoblastic Tumors   209
Victoria J. Dorr

Ovarian Cancer   214
Victoria J. Dorr

Ovarian Germ Cell Tumors   221
Victoria J. Dorr

Adult Soft Tissue Sarcomas   223
John D. Wilkes

Ewing's Sarcoma and Primitive Neuroepithelial Tumors   228
Victoria J. Dorr

Neuroblastoma 230
Victoria J. Dorr

Osteosarcoma 235
Victoria J. Dorr

Retinoblastoma 238
Victoria J. Dorr

Rhabdomyosarcoma 241
Victoria J. Dorr

Wilm's Tumor 246
Victoria J. Dorr

Cancer of Unknown Primary Origin 250
Nasir Shahab and John D. Wilkes

AIDS-Related Malignancies 255
John D. Wilkes

2/Chemotherapy Programs 265
Victoria J. Dorr, John D. Wilkes, and Deborah Morris
AIDS-Related Malignancies 265
Breast Carcinoma 268
Carcinoma of Unknown Primary Site 275
Endocrine Tumors 276
Gastrointestinal Neoplasms 277
Genitourinary Cancers 291
Gynecological Cancers 300
Head and Neck Cancers 308
Leukemia 310
Lung Cancers 321
Lymphoma 327
Melanoma 342
Multiple Myeloma 344
Myelodysplasia 346
Adult Central Nervous System Tumors 346
Pediatric Solid Tumors 347
Sarcoma 348
Performance Scales 354

3/Toxicity Grading 357
John D. Wilkes

4/Chemotherapy Dose Modifications and Precautions 371
John D. Wilkes and Irfan Maghfoor
DNA-Binding Drugs: Alkylating Agents 373
Antimetabolites 380
Antitumor Antibiotics and Related Agents 384
Microtubule-Targeting Drugs 389
DNA Topoisomerase Inhibitors 391
Enzymes 394
Hormonal Agents 395
Biologic Response Modifiers 398
Miscellaneous Agents 399

Section Two / **Chemotherapeutic Agents**

5/Drug Profiles   407

Clay M. Anderson

Altretamine   407
Amifostine   407
Aminoglutethimide   408
Amsacrine   408
Anagrelide   409
Anastrazole   409
L-Asparaginase   410
Pegaspargase   411
Azacytidine   411
Bacillus Calmette-Guérin   412
Bicalutamide   413
Bleomycin   413
Buserelin   414
Busulfan   415
Carboplatin   415
Carmustine   416
Chlorambucil   417
Cisplatin   417
Cladribine   418
Cyclophosphamide   419
Cytarabine   420
Dacarbazine   421
Dactinomycin   422
Daunorubicin   422
Dexamethasone   423
Dexrazoxane   424
Diethylstilbesterol   425
Docetaxel   425
Doxorubicin   426
Edatrexate   427
Erythropoietin   428
Estramustine   428
Etoposide   429
Filgrastim   430
Floxuridine   431
Fludarabine   432
5-Fluorouracil   433
Fluoxymesterone   433
Flutamide   434
Gallium Nitrate   434
Gemcitabine   435
Goserelin Acetate   436
Hydroxyurea   436
Idarubicin   437
Ifosfamide   438
Interferon-α   439
Interferon-γ   440

Interleukin-2   440
Irinotecan   442
Isotretinoin   443
Leucovorin Calcium   443
Leuprolide Acetate   444
Levamisole   445
Lomustine   446
Mechlorethamine   447
Medroxyprogesterone Acetate   447
Megestrol Acetate   448
Melphalan   449
Mercaptopurine   450
Mesna   450
Methotrexate   451
Mitomycin C   452
Mitotane   453
Mitoxantrone   454
Octreotide   454
Oprelvekin   455
Paclitaxel   456
Pamidronate   457
Pentostatin   458
Plicamycin   459
Prednimustine   460
Prednisone   460
Procarbazine   461
Rituximab   462
Sargramostim   463
Streptozocin   463
Suramin   464
Tamoxifen   465
Teniposide   465
Thioguanine   466
Thiotepa   467
Topotecan   468
Toremifene   468
Trastuzumab   469
Tretinoin   470
Trimetrexate   470
Vinblastine   471
Vincristine   472
Vinorelbine   473

Section Three / **Symptom Control**

6/Gastrointestinal Complaints   477
Mary Johnson and Michael C. Perry
Anorexia   477
Constipation   477
Diarrhea   478

Nausea and Vomiting   478
Mucositis   483
Xerostomia   491

7/Pain Control   497
Mary Johnson and Michael C. Perry
General Guidelines   497
Musculoskeletal Pain   500
Neuropathic Pain   500

8/Other Problems   503
Mary Johnson and Michael C. Perry
Cessation of Menses   503
Cough   503
Dyspnea   503
Fatigue   504
Fever   504
Fluid Retention   504
Hiccups   508
Hot Flashes   508
Insomnia   509

Index   511

Section One

Therapy

1
Staging Tables and Treatment Recommendations

Part A

Hematologic Malignancies

Acute Lymphocytic Leukemia

Irfan Maghfoor and Victoria J. Dorr

In 1998 there were 3100 cases of acute lymphocytic leukemia (ALL). In 1998 deaths attributable to ALL were about 1000. Although these cancers are rare, they are the leading cause of cancer death in persons under age 35. The median age of onset for ALL is 10, with a second peak incidence around age 70. Acute leukemia is curable in 50% of good-risk patients.

ETIOLOGY AND RISK FACTORS

Patients with a history of radiation exposure or chemotherapy have an extra risk of developing leukemias. Primarily these secondary leukemias are acute myelogenous leukemia (AML). Post–cancer therapy leukemia tends to be more refractory to treatment than de novo leukemia.

Patients exposed to atomic bomb fallout have an increased risk of leukemia. Tobacco use has a dose-dependent correlation with a risk of leukemia. Viruses are also thought to play a role in the development of hematologic malignancies. Human T-cell lymphoma-leukemia virus-I (HTLV-1) has been associated with the onset of T-cell lymphoma and leukemia. Epstein-Barr virus (EBV) has been associated with B-cell ALL.

Patients with Down's syndrome (trisomy 21) are at increased risk for leukemia, usually M7 or pre-B ALL. Fanconi's anemia, Bloom's syndrome, Wiskott-Aldrich syndrome, and ataxia-telangiectasia are also associated with an increased risk of leukemia. Preleukemic conditions include primary myelodysplasia, myeloproliferative conditions, and paroxysmal nocturnal hemoglobinuria.

SIGNS AND SYMPTOMS

Patients with acute leukemia have a rapid course of general malaise and fatigue. Fever is common. Weight loss and anorexia are common. Patients commonly have bone pain or abdominal pain. Bleeding or bruising may occur. Some leukemia patients have a solitary mass (chloroma) as a presenting sign. Lymphadenopathy and hepatosplenomegaly may occur. Patients may have pancytopenia with symptomatic anemia, neutropenia (infection, fever), or thrombocytopenia (bleeding, petechiae). Abdominal masses and lymphadenopathy may occur in Burkitt's leukemia; mediastinal masses may occur in T-ALL; and central nervous system (CNS) involvement may occur in lymphoblastic T-ALL.

Disseminated intravascular coagulation (DIC) may occur with any subtype of leukemia but is most commonly associated with M3 APL (acute promyelocytic leukemia) subtype. A coagulopathy can also occur with L-asparaginase or vitamin K deficiency. Metabolic abnormalities, including hyperuricemia, acute tumor lysis with hyperkalemia and hypophosphatemia, hypercalcemia, and lactic acidosis, may occur.

DIAGNOSIS

The diagnosis of leukemia is made by obtaining a bone marrow aspirate and biopsy for morphology, cytochemisty, immunophenotyping, and cytogenetic examination. More than 30% blasts should be seen in the bone marrow. Tables 1A.1 and 1A.2 describe some of the characteristics seen with each subtype of leukemia.

Cytogenetics not only may aid in diagnosis but also may have prognostic significance. Patients with normal chromosomes have a 28-month overall survival as compared with 13 months with t(9;22), 11 months with t(4;11), and 5 months with an abnormal 8q24. Patients with other cytogenetic abnormalities and ALL have an overall survival of 18 months.

Favorable features of ALL in children include age 3 to 7, female gender, white race, L1 subtype, common ALL or pre-B ALL classification, white blood cell (WBC) count below 10,000/μL, absence of lymphoma syndrome, absence of CNS involvement, good performance status, hyperdiploidy (fewer than 50 chromosomes), absence of Philadelphia chromosome or t(4;11), and normal or increased serum immunoglobulin (Ig).

Favorable prognostic features of ALL in adults include age below 60 years, WBC fewer than 300,000/μL, T-cell phenotype, mediastinal mass, and absence of t(9;22), t(4;11), and t(8;14) chromosome abnormalities.

Table 1A.1. Pathologic Characterization of Leukemia

FAB Subtype	Morphology	Myelo-peroxidase	Sudan Black	PAS	Nonspecific Esterase	Chloro-acetate Esterase	Acid Phos-phatase	Genetic	Immunophenotype
M0	Large agranular myeloblasts	Neg	Neg						CD13, 33, 34+, HLA-DR
M1	>90% myeloblasts, no maturation	3%+	1–3+	0–1+	0–2+	0–3+	0	occ inv(3)	CD13, 14, 15, 33, 34+, HLA-DR
M2	30–89% myeloblasts, Auer rods	1–3+	1–3+	0–1+	0–2+	0–3+	0	t(8q;21q) in 50%	CD13, 15, 33, 34+, HLA-DR
M3 APL	Heavy azurophilic granulation, nuclei bilobed, Auer rods, >30% blasts and promyelocytes	3+	1–3+	0–1+	0–2+	0–3+	0	t(15q;17q)	CD13, 15, 33+, HLA-DR neg
M4	30–80% myeloblasts, promyelocytes, myelocytes; occasional Auer rod	1–3+	1–3+	1+	2–3+	0–3+	1+		CD13, 14, 15, 33, 34+, HLA-DR
M4Eo	myelomonoblasts with abnormal eosinophils	1–3+	1–3+	1+	2–3+	0–3+	1+	inv 16, t(16:16)	CD13, 14, 15, 33, 34+, HLA-DR

continued

Table 1A.1. Pathologic Characterization of Leukemia *continued*

FAB Subtype	Morphology	Myelo-peroxidase	Sudan Black	PAS	Nonspecific Esterase	Chloro-acetate Esterase	Acid Phos-phatase	Genetic	Immunophenotype
M5	>80% monoblasts, promonocytes, monocytes	0–2+	0–2+	1–2+	3+ Neg with NaF	0	2+	del(11q), t(9;11)	CD 13, 14, 33, 34+, HLA-DR
M6	>50% erythroid	0	0	1+	1+	0	2+		CD 13, 33, 41, 71+, HLA-DR, glycophorin A
M7	Megakaryoblasts, positive for platelet peroxidase, platelet Ab	0	0	1+	1+	0	1+	t(1;22), inv (3), +21, t(9;22)	CD 41, 61
L1	Homogeneous, small lymphoblasts	0	0	0–3+ in blocks	0–1+	0	0–3+	t(9;22), t(4;11), t(1;9)	See Table 1A.2
L2	Heterogeneous, large lymphoblasts	0	0	0–3+ in blocks	0–1+	0	0–3+	t(9;22), t(4;11), t(1;9)	See Table 1A.2
L3	Burkitt's lymphoma, leukemia; large vacuolated cells	0	0	0–3+ in blocks	0–1+	0	0–3+	t(8q;14q), t(2;8), t(8;22)	CD 10, 19, 20, 21, 22+ surface Ig

Table 1A.2. Flow Cytometric and Genetic Abnormalities in Leukemia

Category	FAB	TdT	Ia	CD19	CD10	Clg	SIg	CD7	CD2	Genetic
B-lineage										
Early B-precursor ALL	L1, L2	+	+	+	–	–	–			t(9;22)
Common ALL	L1, L2	+	+	+	+	–	–			t(4;11)
Pre-B ALL	L1	+	+	+	+	+	–			t(1;19)
B-ALL	L3	–	+	+	+/–	–	+			t(8;14), t(2;8), t(8;22)
T lineage										
Early T-precursor ALL	L1, L2	+						+	–	
T-ALL	L1, L2	+						+	+	t(8;14), t(11;14), t(1;14), t(10;14), inv 14, t(7;19), t(1;7)

TREATMENT

Most adult patients with leukemia die of it. The best chance for cure is with initial therapy. Relapse is uncommon more than 2 years after completion of therapy. Supportive care issues are common to all patients with leukemia. This includes appropriate transfusion as clinically indicated. Neutropenic patients with fever should immediately receive broad-spectrum antibiotics. Adequate nutritional intake with consideration of dietary supplements or total parenteral nutrition (TPN) as clinically indicated is necessary. Appropriate infection control procedures (e.g., masks for staff or visitors with infection, careful hand washing) should be followed for patients with neutropenia. Consideration should be given to placement of a Silastic subclavian or internal jugular catheter (i.e., Hickman or Portacath) in all patients. Patients with hyperleukocytosis should be treated with plasmapheresis and hydroxyurea for prompt reduction of blood counts and prevention of stasis. Patients with DIC should be treated with heparin and/or antithrombin-3 as clinically indicated. A cardiac ejection fraction measurement should be completed prior to chemotherapy as a precaution for the use of cardiotoxic chemotherapeutic agents.

ACUTE LYMPHOCYTIC LEUKEMIA

With current treatment options, 70 to 90% of adults achieve a complete remission (CR), and 25 to 50% have long-term disease-free survival. The median disease-free survival is 29 months, and median overall survival is 36 months.

Induction therapy for ALL typically involves a combination of four or five drugs. The addition of daunorubicin to the standard regimen of vincristine, prednisone, and L-aspariginase has been shown to improve CR rates significantly (83% versus 47%). Patients with T-lineage ALL may benefit from chemotherapy with high-dose cytarabine or cyclophosphamide; alternatively, patients with B lineage disease may benefit from chemotherapy that includes high-dose methotrexate.

Consolidation

Current approaches to postremission therapy for adult ALL include short-term, relatively intensive chemotherapy followed by longer-term therapy at lower doses (maintenance), high-dose marrow-ablative chemotherapy, chemoradiation therapy with allogeneic stem cell rescue (alloBMT), or high-dose therapy with autologous stem cell rescue. Several trials of aggressive postremission chemotherapy for adult ALL confirm a long-term disease-free survival rate of approximately 40%. Patents with T-cell

ALL appear to have a favorable prognosis, with long-term survival of 50 to 70%.

The improvement in disease-free survival in patients undergoing alloBMT as primary postremission therapy is offset in part by the increased morbidity and mortality from graft versus host disease (GVHD), veno-occlusive disease of the liver, and interstitial pneumonitis. The results of a retrospective study showed a similar outcome to that for intensive chemotherapy for patients receiving alloBMT in first remission in both the International Bone Marrow Transplant Registry and the German chemotherapy trial (Berlin-Frankfurt-Munster).

Maintenance

While maintenance therapy is routine, its use in patients has not yet been proved useful in adult ALL. Therapy generally lasts 1 to 3 years. Two trials that did not include maintenance therapy did demonstrate relapse rates higher than expected. Unfortunately, both studies can be criticized for suboptimal induction therapy.

Central Nervous System Prophylaxis

The CNS may be a sanctuary site for leukemic cells, as it is frequently involved at the time of relapse. CNS prophylaxis, which generally is given during consolidation therapy, consists of radiation therapy plus intrathecal methotrexate. Alternatively, high-dose methotrexate or cytarabine may be used.

Hematopoietic Growth Factors

Patients receiving induction chemotherapy with granulocyte colony-stimulating factor (G-CSF) in a randomized trial had an insignificant improvement in response rate (91% versus 83%). A significant improvement in time to recovery of granulocytes was seen with G-CSF.

BURKITT'S CELL ALL

Few Burkitt's cell ALL patients receiving standard therapy for ALL have survived. Recent regimens that are undergoing evaluation include 16 to 18 weeks of high-dose methotrexate, cytarabine, and cyclophosphamide. A high response rate with a 30 to 40% disease-free survival appears to be obtained with this approach.

PHILADELPHIA-POSITIVE ALL

Patients with the Philadelphia chromosome have initially high response rates but short durations of response. On average, response lasts about 7 months, and median survival is 11 months. Patients who received an allogeneic bone marrow transplant were found to have a 35% disease-free survival. Additional investigation is centering on the use of interferon as a maintenance agent in this population.

B-CELL ALL

Patents with B-cell ALL and t(4:11) cytogenetic abnormalities may also be candidates for more aggressive treatment at the time of first remission. Aggressive cyclophosphamide-based regimens similar to those used in aggressive non-Hodgkin's lymphoma have shown improved outcome and prolonged disease-free status for patients with B-cell ALL (L3 morphology, surface immunoglobulin positive).

RELAPSED OR REFRACTORY DISEASE

Most patients with ALL have relapsed within 2 years of diagnosis. High response rates have been seen with salvage therapy, including treatment with high-dose cytarabine. The average disease-free survival is only 6 months, with only a few long-term survivors seen. Thus, consideration should be given to allogeneic bone marrow transplant in patients at the time of second remission.

BIBLIOGRAPHY

Adult acute lymphocytic leukemia. PDQ Treatment for Health Professionals. National Cancer Institute. http://cancernet.nci.nih.gov/clinpdq/soa/Adult_acute_lymphocytic_leukemia_Physician.html; 1/18/98.

Landis SH, Murray T, Bolden S, Wingo PA. Cancer Statistics 1998. CA Cancer J Clin 1998;48:6–29.

Scheinberg DA, Maslak P, Weiss M. Leukemias. In: DeVita VT, Hellman S, Rosenberg SA, eds. Cancer: principles & practice of oncology. 5th ed. Philadelphia: Lippincott-Raven, 1997;2285–2396.

Zent CS, Larson RA. Chemotherapy of acute leukemias in adults. In: Perry MC, ed. The chemotherapy source book. 2nd ed. Baltimore: Williams & Wilkins, 1997;1379–1198.

Acute Myelogenous Leukemia

Irfan Maghfoor and Victoria J. Dorr

In 1998 there are expected to be 9400 cases of acute myelogenous leukemia (AML). In 1998 deaths attributable to AML are expected to number 6600. Although these cancers are rare, they are the leading cause of cancer death in persons under age 35. The median age of onset is 65 years. It is unusual to see AML in a patient under age 45. Acute leukemia is now curable in 50% of good-risk patients.

ETIOLOGY AND RISK FACTORS

Patients with a history of radiation exposure or chemotherapy are at an increased risk for developing subsequent leukemias. Primarily these secondary leukemias are AML. Post–cancer therapy leukemia tends to be more refractory to treatment than de novo leukemia. Most treatment-related leukemia appears to occur 2 to 10 years after the initial cancer therapy. Epidophyllotoxins used in the treatment of childhood ALL are associated specifically with 11q23 abnormalities and AML occurring approximately 6 years after the initial chemotherapy. Patients with therapy-related AML may have cytogenetic abnormalities composed of loss of 5 or 5q, loss of 7 or 7q, abnormal 11q23, or t(3;21)(q22;q13).

Patients exposed to fallout from an atomic bomb have an increased risk of leukemia. Tobacco use has a dose-dependent correlation with risk of leukemia. Patients with Down's syndrome (trisomy 21) are at an increased risk for leukemia (usually M7 or pre-B ALL). Fanconi's anemia, Bloom's syndrome, Wiskott-Aldrich syndrome, and ataxia-telangiectasia are also associated with an increased risk of leukemia. Preleukemic conditions include primary myelodysplasia, myeloproliferative conditions, and paroxysmal nocturnal hemoglobinuria.

SIGNS AND SYMPTOMS

Patients with acute leukemia have a rapid course of general malaise and fatigue. Fever is common. Weight loss and anorexia are common. Patients frequently have bone pain or abdominal pain. Bleeding or bruising may occur. Some leukemia patients have a solitary mass (chloroma) as a presenting sign. Lymphadenopathy and hepatosplenomegaly may occur. Patients may have pancytopenia with symptomatic anemia, neutropenia (infection, fever), or thrombocytopenia (bleeding, petechiae). Skin and gingival infiltration may occur and is usually associated with M5 AML. CNS involvement may occur in M5 or lymphoblastic T-ALL; and orbital involvement may occur in M2 disease with t(8;21) genetic abnormalities.

Hyperleukocytosis occurs when the WBC is above 100,000/μL. Leukostasis with vascular injury and hypoxic injury to multiple end organs, especially lung and brain, may follow. The treatment of choice for this hematologic emergency is leukapheresis and immediate chemotherapy to decrease blood counts.

DIC may occur with any subtype of leukemia but is most commonly associated with M3 APL (acute promyelocytic leukemia) subtype. The treatment for this complication is to treat the underlying malignancy and then treat with heparin as clinically indicated. A coagulopathy can also occur with L-asparaginase or vitamin K deficiency.

Possible metabolic abnormalities include hyperuricemia, acute tumor lysis with hyperkalemia and hypophosphatemia, hypercalcemia, and lactic acidosis.

DIAGNOSIS

The diagnosis of leukemia is made by obtaining a bone marrow aspirate and biopsy for morphology, cytochemistry, immunophenotyping, and cytogenetic examination. Greater than 30% blasts should be seen in the bone marrow. Tables 1A.1 and 1A.2 show characteristics seen with each subtype of leukemia. Electron microscopy may be required in M7 AML subtype.

Cytogenetics not only may aid in diagnosis, but also may have prognostic significance. In AML, patients with t(8;21) translocations tend to have high complete remission rates with durable long remissions. Patients with inv(16)(p13q22), t(16;16), or t(15;17) have a high complete remission rate with an intermediate-to-long duration of remission. Patients with t(9;11) tend to have high complete response rates, but a short duration of response. Finally, patients with del(5q), +13, +8, inv 3 or del(12 p) have a poor prognosis and are unlikely to obtain or sustain a remission.

Favorable prognostic factors for AML include young age, no concurrent infection or fever, no antecedent hematologic disorder, a low WBC, presence of Auer rods, and low circulating immune complexes.

TREATMENT

Most adult patients with leukemia die of it. The best chance for cure is with initial therapy. Relapse is uncommon more than 2 years after completion of therapy.

Supportive care issues are common to all patients with leukemia. This includes appropriate transfusion as clinically indicated. Institution of broad-spectrum antibiotics in neutropenic patients with fever should rapidly be performed. Adequate nutritional intake with consideration of dietary supplements or TPN as clinically indicated is necessary. Patients with neutropenia need appropriate infection control procedures (e.g., masks for staff or visitors with ongoing infection, careful hand washing). Placement of a Silastic subclavian or internal jugular catheter (i.e., Hickman or Portacath) should be considered for all patients. Patients with hyperleukocytosis should be treated with plasmapheresis and hydroxyurea for prompt reduction of blood counts and prevention of stasis.

Patients with DIC should be treated with heparin and/or antithrombin-3 as clinically indicated. A cardiac ejection fraction measurement should be completed prior to chemotherapy as a precaution for the use of cardiotoxic chemotherapeutic agents.

ACUTE MYELOGENOUS LEUKEMIA

The most common remission induction regimen for AML is cytarabine given by continuous infusion for 7 days plus daunorubicin for 3 days. Depending on age and other prognostic factors, 60 to 80% of patients are expected to achieve a complete remission (CR). Overall, 20 to 45% are expected to have a clinical CR at 2 years. The use of high-dose cytarabine has been investigated in patients under 60 years of age and has response rates of 83 to 90%. While the initial CR appears to be slightly improved, the 2-year clinical CR is 35 to 40%. No difference in survival, response, or cardiotoxicity has been seen with the substitution of idarubicin for daunorubicin. The addition of etoposide to the standard protocol has been investigated. Patients receiving etoposide apparently had a longer response but no difference in survival. Patients in poor prognostic categories as defined earlier should be candidates for experimental approaches if available. The median duration of remission is 4 to 8 months with induction therapy alone; therefore patients should receive additional consolidation chemotherapy.

For patients over age 60 years a randomized trial of observation and supportive care versus induction therapy was performed. Patients who underwent induction therapy had a significantly improved survival. No difference in survival was seen in a separate study comparing low-dose subcutaneous cytarabine with induction therapy, although more CRs were observed with the induction therapy. Patients with no competing comorbidities and with good prognostic factors possibly should receive aggressive induction therapy.

APL (FAB M3)

APL (FAB M3) (acute promyelocytic leukemia) is a biologically distinct disease. DIC can occur in up to 40% of patients, and DIC parameters should be monitored regularly. All-trans retinoic acid (ATRA) has been proven to be an effective agent for induction of remission. ATRA appears to work by inducing the terminal differentiation of malignant promyelocytes to mature WBC. ATRA induction therapy has initial CR rates of 80 to 95%; the time to CR varies from 38 to 90 days. The recommended daily dose is 45 mg/m^2. ATRA use has been associated with the retinoic acid syndrome, which is described as fever, peripheral edema, pulmonary infiltrates, respiratory distress, hypertension, renal or liver dysfunction, and serositis. Treatment is cessation of ATRA until symptoms resolve (ATRA can be restarted) and therapy with high-dose steroids.

The initial management of APL has been investigated in a randomized trial of ATRA versus the routine induction chemotherapy. Response rates were the same, but patients treated initially with ATRA had a longer response duration. The duration of response of a CR with ATRA alone is only 3.5 months; therefore consolidation therapy is routinely indicated.

CONSOLIDATION THERAPY FOR AML

The addition of consolidation chemotherapy to induction therapy appears to improve survival to 35 to 50% at 2 to 3 years for patients younger than 60 years. Nontransplant consolidation therapy using cytarabine-containing regimens has treatment-related death rates that are usually less than 10 to 20%. Four cycles of high-dose cytarabine (2 to 3 g/m^2 intravenously every 12 hours on days 1, 3, and 5) appear to produce a response superior to that of other consolidation regimens. In a recent study, patients who received high-dose cytarabine had a 46% 3-year disease-free survival, patients receiving an intermediate dose had a response rate of 35%, and patients receiving the low-dose therapy had a response rate of 31%. The high-dose therapy arm did have increased toxicity, with a 5% mortality attributable to therapy. For elderly patients (age above 60), consolidation with 2 cycles of standard-dose cytarabine and daunorubicin is recommended.

Because of the substantial risk of relapse, consideration may be given to autologous or allogeneic transplant of bone marrow or peripheral blood stem cells in patients with no competing comorbidities or with poor prognostic factors. Few studies have addressed the question of transplant in patients at the time of first remission. One European study demonstrated an improved disease-free survival but not overall survival with the use of transplant.

SALVAGE THERAPY FOR AML

A 50 to 60% reinduction rate is seen when patients whose disease recurs more than 1 year from original diagnosis are rechallenged with standard cytarabine and daunorubicin. High-dose cytarabine may be a reasonable choice as well. Alternative regimens with mitoxantrone and etoposide or etoposide and cyclophosphamide are also a consideration. The second remission is usually shorter than the first. Transplantation may be considered at this juncture. Allogeneic bone marrow transplantation in early first relapse or in second complete remission provides a disease-free survival rate of approximately 30%.

HEMATOPOIETIC GROWTH FACTOR SUPPORT

Patients treated either with G-CSF or granulocyte-macrophage colony-stimulating factor (GM-CSF) after induction therapy appear to have a more rapid recovery of neutrophils. Stimulation of leukemic cell lines has not been demonstrated. Survival has not been effected by the use of cytokine support.

BIBLIOGRAPHY

Adult acute myeloid leukemia. PDQ treatment for health professionals. National Cancer Institute. http://cancernet.nci.nih.gov/clinpdq/soa/Adult_acute_myeloid_leukemia_Physician.html; 1/18/98.

Landis SH, Murray T, Bolden S, Wingo PA. Cancer Statistics 1998. CA Cancer J Clin 1998;48:6–29.

Scheinberg DA, Maslak P, Weiss M. Leukemias. In: DeVita VT, Hellman S, Rosenberg SA, eds. Cancer: principles & practice of oncology. 5th ed. Philadelphia: Lippincott-Raven, 1997;2285–2396.

Zent CS, Larson RA. Chemotherapy of acute leukemias in adults. In: Perry MC, ed. The chemotherapy source book. 2nd ed. Baltimore: Williams & Wilkins, 1997;1379–1398.

Chronic Lymphocytic Leukemia

Nasir Shahab and Victoria J. Dorr

BACKGROUND

Chronic lymphocytic leukemia (CLL) is a clonal expansion of neoplastic B-lymphocytes with low proliferative index but prolonged survival. In 1998 CLL is expected to affect 7300 persons in the United States and to result in 4800 deaths.

EPIDEMIOLOGY

CLL is the most common form of adult leukemia in the Western world. The incidence is age dependent. The median age of patients at diagnosis is 65. Fewer than 15% are under 50 years of age. The male to female ratio is 2:1.

ETIOLOGY AND PATHOGENESIS

The cause of CLL is unknown. Although preliminary data support a genetic basis, no definitive gene has yet been identified. Evidence suggests that overexpression of *bcl-2* leads to accumulation of neoplastic B cells because of inhibition of apoptosis. About 50% of patients have cytogenetic abnormalities, such as trisomy 12, 14q+, deletions of chromosomes 6 and 11, and abnormalities of 13q14. The significance of these abnormalities at the molecular level is unclear. With disease progression, overexpression of *-myc* oncogene, deletion of *RB1* gene, and mutations of p53 gene have been observed.

CLINICAL PRESENTATION

The spectrum of symptoms and signs ranges from asymptomatic lymphocytosis discovered on a routine blood cell count to massive lymphadenopathy and hepatosplenomegaly. If diagnosed at an advanced stage, constitutional symptoms (fever, night sweats, and weight loss) are the major complaints.

DIAGNOSTIC CRITERIA

Bone marrow is generally not required to make a diagnosis but may be necessary if the diagnosis is uncertain. An NCI-sponsored working group has established the following revised criteria for diagnosis of CLL:

1. Absolute lymphocyte count must be more than 5,000/mL in the peripheral blood.
2. The lymphocytes must appear morphologically mature. If atypical lymphocytes are present, their percentage should be less than 55%.

3. Immunophenotyping should reveal B-cell markers (CD19, CD20, and CD23) along with CD5 antigen.
4. Monoclonality is established either by l or k surface markers.
5. There must be lymphocytes in the bone marrow.

The French-American-British classification proposed three morphologic subtypes of CLL based on the population of atypical lymphocytes in blood:

Typical CLL, in which more than 90% of lymphocytes are small
Atypical CLL, with 10% prolymphocytes
CLL-PLL (CLL-prolymphocytic leukemia), with 10 to 55% prolymphocytes

STAGING

Staging for CLL is shown in Table 1A.3.

NATURAL HISTORY

A distinctive feature of CLL is that the neoplastic B cells accumulate over time. In early-stage CLL the disease is indolent, with a median survival of 10 years. A subset of these patients have smoldering CLL and have a median survival duration equal to that of a control population. At the other end of the spectrum patients with stage III or IV disease have a median survival of 2 years. Also, patients with CLL-PLL subtype have a worse prognosis than that of typical CLL.

COMPLICATIONS

CYTOPENIAS

Anemia, although a feature of advanced disease, may also be the result of autoimmune hemolysis (10 to 25%), pure red cell aplasia (0.5%), and/or hypersplenism. Autoimmune thrombocytopenia and neutropenia are seen in 2% and 0.5% of patients, respectively.

Table 1A.3. Staging for CLL

Rai Stage	Modified Rai	Description
Stage 0	Low risk	Lymphocytosis
Stage I	Intermediate risk	Lymphadenopathy
Stage II		Clinical splenomegaly or hepatomegaly
Stage III	High risk	Anemia[a]
Stage IV	High risk	Thrombocytopenia[a]

[a]*Secondary to bone marrow failure.*

INFECTIONS

The most common infections are *Streptococcus pneumoniae* and *Haemophilus. influenzae,* but the rare opportunistic infections, such as *Pneumocystis carinii* and *Listeria,* are a major concern. Hypogammaglobulinemia, which occurs in up to 60% of patients, is a major predisposing factor.

TRANSFORMATION

Clonal evolution to prolymphocytic leukemia occurs in 10%; transformation to large cell lymphoma (Richter's syndrome) occurs in 3 to 5%. Transformation to acute leukemia or multiple myeloma, which is rare (fewer than 1%), signals a bad prognosis.

TREATMENT

At present there is no curative treatment for CLL. Therefore, patients with early asymptomatic nonbulky disease, because of the disease's indolent nature, should not be treated. *The absolute indications for treatment are as follows:*

1. Marrow failure; that is, stage III or IV
2. Bulky disease (lymph nodes larger than 10 cm or splenomegaly larger than 6 cm)
3. Progressive lymphocytosis with doubling time of less than 12 months
4. Absolute lymphocyte count above 250×10^9/L
5. Constitutional symptoms as noted earlier

Suggestive indications:

1. Autoimmune anemia refractory to steroids
2. Autoimmune thrombocytopenia refractory to steroids

THERAPEUTIC OPTIONS

Because of the indolent nature of stage 0 and I CLL, treatment is generally not indicated. A study randomizing patients to immediate treatment with chlorambucil or obsevation has shown no significant difference in survival; however, in another study the use of fludarabine resulted in some durable long-term remissions. Studies addressing the use of fludarabine in early-stage CLL are under way. For symptomatic disease, localized radiation therapy or chemotherapy may be considered. Chemotherapy with an alkylating agent with or without an oral steroid produces a 40 to 50% response. Usually chlorambucil is the drug of choice. More recent data—the few durable long-term remissions that have been seen—suggest a benefit to the use of fludarabine. However, chlorambucil can still be considered standard therapy for advanced CLL, since polychemotherapy protocols as well as newer agents such as fludarabine have failed to show an improvement in survival over that produced with chlorambucil.

A study comparing chlorambucil to COP (cyclophosphamide, vincristine, and prednisone) demonstrated identical results with either drug regimen. Treatment should be continued until time of maximal response. Chemotherapy is discontinued once a response has been achieved and is restarted when the disease progresses.

Splenectomy is indicated for severe symptomatic hypersplenism. The role of radiation at present is limited to palliation in patients with large symptomatic splenomegaly and/or lymphadenopathy. Symptomatic refactory patients may receive some benefit from total body irradiation. Transplantation, monoclonal antibodies, interleukin-2 (IL-2) and α-interferon (α-IFN) α are all promising investigational options.

BIBLIOGRAPHY

Adult acute lymphocytic leukemia. PDQ treatment for health professionals. National Cancer Institute. http://cancernet.nci.nih.gov/clinpdq/soa/Adult_acute_lymphocytic_leukemia_Physician.html; 1/18/98.

O'Brien S, del Giglio A, Keating M. Advances in the biology and treatment of B-cell chronic lymphocytic leukemia. Blood 1995;85:307–318.

Rai KR, Keating MJ. Chronic lymphocytic leukemia. In: Holland JF, Frei E, Bast RC, et al, eds. Cancer medicine. 4th ed. Baltimore: Williams & Wilkins, 1997;2697–2718.

Rai KR, Patel DV. Chemotherapy of chronic lymphocytic leukemia and hairy cell leukemia. In: Perry MC, ed. The chemotherapy source book. Baltimore: Williams & Wilkins, 1997;1399–1408.

Rozman C, Montserrat E. Chronic lymphocytic leukemia. N Engl J Med 1995;333:1052–1057.

Sorensen JM, Vena DA, Fallavollita A, et al. Treatment of refractory CLL with fludarabine phosphate: 5 year follow-up report. J Clin Oncol 1997;15:458–465.

Hairy Cell Leukemia

Nasir Shahab and Victoria J. Dorr

BACKGROUND

Hairy cell leukemia (HCL), or leukemic reticuloendotheliosis, was first described as a distinctive entity in 1958. It is a rare chronic B-cell lymphoproliferative disorder characterized by cells with large cytoplasmic projections.

EPIDEMIOLOGY

HCL has a wide geographic distribution and is reported in all ethnic groups. The incidence has been stable over the past several years in the United States, with only 600 new cases per year. Median age at diagnosis is 50 years. In contrast to CLL, it is also seen in young adults. Male to female ratio is 4:1.

ETIOLOGY

Exposure to benzene, radiation, agricultural chemicals, wood dusts, and solvents and related products has been implicated as causative. Familial cases of HCL have rarely been reported.

CLINICAL PRESENTATION

Nonspecific symptoms such as weakness, weight loss, and dyspnea as well as abdominal distention are the most common presentation. Symptoms attributable to infection or hemorrhage are complaints in other patients. Occasionally, however, HCL is diagnosed as an incidental finding on a routine blood count done for unrelated reasons.

Physical examination may reveal pallor and splenomegaly. Hepatic enlargement is much less common. Although lymph nodes are not clinically enlarged, microscopic involvement with hairy cells is a common finding at autopsy.

LABORATORY FEATURES

Peripheral cytopenias with circulating hairy cells are frequently seen. The anemia is normocytic and normochromic, with a mean hemoglobin of approximately 10 g/dL. Thrombocytopenia is rarely severe and if it occurs the splenic sequestration of platelets is an important contributor. Because of variable leukopenia, the percentage of circulating hairy cells ranges from 0 to 100%. These cells have blue-gray cytoplasm with fine to broad fingerlike projections. The cytoplasm stains strongly positive for tartrate-resistant acid phosphatase (TRAP). The nucleus is oval, indented, and with fine chromatin. Profound monocytopenia is commonly seen. A polyclonal hypergammglobuline-mia is seen in up to 30% of patients.

The bone marrow is invariably involved with hairy cells. Bone marrow aspiration is usually impossible because of "dry" marrow secondary to an increased percentage of reticulin fibers. The bone marrow biopsy reveals a normocellular to hypercellu-lar marrow with immature cells. The diagnostic hairy projec-tions, however, are not apparent on tissue sections.

IMMUNOPHENOTYPING

There are no specific cell surface antigens for HCL. The HCL cells commonly bear the classic B-cell markers (CD 19, CD 20, CD 22, monoclonal immunoglobulin), as well as CD 11c, CD 25, and CD 103 on their surface.

DIAGNOSIS

The diagnosis is easy in the presence of splenomegaly, pan-cytopenia, and the "pathognomonic" circulating TRAP positive hairy cells bearing the distinctive immunphenotype (CD 11c, CD 25, CD 103). In cases where few circulating cells are present, a bone marrow aspiration and biopsy is required.

DIFFERENTIAL DIAGNOSIS

Hairy Cell Variant

Advanced age at presentation, leukocyte count about 50 to $100 \times 109/L$, no monocytopenia, TRAP-negative hairy cells, and preserved bone marrow differentiate this disease from the typi-cal HCL. The median survival is approximately 4 years. This variant has a poor response to therapy.

Japanese Form

The approximate age at presentation is 65 years, with a slight female predominance. Malignant cells have aggregated nuclear chromatin instead of the fine pattern of typical hairy cells.

Splenic Villous Lymphoma

Splenomegaly without lymphadenopathy and weakly TRAP-positive villous lymphocytes make the distinction from HCL very difficult. However, leukocytosis instead of leukope-nia and the absence of CD 103 surface antigen help in the differ-entiation.

NATURAL HISTORY

Without proper treatment, the median survival is 4 months for HCL. However, some patients have indolent disease and do not need treatment for several years. Spontaneous remissions are rare. With the advent of purine analogues, the natural history of this disease has changed. It is now considered a curable malignancy.

TREATMENT

2-Chlorodeoxyadenosine (2-CDA) is the standard treatment. A single 7-day continuous infusion at 0.1 mg/kg per day induces complete remissions in 95 to 100% of patients. Relapses are observed in approximately 20%. Long-term follow-up studies have shown a better than 80% 4-year survival. Other options for treatment include IFN-α, splenectomy, and 2'-deoxycoformycin. For years the indications for the initiation of treatment in HCL have been as follows:

1. Symptomatic splenomegaly
2. Anemia (Hgb below 10 g/mL)
3. Thrombocytopenia (platelet count below 100,000/mL)
4. Neutropenia (fewer than 1,000/mL)
5. Leukemic phase of HCL (more than 20,000/mL)

These guidelines were outlined in the pre-2-CDA era, when the disease was incurable and significant morbidity was associated with the available treatments. Now there is a trend among physicians for earlier treatment secondary to the excellent results after 2-CDA.

BIBLIOGRAPHY

Burthem J, Cawley JC, eds. Hairy cell leukemia. Springer-Verlag, 1996.

Golomb HM, Vardiman J. Hairy-cell leukemia. In: Holland JF, Frei E, Bast RC, et al., eds. Cancer medicine. 4th ed. Baltimore: Williams & Wilkins, 1997;2719–2728.

Hoffman MA, Johnson D, Rose E, Rai K. Treatment of hairy cell leukemia with cladarabine: response, toxicity and long term follow-up. J Clin Oncol 1997;15: 1138–1142.

Rai KR, Patel DV. Chemotherapy of chronic lymphocytic leukemia and hairy cell leukemia. In: Perry MC, ed. The chemotherapy source book. 2nd ed. Baltimore: Williams & Wilkins, 1997;1399–1408.

Saven A, Piro L. Newer purine analogues for the treatment of hairy cell leukemia. N Engl J Med 1994;330:691–697.

Chronic Myelogenous Leukemia

Nasir Shahab and Victoria J. Dorr

BACKGROUND

Chronic myelogenous leukemia (CML) is a clonal myeloproliferative disorder resulting from the neoplastic transformation of the primitive hematopoietic stem cell. In 1998 there are expected 4300 cases of CML and 2400 deaths.

EPIDEMIOLOGY

CML accounts for 7 to 20% of all leukemias in adults. The incidence of CML is approximately 1 to 1.5 cases per 100,000 population. The median age at presentation is 50 to 60 years, and it is uncommon in anyone under age 20 years. There is a male predominance.

ETIOLOGY

The causation is not known. Familial cases are very rare. Survivors of Hiroshima and Nagasaki atomic irradiation have a high incidence of CML. There is no known association with chemicals.

PATHOGENESIS

Up to 95% of CML patients have the well-known Philadelphia chromosome. This involves the balanced translocation between chromosomes 9 and 22, t(9;22) (q34;q11). The result is rearrangement of *bcr-abl* genes. This new gene is detected by polymerase chain reaction even in those who do not have the Philadelphia chromosome. The *bcr-abl* fusion gene encodes for a new 210 kD tyrosine kinase that has increased autophosphorylating activity and transforms the transfected cells to leukemic cells.

CLINICAL PRESENTATION

In the initial stages patients are asymptomatic, but in later stages, fatigue, lethargy, malaise, abdominal pain, bone pain, early satiety, fever, and weight loss predominate. Prominent physical findings include splenomegaly, pallor, and bone tenderness. Formation of chloromas (granulocytic sarcomas) are seen in advanced cases. When the WBC is above 300,000/mL, patients have symptoms and sign of leukostasis.

LABORATORY FINDINGS

PERIPHERAL BLOOD

There is a moderate to markedly elevated WBC with complete left shift. The absolute basophil count is also increased.

The platelet count is usually more than 600,000/mL, although in advanced disease thrombocytopenia with counts below 100,000/mL may be observed. Mild to severe anemia is present in all stages of the disease. The peripheral smear reveals giant and agranular blue platelets with hypersegmentation of neutrophils. Serum levels of lactate dehydrogenase (LDH), uric acid, vitamin B_{12}, and transcobalamin can be increased. The leukocyte (neutrophil) alkaline phosphatase (LAP) score is usually low.

BONE MARROW

The bone marrow is hypercellular, with an increased myeloid to erythroid ratio. All cell lines are increased in number with a predominance of myelocytes.

DIAGNOSIS

CML is usually diagnosed by a careful evaluation of cell count and peripheral blood smear. Formal cytogenetic analysis of bone marrow aspirate to assess for the Philadelphia (Ph) chromosome should be routine. If Ph is not visible, the *bcr-abl* gene should be sought by polymerase chain reaction testing. The presence of either the Ph chromosome or the *bcr-abl* gene is mandatory for making a correct diagnosis.

NATURAL HISTORY

CML usually is diagnosed in its chronic indolent phase. WBC and platelets gradually increase in numbers and the spleen enlarges. After a median of 4 to 5 years, CML transforms to an accelerated phase. The criteria for accelerated-phase CML includes a marked increase in WBC count despite adequate treatment, a decrease in the platelet count to fewer than 100,000/mL, an increase in the number of circulating blasts (above 15%), an increase in circulating basophils, and development of new chromosomal abnormalities. After a median of less than 18 months, the disease may enter into its final phase, the blast crisis. About 20 to 40% of patients develop blast crisis without the intermediate accelerated phase. The number of blasts is fewer than 30% in the bone marrow or peripheral blood. Morphologically this phase is indistinguishable from acute leukemia. Although the majority of blasts are of myeloid origin, lymphoid or undifferentiated forms are also seen.

TREATMENT

The goal of treatment is to induce a complete and durable cytogenetic remission. The best results are obtained if patients are treated in the chronic phase. Conventional chemotherapy with hydroxyurea is very successful in producing hematologic remission in more than 90% of patients. The dosage depends upon the total WBC count. Initially higher doses (2 to 6 g/day orally) are required. Once the counts are reduced, the maintenance dosage of hydroxyurea is titrated to keep the WBC count to fewer than 25,000/mL. However, hydroxyurea does not induce cytogenetic remission. All patients eventually evolve to blast crisis and die.

AlloBMT remains the only curative treatment of this disease. However, it is an option only in patients under age 55 years who have a matched donor. Recent trials have demonstrated a benefit to therapy with IFN. Treatment with IFN-α at 3 million to 5 million units subcutaneously three times a week have produced hematologic remissions in up to 70% and cytogenic remissions in up to 40% of patients. Whether this will produce long-term survivors remains to be seen. The addition of low-dose cytarabine to IFN-α to improve response rates is under investigation in clinical trials. In patients with hyperleukocytosis, leukapheresis and hydroxyurea should be used to bring the count down rapidly. Irradiation to the spleen or chloromas may produce symptomatic relief. The treatment of blast crisis should be the same as the treatment of acute leukemia.

BIBLIOGRAPHY

Chronic myeloid leukemia. Baillieres clinical hematology. 1997;10:2–97.

Doll DC, ed. Myeloproliferative disorders. Semin Oncol 1995;22–24.

Kamtarjian H, Deisseroth A, Kurzrock R, et al. CML: a concise update. Blood 1993;82:691–703.

Landis SH, Murray T, Bolden S, Wingo PA. Cancer statistics 1998. CA Cancer J Clin 1998;48:6–29.

Silver RT. Chronic myeloid leukemia. In: Holland JF, Frei E, Bast RC, et al, eds. Cancer medicine. 4th ed. Baltimore: Williams & Wilkins, 1997;2651–2662.

Weick JK. Chemotherapy of myeloproliferative disorders. In: Perry MC, ed. The chemotherapy source book. 2nd ed. Baltimore: Williams & Wilkins, 1997; 1423–1431.

Myelodysplastic Syndromes

Irfan Maghfoor and Victoria J. Dorr

INTRODUCTION

Myelodysplastic syndromes (MDS) are a group of clonal hematopoietic stem cell disorders associated with abnormalities of cellular differentiation and maturation leading to varying degrees of bone marrow failure and peripheral blood cytopenias. The term MDS is used to describe the disorders previously called preleukemia, smoldering acute leukemia, and subacute leukemia. Myelodysplastic syndromes can be *primary* (arising de novo) or *secondary* (following exposure to chemotherapeutic agents or ionizing radiation). Approximately 50 to 90% of cases of MDS are associated with chromosomal abnormalities, and up to 30% may evolve into acute leukemia.

ETIOLOGY

Reports of familial occurrence of MDS and development of MDS in children with Down's syndrome and Fanconi's anemia associated with trisomy 7 suggest a genetic predisposition. A stronger causative association is seen with environmental or occupational exposure to certain chemicals and to ionizing radiation. Exposure to benzene and ionizing radiation, especially in low doses, are well-known risk factors for the development of acute leukemia. These secondary acute leukemias are preceded by a cytopenic state with morphologic characteristics similar to those of MDS. Patients with de novo MDS with a history of exposure to certain chemicals and insecticides sometimes have abnormalities of chromosomes 5 and 7 characteristic of MDS associated with alkylating agent chemotherapy.

THERAPY-RELATED MDS

Chemotherapy with alkylating agents increases the risk of developing MDS and acute leukemia. The risk starts to increase immediately after initiation of alkylating agent therapy and peaks at 4 years. The development of acute leukemia is preceded by MDS for 6 months to a year. The cumulative risk of developing MDS and acute leukemia is 13% at 10 years in patients who have received MOPP (mechlorethamine, vincristine, procarbazine, prednisone) chemotherapy for Hodgkin's disease. Alkylator-induced MDS and acute leukemias frequently have unbalanced abnormalities of chromosomes 5 and 7. In recent years the epidophyllotoxins (etoposide [VP-16] and teniposide [VM-26]) have emerged as important causes of secondary acute leukemia.

Table 1A.4. Morphologic Features of Myelodysplastic Syndromes According to FAB Types

FAB subtype	Blasts in Bone Marrow	Ringed Sideroblasts	Peripheral Blood Morphology	Dysplasia
RA	<5%	<15%	Variable	+
RARS	<5%	>15%	Variable	+
RAEB	5–20%	Variable	Variable	++
CMML	1–20%	Variable	AMC>1000	++
RAEB-T	21–30%	Variable	Variable	++

AMC, absolute monocyte count.

Table 1A.5. Dysplastic Changes Found in Peripheral Blood and Bone Marrow

	Peripheral Blood	Bone Marrow
Dyserythropoiesis	Macrocytosis	Nuclear budding
	Basiphilic stippling	Internuclear bridging
	Acanthocytes	Multinuclearity
		Ringed sideroblasts
		Vacuoles
Dysmyelopoiesis	Hypogranularity	Abnormal localization of
	Hyposegmentation	immature precursors
	Pelger-Huet–like anomaly	
Dysmegakaryopoiesis	Giant platelets	Micromegakaryocytes
	Hypogranular platelets	Separated nuclei
	Megakaryocyte fragments	Decreased number of nuclei

These leukemias are associated with balanced aberrations of bands 11q23 and 21q22 and are usually not preceded by MDS.

PATHOLOGY AND MORPHOLOGY

In 1982, the French-American-British group classified MDS into five distinct types based on morphologic characteristics of peripheral blood and bone marrow (Table 1A.4). These are refractory anemia (RA), refractory anemia with ringed sideroblasts (RARS), refractory anemia with excess blasts (RAEB), chronic myelomonocytic leukemia (CMML), and refractory anemia with excess blasts in transformation (RAEB-T). The diagnosis of MDS depends on establishing morphologic evidence of dysplasia in peripheral blood and bone marrow. All three cell lines may show evidence of dysplasia (Table 1A.5).

CLINICAL PRESENTATION

Myelodysplastic syndromes are uncommon before age 50 years unless caused by exposure to chemotherapy or radiation. The patients may be asymptomatic or may have weakness, decreased exercise tolerance, dyspnea on exertion, and pallor. Some patients may develop infection due to granulocytopenia or bleeding due to thrombocytopenia. Nonspecific symptoms of arthralgias and fever unrelated to infection may be present. Hepatomegaly and splenomegaly may affect 5% and 10% of the patients, respectively.

Acute neutrophilic dermatosis (Sweet's syndrome) is associated with blood neutrophilia and erythematous patches on face, arms, and legs. Approximately 10% of these patients develop acute leukemia or other stem cell disorders, such as paroxysmal nocturnal hemoglobinuria (PNH). Coomb's positive hemolytic anemia and monoclonal gammopathy are rarely seen in patients with MDS. Patients with MDS associated with monosomy 7 may also develop hypothalamic–posterior pituitary insufficiency.

LABORATORY FEATURES

In addition to these morphologic abnormalities, there may be elevations of serum iron, ferritin, and transferrin. Ineffective hematopoiesis and intramedullary cell death may lead to elevations in lactate dehydrogenase, uric acid, and serum indirect bilirubin.

CYTOGENETICS

Abnormalities of almost every chromosome have been described. Common abnormalities include trisomy 8, loss of long arm of chromosome 5, 7, 9, 20, 21, and monosomy 7.

Patients with 5q-syndrome may have unique clinical features. Most of these patients are elderly women with macrocytic anemia and FAB type of RA. Thrombocytosis with platelet counts approaching 1 million may be present.

THERAPY

Management options tried in MDS include induction of differentiation, hematopoietic growth factors, and cytotoxic chemotherapy. Hormonal agents, such as androgens and corticosteroids, have been tried in MDS, but randomized trials have failed to show significant benefit, and only minimal increments in hemoglobin were produced. In addition, long-term therapy with corticosteroids increases the risk of opportunistic infections.

The use of differentiating agents is a very attractive concept in the treatment of MDS because of the low toxicity profiles of these agents. The agents studied include vitamin D_3, 13-*cis* retinoic acid, IFN-α, IFN-γ, and growth factors. Although encouraging results have been obtained with differentiating agents in vitro, clinical trials of the same agents have produced disappointing results, with minimal improvement in cytopenias and no improvement in survival. Cancer and Leukemia Group B recently closed a large randomized trial evaluating the effect of 5-azacytidine on cytopenias and quality of life of patients with MDS after treatment. Preliminary results demonstrate very encouraging results in this phase II trial. Complete remissions were seen in 11% and partial remissions in 25%.

Hematopoietic growth factors have been used in an attempt to induce differentiation of the abnormal clone or to stimulate the normal hematopoietic cells. There is, however, a theoretic and hitherto unproven risk of inducing the abnormal clone to grow and accelerating the progression to acute leukemia. Small clinical studies show that G-CSF and GM-CSF may increase neutrophil counts and improve neutrophil function. Hematopoietic growth factors have also been used in combination with cytotoxic chemotherapy, such as cytosine arabinoside (Ara-C). Randomized trials comparing Ara-C alone with Ara-C and growth factors have shown no difference in response rates and survival between the two groups. The use of erythropoietin has similarly shown inconsistent results, with minimal elevations in hemoglobin in a minority of patients. The doses required are high (10,000 to 60,000 units per week). Furthermore, low levels of endogenous erythropoietin do not predict a response to exogenous erythropoietin. The completion of large multicenter randomized trials is required to clarify the role of hematopoietic growth factors in MDS. At present the use of hematopoietic growth factors cannot routinely be recommended in MDS because of their high cost and lack of demonstrable efficacy.

Cytotoxic chemotherapy trials in MDS have ranged from low-dose single agents to intensive antileukemia therapy and allogeneic bone marrow transplantation. Low-dose Ara-C has been studied extensively in MDS. In one study of 250 patients, low-dose Ara-C produced response rates of 36% with 17% complete responses and 19% partial responses. Some 88% of the patients had myelosuppression, fatal in 15%. In the only randomized trial comparing low-dose Ara-C with supportive care only, there was no difference in survival and time to progression to acute leukemia. Low-dose Ara-C should be reserved for select populations of patients. Intensive antileukemia therapy in MDS is difficult to evaluate because all of the studies completed to date are small and have used a variety of chemotherapy regimens. The response rates with intensive chemotherapy ranged from 15 to 64%, but treatment-related mortality has been higher (20%) than with de novo acute leukemia. This higher mortality rate is thought to be due to advanced age of these patients and prolonged cytopenias after chemotherapy.

Allogeneic bone marrow transplantation remains the only potentially curative treatment for MDS, but it is not available to the majority of patients because of advanced age and lack of appropriately matched donor.

TREATMENT SUMMARY

It is evident from this discussion that standard therapy for MDS is supportive care with transfusion of blood products and antibiotics when required. If the marrow blast population exceeds 30%, a diagnosis of acute leukemia can be made and appropriate treatment initiated, although the response rates are lower than with de novo acute leukemias. Every effort should be made to enroll newly diagnosed patients with MDS in available clinical protocols or if the patient is eligible, to make a referral for bone marrow transplantation.

BIBLIOGRAPHY

Anderson JF, Appelbaum FR, Ficher LD, et al. Allogeneic bone marrow transplantation for 93 patients with myelodysplastic syndromes. Blood 1993:82;677–681.

Anderson JF, Appelbaum FR. Myelodysplasia and myeloproliferative disorders. Curr Opin Hematol 1997:4;261–267.

Bennett JM, Catovsky D, Daniel MT, et al. Proposals for classification of myelodysplastic syndromes. Br J Haematol 1982:51;189–199.

Cheson BD. Chemotherapy of the myelodysplastic syndromes. In: Perry MC, ed. The chemotherapy source book. Baltimore: Williams & Wilkins, 1997; 1409–1423.

Farrow A, Jacobs A, West PR. Myelodysplasia, chemical exposure and other environmental factors. Leukemia 1989:3;33–35.

Foucar K, Langdon RM II, Armitage JO. Myelodysplastic syndromes: a clinical and pathologic analysis of 109 cases. Cancer 1985:56;553–561.

Hirst WJ, Mufti GJ. Management of myelodysplastic syndromes. Br J Haematol 1993:84;191–196.

Mattijssen V, Schattenberg A, Schaap N, et al. Outcome of allogeneic bone marrow transplantation with lymphocyte depleted marrow graft in adult patients with myelodysplastic syndrome. Bone Marrow Transplant 1997:19;791–794.

Tricot G, De Wolf-Peeters C, Hendrickz B, et al. Bone marrow histology in myelodysplastic syndromes: 1. Histological findings in myelodysplastic syndromes and comparison with bone marrow smears. Br J Haematol 1984:57; 423–430.

Tricot G, De Wolf-Peeters C, Vlientinck R, et al. Bone marrow histology in myelodysplastic syndromes: 2. Prognostic value of abnormal localization of immature precursors in MDS. Br J Haematol 1984:58;217–225.

Tricot G, Boogaerts MA. The role of aggressive chemotherapy in the treatment of myelodysplastic syndromes. Br J Haematol 1986:63;477–483.

Plasma Cell Dyscrasias

Somasekhara Bandi and John D. Wilkes

BACKGROUND

The plasma cell disorders are a varied collection of diseases characterized by an abnormal proliferation of plasma cells. Clinically, these entities may be benign (benign monoclonal gammopathy [MGUS, or monoclonal gammopathy of undetermined significance], Castleman's disease) or overtly malignant (multiple myeloma, Waldenstrom's macroglobulinemia).

Plasma cell disorders include the following:

1. MGUS
2. Heavy chain disease (α, γ, θ)
3. Castleman's disease
4. Waldenstrom's macroglobulinemia
5. Indolent myeloma
6. Plasmacytoma
7. Multiple myeloma

This part of the chapter deals primarily with multiple myeloma, the most common malignant expression of plasma cell diseases. This disease is characterized by a clonal expansion of malignant plasma cells, monoclonal immunoglobulin production, decreased normal immunoglobulins, anemia, renal failure, and osteolytic bone disease.

EPIDEMIOLOGY

There were an estimated 13,800 new cases and 11,300 deaths from multiple myeloma in 1998 (1% of all cancer-related deaths in the United States). In contrast to myeloma, MGUS is a relatively common condition, with an incidence of 0.15%, occurring in nearly 1% of the population over the age 30. Multiple myeloma develops in approximately 16% of patients with MGUS, carrying an annual risk of 0.8%. The incidence of both MGUS and multiple myeloma increases with age, and myeloma is more frequent in men and African-Americans than in women and whites.

ETIOLOGY

Although the precise causation of myeloma remains unknown, a number of risk factors appear to predispose to the development of the disease. These include MGUS and exposure to chemicals, radiation, and petroleum products. Recent identification of herpesvirus DNA in the dendritic cells of myeloma pa-

Table 1A.6. Diagnostic Criteria for Multiple Myeloma

Major criteria
   1. Soft tissue tumor biopsy revealing plasmacytoma
   2. Bone marrow plasma cells >30%
   3. Ig paraprotein of IgG >3.5 g/dL, Ig A >2 g/dL, or urine k or l excretion >1 g/day

Minor criteria
   a. Bone marrow plasma cells 10–30%
   b. Ig spikes less than in major criteria
   c. Lytic bone lesions
   d. Normal IgM < 50 mg/dL, IgA < 100 mg/dL, IgG < 600 mg/dL

Diagnostic criteria
   • Any 2 major criteria
   • Major #1 *or* #2 + minor b, c, or d
   • Major #3 + minor a, c, or d
   • Minor a, b, and c or a, b, and d

Table 1A.7. Durie-Salmon Staging System for Multiple Myeloma

	5-Year Survival
Stage I	25–40%
Hemoglobin > 10 gm/dL	
Normal serum calcium	
Normal skeletal survey	
Low M-protein production (IgG < 5 g/dL, IgA < 3 g/dL, urinary κ or λ < 4 g/24 hr)	
Estimated myeloma cell mass < 0.6×10^9 cells/m² (low burden)	
Stage II	15–30%
Myeloma that fits neither stage I or stage III	
Estimated myeloma cell mass $0.6 - 1.2 \times 10^9$ cells/m² (intermediate burden)	
Stage III	10–25%
Hemoglobin < 8.5 gm/dL	
Serum calcium > 12 mg/dL	
More than 3 lytic lesions	
High M-protein values (IgG > 7.5 g/dL, IgA > 5 g/dL, urinary κ or λ ≥ 12 g/24 hr)	
Estimated myeloma cell mass >1.2×10^9 cells/m² (high burden)	

The following subclassifications of stages are used:
   A. Serum creatinine < 2 mg/dL
   B. Serum creatinine ≥ 2 mg/dL

tients has generated significant interest. Rarely, myeloma is diagnosed in more than one family member, suggesting a possible genetic predisposition, though this remains unclear.

CLINICAL MANIFESTATIONS

The major clinical manifestations of multiple myeloma result from the expansion of malignant plasma cells in the marrow and the systemic effects of the excess paraproteins. Approximately 20% of patients are asymptomatic at diagnosis. Bone pain is the most frequent presenting symptom. Other common clinical features include osteolytic lesions, anemia, renal failure, recurrent bacterial infections, fatigue, and hypercalcemia. Less common clinical findings include neuropathies, hyperviscosity syndrome, bleeding, and thrombosis. The bone lesions, hypercalcemia, and anemia, which correlate with total myeloma cell mass, have prognostic value. The most common causes of death in myeloma patients are infections and/or renal failure.

DIAGNOSIS AND STAGING

To make the diagnosis of multiple myeloma, the clinician must perform the appropriate clinical, laboratory, radiographic, and pathologic evaluations (Table 1A.6). Staging for multiple myeloma appears in Table 1A.7.

PROGNOSIS

The 5-year survival rates for myeloma are given in Table 1A.7. However, multiple myeloma is a heterogeneous disease with a survival range of 1 to 10 years. There are two major prognostic categories:

1. *Tumor burden,* represented by increased bone marrow plasma cells, lytic bone lesions, serum calcium level, and low hemoglobin level
2. *Proliferation rate,* represented by high plasma cell labeling index and elevated C-reactive protein and interleukin-6 levels

TREATMENT

The treatment of multiple myeloma is directed at the reduction of tumor burden and reversal of complications of the disease. Thus, asymptomatic patients do not need immediate chemotherapy. Clinicians must be mindful of a wide range of supportive measures.

The asymptomatic patient with myeloma should be monitored carefully with routine examinations, measurement of serum calcium, creatinine, and M-protein, and complete blood counts, in addition to skeletal radiographs. At present treatment of asymptomatic (smoldering) myeloma has not been demonstrated to be useful.

As infectious complications are potentially life-threatening, pneumococcal vaccination is recommended to all patients, although the host immune response to the vaccine may be incomplete and/or short lived. In an effort to avoid renal complications, nephrotoxic agents such as intravenous contrast should be avoided entirely. Bisphosphonates are extremely effective for the treatment of hypercalcemia, and pamidronate has been shown to reduce the incidence of skeletal complications, need for radiation treatments, and spinal cord compressions. Erythropoietin may be used to treat anemia of multiple myeloma. Response is significantly better in patients with low levels of erythropoietin. Radiation therapy may provide effective palliation of symptomatic bone disease.

CHEMOTHERAPY

A small fraction of patients with myeloma may have an indolent disease process that requires treatment only in the event of symptoms. As mentioned previously, routine surveillance is indicated.

For the patient with symptomatic disease progression, systemic chemotherapy with single-agent alkylators (melphalan) with prednisone or combination regimens may be appropriate (discussed later). A variety of treatments have been demonstrated to prolong survival of patients with symptomatic myeloma. The melphalan and prednisone (MP) combination was introduced in the 1960s and has long been the standard therapy for myeloma. However, there is no evidence that any one alkylating agent is superior to another. It must be remembered that the pharmacologic properties of some alkylating agents may favor their use in certain patients. The oral bioavailability of melphalan is extremely variable, and food may interfere with absorption. For this reason, melphalan should be administered on an empty stomach and with aggressive oral hydration. The clearance of melphalan from the blood is delayed in patients with renal insufficiency; this may result in increased toxicity. Thus, the dose of melphalan should be reduced in patients with a serum creatinine above 2 mg/dL. (See Chapter 4, Chemotherapy Dose Modifications.) Cumulative bone marrow toxicity may develop with repeated courses of melphalan. Bone marrow recovery following melphalan is often prolonged. If hematologic toxicity results in treatment delays of more than 6 weeks, one should consider switching to cyclophosphamide, which may allow for more rapid marrow recovery. In contrast to melphalan, oral cyclophosphamide is well absorbed, and renal function does not affect toxicity. Cyclophosphamide is also the drug of choice for patients who are candidates for autologous bone marrow transplantation, as melphalan has significant adverse effects on hematopoietic stem cells and should be avoided in these patients.

The MP regimen induces responses in 50 to 60% of patients with multiple myeloma; however, complete disappearance of the M-component occurs in only 5 to 10% of patients. Failure of M-component to decrease and persistence of Bence Jones proteinuria indicate MP resistance and consideration of alternative therapies. In addition to the standard MP, many combination regimens have been tried; they may produce higher response rates but have yet to demonstrate significant prolongation of survival. These regimens often prove to be more toxic than MP.

Alternative regimens for the treatment of symptomatic myeloma include CP (cyclophosphamide and prednisone), VBMCP (vincristine, carmustine, melphalan, cyclophosphamide, and prednisone), alternating VMCP (vincristine, melphalan, cyclophosphamide, and prednisone), VBAP (vincristine, carmustine, doxorubicin [Adriamycin], prednisone), high-dose dexamethasone, and VAD (vincristine, doxorubicin, dexamethasone). A meta-analysis comparing MP against combination regimens concluded that MP and combination chemotherapy were equivalent treatments. However, survival varied widely in the MP-treated patients, and combination regimens appeared to have an advantage over MP in studies that accrued patients with poor risk factors.

Some clinical investigators have suggested that the VAD regimen may be the best salvage treatment for patients who are refractory to alkylating agents or who have relapsed following an initial remission. Although the time to response (about 6 weeks) for VAD is superior to that of MP, VAD has not been demonstrated to be superior to MP as first-line therapy.

For younger patients who are healthy enough to undergo intensive approaches, high-dose therapy with allogeneic or autologous bone marrow and stem cell support should be considered. Retrospective analysis of bone marrow registry data from 162 patients who underwent allogeneic matched sibling donor transplants for myeloma has demonstrated an actuarial 7-year survival rate of 28%. In this review, favorable prognostic features included low tumor burden and chemosensitive disease at the time of transplant and application of transplantation after first-line therapy. Unfortunately, significant transplant-related mortality remains a major obstacle to the routine use of this aggressive approach.

With regard to autologous transplantation, a randomized

study of patients less than 65 years of age with newly diagnosed myeloma was performed. The patients were treated with combination chemotherapy, then randomized to receive high-dose therapy with autologous bone marrow transplant or ongoing chemotherapy. The overall and disease-free survival were significantly improved in the high-dose arm. The estimated 5-year survival for those receiving high-dose therapy was 52% versus 12% in the control group. At present the standard application of myeloablative therapy with autologous transplant requires confirmation by ongoing randomized phase III trials.

Multiple myeloma patients who are responding to therapy show a progressive fall in M-protein until a plateau is reached. At this time further treatment does not add any benefit. Most clinicians continue induction chemotherapy for at least 12 months; others discontinue induction after the M-protein reaches a plateau for 4 months.

Several clinical trials have evaluated the role of maintenance therapy in myeloma and found no improvement in survival with chemotherapy. Maintenance therapy with IFN-α has been reported to prolong remission duration in several studies. An initial Italian report even showed a slight prolongation in overall survival with IFN-α. Unfortunately, this benefit disappeared on further follow-up. Additional randomized studies of IFNmaintenance have also demonstrated longer response. However, overall survival was not improved in any of the studies, and the use of IFN-maintenance therapy remains investigational.

ISOLATED PLASMACYTOMA AND EXTRAMEDULLARY PLASMACYTOMA

An isolated plasmacytoma is defined as a single lytic bone lesion of plasma cells in an otherwise asymptomatic patient who has marrow plasma cells less than 5%. An extramedullary plasmacytoma is an isolated soft tissue mass of plasma cells often occurring in the paranasal sinuses or tonsils. Approximately 25% of these patients have an elevated paraprotein in the serum. Irradiation of the plasmacytoma may be curative, with 50% overall survival at 10 years. Although many patients are eventually shown to have overt myeloma, those with low paraprotein levels that disappear following radiation have an excellent prognosis.

MACROGLOBULINEMIA

Disorders associated with macroglobulinemia include MGUS, Waldenstrom's macroglobulinemia, IgM myeloma, CLL, non-Hodgkin's lymphoma, and cold agglutinin disease. The clinical manifestations of macroglobulinemia include lymphadenopathy, hepatosplenomegaly, and the hyperviscosity syndrome. In contrast to myeloma, bony lesions are rare. The most common symptoms, which relate to the hyperviscosity syndrome, include fatigue, headache, epistaxis, visual disturbances, and neurologic complaints, including lethargy and coma.

The increased concentration of IgM, which is largely confined to the intravascular space, produces an expansion of the plasma volume that in extreme cases may result in congestive heart failure. Sludging of the blood can be seen in conjunctival and retinal veins, with dilation and segmentation of retinal hemorrhages, and papilledema. Hyperviscosity of the CNS circulation may result in a variety of neurologic signs and symptoms.

The recommendations for the treatment of patients with macroglobulinemia are similar to those for myeloma. Patients must be observed carefully for hyperviscosity syndrome. The median survival of patients with macroglobulinemia is approximately 5 years. Treatment options include expectant management for asymptomatic patients with initiation of an alkylating agent, such as chlorambucil, at the time of progression of symptoms. Favorable results have been reported with combination regimens such as M2 (melphalan, vincristine, cyclophosphamide, carmustine, and prednisone) and the nucleoside analogues, 2-CDA, and fludarabine. In contrast to the unproven benefit seen in patients with myeloma, interferon-α appears to have some activity in macroglobulinemia.

Plasmapheresis is the treatment of choice for patients with symptomatic hyperviscosity; 2 to 3 L of plasma can be pheresed at each setting and replaced by saline and 5% albumin. Clotting studies should be monitored carefully during the initial management of hyperviscosity, with administration of fresh frozen plasma as needed. Plasmapheresis should be repeated two or three times a week until symptoms of hyperviscosity syndrome are adequately controlled.

The therapy for patients with IgM paraprotein in association with chronic lymphocytic leukemia (CLL) or non-Hodgkin's lymphoma is no different from that for other patients with these malignant disorders; it is reviewed elsewhere in this chapter. Therapy of chlorambucil with or without prednisone may be required to correct the hemolytic anemia in patients with cold agglutinin disease.

MONOCLONAL GAMMOPATHY OF UNKNOWN SIGNIFICANCE

Patients with MGUS have a serum monoclonal protein in the absence of findings to suggest another diagnosis such as myeloma, lymphoma, amyloidosis, or macroglobulinemia. No treatment is indicated, but these patients must be followed closely for the development of a malignant lymphoproliferative disorder. In a longitudinal study of patients with MGUS, nearly 25% of patients were diagnosed with a lymphoproliferative disorder after a median follow-up of 22 years.

BIBLIOGRAPHY

Alexanian R, Dimopoulos M. The treatment of multiple myeloma. N Engl J Med 1994;330:484–489.

Barlogie B, Vesole DH, Jagannath S. Salvage therapy for multiple myeloma: the University of Arkansas experience. Mayo Clin Proc 1994;69:787–795.

Bataille R, Harousseau J. Multiple myeloma. N Engl J Med 1996;336:1657–1664.

Berenson JR, Lichtensein A, Porter L, et al. Efficacy of pamidronate in reducing skeletal events in patients with advanced multiple myeloma. N Engl J Med 1996;334:488–493.

Blade J, Kyle RA, Greipp PR. Presenting features and prognosis in 72 patients with multiple myeloma who were younger than 40 years. Br J Hematol 1996;93:345–351.

Browman GP, Bergsagel DE, Sicheri D, et al. Randomized trial of interferon maintenance in multiple myeloma: a study of the National Cancer Institute of Canada Trials Group. J Clin Oncol 1996;13;2354–2360.

Hodgkin's Disease

Irfan Maghfoor and John D. Wilkes

INTRODUCTION

Hodgkin's disease was first described by Thomas Hodgkin in 1832 in the historic paper "On Some Morbid Appearances of the Absorbent Glands and Spleen," which was read before the Medical and Chirurgical Society in London. However, it was not until 1865 that the entity was named Hodgkin's disease by Sir Samuel Wilks. Physicians Carl Sternberg and Dorothy Reed provided the first microscopic descriptions of Hodgkin's disease; hence the name Reed-Sternberg cell, found on microscopic examination of pathologic specimens.

Once uniformly fatal, Hodgkin's disease now is an extremely treatable malignancy, curable in most patients. This dramatic change in prognosis for patients with Hodgkin's disease has resulted from the successful application of combination chemotherapy as well as radiation therapy. Current efforts are aimed at refining the therapy for Hodgkin's disease in an effort to decrease toxicity without compromising disease-free survival.

EPIDEMIOLOGY AND ETIOLOGY

Approximately 7500 new cases of Hodgkin's disease are diagnosed each year in the United States. The male to female ratio is 1.4:1, and there is an age-related bimodal incidence. The first peak occurs in the third decade of life and the second occurs after age 50. Lymphocyte-depleted (LD) and mixed-cellularity (MC) histologies are more common in patients at least 40 years of age, while lymphocyte-predominant (LP) and nodular-sclerosing (NS) Hodgkin's disease occur more frequently in patients under age 40. LP Hodgkin's disease is also more common in patients under age 16.

The cause of Hodgkin's disease remains unknown, although several theories have been proposed. The most compelling epidemiologic and serologic data link Epstein-Barr virus (EBV) to Hodgkin's disease. The EBV genome can be found in up to 80% of tumor specimens. Recent studies of monozygotic and dizogotic twins suggest a genetic predisposition. Other risk factors for the development of Hodgkin's disease include a variety of familial and socioeconomic factors, human immunodeficiency virus (HIV), and exposure to illness in childhood.

PATHOLOGY

Hodgkin's disease has a distinct microscopic appearance characterized by the aforementioned Reed-Sternberg cells and

Table 1A.8. Rye Classification of Hodgkin's Disease

Histology	Frequency (%)	Clinical Features
Lymphocyte Predominant	5–10	Tendency to be limited
Mixed Cellularity	20–40	Intermediate in stage at presentation between NSHD and LDHD
Nodular Sclerosis (NSHD)	30–60	Common mediastinal presentation, young women
Lymphocyte Depleted (LDHD)	5–10	Usually, advanced disease with marrow and retroperitoneal involvement

NSHD, nodular sclerosis Hodgkin's disease; LDHD, lymphocyte depleted Hodgkin's disease.

varying degrees of normal and inflammatory cells. The Reed-Sternberg cell, however, is neither diagnostic of Hodgkin's disease nor a clonal malignant cell. These cells can be found in infectious mononucleosis, carcinomas, and sarcomas. The Rye classification divides Hodgkin's disease into four distinct histologic subtypes (Table 1A.8).

CLINICAL PRESENTATION

The typical presentation of a patient with Hodgkin's disease is characterized by painless lymphadenopathy in a young adult. Some 40% of patients have the classic B-symptoms of unexplained fever (above 38°C, or 100.4°F), drenching night sweats, and weight loss (more than 10% of body weight). Hodgkin's disease spreads in a predictable fashion involving contiguous lymph node areas. Approximately 80% of patients will present with lymphadenopathy above the diaphragm, and widespread adenopathy is rare at presentation. Extranodal involvement is usually a result of contiguous extension, although in rare cases Hodgkin's disease spreads hematogenously to the lungs, liver, and bone marrow.

To establish a diagnosis, the largest and most central lymph node of an involved group should be removed with the capsule intact. As nodal architecture is crucially important in establishing the diagnosis, needle biopsies should generally be avoided.

Table 1A.9. Cotswold Modification of the Ann Arbor Staging System for Hodgkin's Disease

Stage	Substage
Stage I	
Involvement of a single lymph node region	I
Localized involvement of a single extralymphatic site or organ	I^E
Stage II	
Two or more nodal regions on the same side of diaphragm	II
Localized involvement of a single associated extralymphatic site or organ and its regional nodes with or without other lymph node regions on the same side of the diaphragm	IIE
Stage III	
Nodal regions on both sides of diaphragm	III
Nodal regions on both sides of diaphragm and localized involvement of an extralymphatic site or organ	IIIE
Including the spleen	III^S
Or both the spleen and an extralymphatic site	III^{E+S}
Stage IV	
Disseminated (multifocal) involvement of one or more extralymphatic sites or organs with or without associated lymph node involvement or isolated extralymphatic organ involvement with distant lymph node involvement	IV

The number of lymph node groups involved may be indicated by a subscript (e.g., II^3).
Patients may be further subclassified as A (absence) or B (presence) of systemic symptoms (weight loss > 10% in 6 months, fevers, drenching night sweats). Subscript X indicates bulky disease.

STAGING

The staging system for Hodgkin's disease (Table 1A.9), a modification of the well-established Ann Arbor system, was proposed in 1989 at Cotswold, England.

STAGING PROCEDURES

The following procedures are recommended for proper staging of Hodgkin's disease:

Adequate surgical biopsy reviewed by an expert hematopathologist

Detailed history with particular attention to presence or absence of B symptoms

Careful physical examination with attention to nodal sites and splenomegaly

Laboratory tests: blood counts, erythrocyte sedimentation

rate (ESR), liver function tests, uric acid, and lactate dehydrogenase (LDH)

Chest and abdominal computed tomography

Bipedal lymphangiograms; may be useful in select patients
when a radiologist who routinely performs and interprets
these studies is available

Bone marrow aspiration with bilateral biopsies for patients
with advanced disease or systemic symptoms

Staging laparotomy is indicated in clinical stages I and II if
negative bone marrow aspiration and biopsy and only if a therapeutic decision depends on detection of occult abdominal disease. The clinical utility of staging laparotomies remains controversial, and most major institutions are abandoning that
once-routine practice.

TREATMENT

Hodgkin's disease is an extremely radiosensitive and
chemosensitive malignancy, and all patients should be treated
with curative intent. A complete discussion of treatment of
Hodgkin's disease is beyond the scope of this chapter, and many
areas remain controversial.

As is always the case with oncology, therapy depends on the
stage of the disease. In this chapter, treatment recommendations
are for patients who are clinically staged as well as those who
undergo formal staging laparotomy (pathologic staging). With a
few exceptions radiation therapy alone is used only if the patient
had a staging laparotomy. Exploratory laparotomy changes the
stage of disease in approximately 30% of patients. However,
subsets of patients who have a very low risk (6 to 9%) of occult
abdominal disease can be offered radiation therapy alone without a staging laparotomy. These groups include female patients
with stage IA lymphocyte predominant disease, female patients
under age 26 with stage IIA nodular sclerosing disease, and male
patients with stage IA nodular sclerosing Hodgkin's disease.

RADIATION THERAPY

In general, megavoltage radiation therapy is used for patients
with Hodgkin's disease. Standard total doses are 36 to 40 Gy to
each field, with boosts up to 45 Gy to involved sites. Lower doses
may be employed if chemotherapy is also given. Common fields
include the mantle, para-aortic, pelvic, and inverted Y.

CHEMOTHERAPY

The classic MOPP regimen resulted in complete remission
rates of 70 to 80% in advanced Hodgkin's disease, with 50 to 60%

Table 1A.10. Treatment Guidelines for Hodgkin's Disease

Stage IA	
Pathologic	Radiation therapy
Clinical	Chemotherapy
	or
	Radiation therapy for patients with peripheral stage IA, women, LP histology or NS in a male, or isolated small-volume mediastinal disease
	or
	Radiation therapy and chemotherapy for patients with less favorable clinical features
Stage IB	
Pathologic	Radiation therapy
Clinical	Chemotherapy
	or
	Radiation therapy + chemotherapy for patients with less favorable clinical features
Stage IIA	
Pathologic	Radiation therapy
Clinical	Chemotherapy
	or
	Radiation for female patients < age 26 with NS histology
	or
	Radiation therapy + chemotherapy for patients with less favorable clinical features
Stage IIB	
Pathologic	Radiation therapy
Clinical	Chemotherapy
Stages IIIA and IIIB	Chemotherapy
Stages IVA and IVB	Chemotherapy
Large mediastinal mass	Radiation therapy + chemotherapy without staging laparotomy

of complete responders being relapse free at 5 years. Bonadonna and colleagues introduced a new drug combination, doxorubicin plus bleomycin, vinblastine, and dacarbazine (ABVD) for the treatment of Hodgkin's disease. Compared with MOPP for patients with stages IIB, III, and IV, ABVD resulted in similar response rates with less long-term toxicity. Further modifications in the chemotherapy of advanced Hodgkin's disease include alternating MOPP and ABVD; MOPP-ABV hybrid; and the Stanford V regimen. These newer regimens, which are designed to minimize acute and long-term toxicities without reducing survival, provide response rates comparable with those of MOPP. Routinely six cycles of therapy are administered to patients with advanced disease, although more cycles may be necessary in up to 20% of patients. The treatment recommendations for various stages of Hodgkin's disease are given in Table 1A.10.

COMPLICATIONS OF THERAPY

In addition to successful treatment of the malignancy, one of the most important factors in determining the primary therapeutic modality for the management of Hodgkin's disease relates to the concern about long-term toxicity of treatment. The gravest complication of chemotherapy is acute nonlymphocytic leukemia. The cumulative incidence of acute leukemia 10 years after starting chemotherapy for Hodgkin's disease is 10 to 13%. The risk of developing acute leukemia is directly related to the cumulative dose of alkylating agents, age over 40, and splenectomy. There is also a higher incidence of myelodysplasia and solid tumors (lung, breast, thyroid, non-Hodgkin's lymphoma, melanoma) following treatment.

Long-term toxicities of mediastinal radiation may include restrictive pericarditis, radiation pneumonitis, premature coronary artery disease, and/or cardiomyopathy. Mantle radiation results in hypothyroidism in 5 to 10% of patients. Cardiac toxicity and pulmonary toxicity from doxorubicin and bleomycin respectively are well known. Male and female infertility are also important long-term toxicities, particularly with MOPP. ABVD therefore offers a more attractive alternative for patients in whom fertility is an important issue.

RELAPSED DISEASE

MOPP or ABVD may salvage up to 60% of patients who relapse after radiation treatment for early-stage Hodgkin's disease. Unfortunately, salvage therapy of MOPP failures is less successful, with only 30% of patients achieving complete remissions and only 50% of these complete responders remaining in long-term remission. Complete remission with third-line regimens occurs in only 10 to 15% of patients. Autologous bone marrow transplant offers a 50% chance of disease-free survival at 3 years if offered promptly after failure from MOPP or ABVD

BIBLIOGRAPHY

Bartlett NL, Rosenberg SA, Hoppe RT, et al. Brief chemotherapy, Stanford V, and adjuvant radiotherapy for bulky or advanced-stage Hodgkin's disease: a preliminary report. J Clin Oncol 1995;13:1080–1088.

DeVita VT, Hubbard SM. Hodgkin's disease. N Engl J Med 1993;328:560–565.

Hagemeister FB. Hodgkin's disease: the next decade. Leukemia Lymphoma 1996;21:53–61.

Mauch PM. Management of early stage Hodgkin's disease: the role of radiation therapy and/or chemotherapy. Ballieres Clin Haematol 1996;9:531–541.

Straus, DJ. Treatment of Hodgkin's disease: the role of radiation and/chemotherapy in advanced stages. Ballieres Clin Haematol 1996;9:553–558.

Urba WJ, Longo DL. Hodgkin's disease. N Engl J Med 1992;326:678–687.

Viviani S, Bonadonna G, Santoro A, et al. Alternating versus hybrid MOPP and ABVD combinations in advanced Hodgkin's disease: ten-year results. J Clin Oncol 1996;14:1421–1430.

Yuen AR, Horning SJ. Recent advances in the treatment of Hodgkin's disease. Curr Opin Hematol 1997;4;286–290.

Non-Hodgkin's Lymphoma

Haleem J. Rasool and John D. Wilkes

BACKGROUND

The non-Hodgkin's lymphomas (NHLs) are a group of lymphoid neoplasms comprising numerous distinct entities defined by various clinical, histologic, immunologic, molecular, and genetic characteristics. These diseases are extremely diverse in their clinical manifestations and therapeutic options. Current treatment approaches center on the use of systemic chemotherapy; they are curative in approximately half of diagnosed patients. The management of acquired immunodeficiency syndrome (AIDS)-related NHL and primary CNS lymphoma are reviewed in Chapter 1B (see AIDS-related malignancies).

EPIDEMIOLOGY

Approximately 55,400 cases of non-Hodgkin's lymphomas were diagnosed in 1998 in United States. Since 1950 the incidence of NHL has been increasing steadily, and NHL now accounts for approximately 4% of all cancer diagnoses. Men are affected approximately 50% more frequently than women. There were an estimated 24,900 deaths from NHL in 1998.

ETIOLOGY

Although precise molecular abnormalities have been identified for many NHL subtypes, the exact cause of these diseases remains unclear. Specific populations at relatively high risk include patients with congenital or acquired immunodeficiency syndromes (ataxia-telangiectasia, Wiskott-Aldrich syndrome, X-linked lymphoproliferative disease, autoimmune diseases, AIDS) and those who have received immunosupressive therapy (recipients of organ or bone marrow transplants). Environmental factors appear to play some role, as exposures to radiation and/or chemicals (herbicides, solvents, pesticides) increases the risk of NHL. Viruses (EBV, HTLV-I, Kaposi Sarcoma-Associated Herpes Virus [KSHV], Hepatitis C Virus [HCV]) have also been implicated in the pathogenesis of certain types of non-Hodgkin's lymphomas. *Helicobacter pylori* infection has been associated with mucosa-associated lymphoid tissue (MALT) lymphomas of the GI tract.

CLINICAL MANIFESTATIONS

The varied clinical features of non-Hodgkin's lymphoma depend on the histologic subtype, the stage, and the primary site or sites of tumor. Systemic (B) symptoms may include unexplained fevers or weight loss and/or drenching night sweats. Many patients have a painless slowly enlarging mass. In addition to palpable adenopathy, splenomegaly may be appreciated. Patients with lymphoblastic lymphoma may have superior vena cava syndrome and hypercalcemia. Those with high-grade NHL (Burkitt's, lymphoblastic lymphoma) may have neurologic deficits and CNS involvement. In contrast to Hodgkin's disease, the non-Hodgkin's lymphomas have a much less predictable pattern of spread and often disseminate early and/or involve extranodal sites.

CLASSIFICATION

With today's therapies nearly half of patients with NHL can be cured. In contrast, some patients with NHL are probably incurable by virtue of their histologic subtype, and for them the goals of therapy are palliative. Thus it is necessary to divide non-Hodgkin's lymphoma into clinically relevant subgroups.

Earlier systems (Rappaport) to classify non-Hodgkin's lymphomas were based on morphology. Subsequently, both the Lukes-Collins and the Kiel (Lennert) classifications expanded the Rappaport system with immunophenotypic subgrouping. The Working Formulation (Table 1A.11) was devised to incor-

Table 1A.11. The International Working Formulation of Non-Hodgkin's Lymphoma

Low grade
  A. Small lymphocytic (consistent with chronic lymphocytic leukemia) (SL)
  B. Follicular, predominantly small cleaved cell (FSC)
  C. Follicular, mixed small cleaved and large cell (FM)
Intermediate grade
  D. Follicular, predominantly large cell (FL)
  E. Diffuse, small cleaved cell (DSC)
  F. Diffuse mixed, small and large cell (DM)
  G. Diffuse, large cell cleaved or noncleaved cell (DL)
High grade
  H. Immunoblastic, large cell (IBL)
  I. Lymphoblastic, convoluted or nonconvoluted cell (LL)
  J. Small noncleaved cell, Burkitt's or diffuse undifferentiated, non-Burkitt's (SNC)
Unclassifiable
  K. Composite lymphoma, mantle cell lymphoma, monocytoid B-cell lymphoma, MALT-oma, anaplastic large cell lymphoma, mycosis fungoides (CTCL), angiocentric lymphoma, angiotropic lymphoma, AILD, T-cell rich B-cell lymphoma, adult T-cell leukemia or lymphoma

porate information from the various systems in use at the time. This classification system has significant clinical utility but is limited by the identification of newer clinically significant subtypes of NHL that were unclassifiable by the Working Formulation. In addition, improved understanding of the biology and treatment of certain NHL subtypes prompted the revised European-American Classification (REAL) of lymphoid neoplasms (Table 1A.12). An attempt to categorize the lymphomas using the REAL classification as indolent (I), aggressive (A), or controversial (C) has been made. However, the clinical utility of the REAL classification remains under investigation.

STAGING EVALUATION

After the diagnosis of NHL is established, the appropriate staging should begin with a careful history and physical examination with attention to B symptoms, associated risk factors, and nodal and extranodal sites. Laboratory evaluation should include a hemogram, a chemistry profile that includes a serum LDH level, serum b-2 microglobulin, serum protein electropheresis, and HIV test. Staging studies should include chest radiograph; computed tomographys of the chest, abdomen, and pelvis; and a bone marrow biopsy. In certain cases additional information may be obtained with nuclear medicine studies (gallium scan, bone scan, positron emission tomography), spinal tap, magnetic resonance imaging, or gastrointestinal series. As with Hodgkin's disease, the Ann Arbor staging system (Table 1A.13) is used for the staging of patients with NHL.

PROGNOSIS

Histologic subtype (indolent versus aggressive) remains the most significant predictor of survival in NHL. The International Non-Hodgkin's Lymphomas Prognostic Factors Project has reported a predictive model for aggressive non-Hodgkin's lymphoma based on an analysis of presenting features and outcome in 2031 patients. Four risk groups were identified according to age (above or below age 60 years), stage (I, II or III, IV), serum lactic acid dehydrogenase (LDH) levels (normal or elevated), performance status (0 to 1 or 2 to 4), and number of extranodal sites (0 to 1 or 2 to 4). In the low-risk group (35% of patients), the CR rate was 87%, and overall survival at 5 years was 73%. In the high-risk group the CR rate was 44%, and the overall survival at 5 years was only 26%. The International Prognostic Index appears to apply also to indolent lymphomas.

TREATMENTS

For clinical purposes the non-Hodgkin's lymphomas are divided into indolent and aggressive subtypes. Indolent NHL has

Table 1A.12. Revised European-American Classification of Lymphoid Neoplasms

B-cell neoplasms

I. Precursor B-cell neoplasm: Precursor B-lymphoblastic leukemia or lymphoma[A]
II. Peripheral B-cell neoplasms
    A. B-cell CLL[I], prolymphocytic leukemia[A], small lymphocytic lymphoma[I]
    B. Lymphoplasmacytoid lymphoma[I], immunocytoma[I]
    C. Mantle cell lymphoma[AI]
    D. Follicle center lymphoma, follicular[I]
        1. Provisional cytologic grades: I (small cell[I]), II (mixed small, large cell[I]), III (large cell[C])
        2. Provisional subtype: diffuse, predominantly small cell type[I]
    E. Marginal zone B-cell lymphoma[I]
        1. Extranodal (MALT type[I] with or without monocytoid B-cells[I])
        2. Provisional subtype: nodal with or without monocytoid B cells[I]
    F. Provisional entity: splenic marginal zone lymphoma[I] with or without villous lymphocytes
    G. Hairy cell leukemia[I]
    H. Plasmacytoma, plasma cell myeloma[I]
    I. Diffuse large B-cell lymphoma[A]
        1. Subtype: Primary mediastinal (thymic) B-cell lymphoma[A]
    J. Burkitt's lymphoma[A]
    K. Provisional entity: high-grade B-cell lymphoma, Burkitt's-like[A]

T-cell and Putative NK-cell Neoplasms

I. Precursor T-cell neoplasm: precursor T-lymphoblastic lymphoma, leukemia[A]
II. Peripheral T-cell and NK-cell neoplasms
    A. T-cell chronic lymphocytic leukemia[A], prolymphocytic leukemia[A]
    B. Large granular lymphocyte leukemia (LGL)
        1. T-cell type[I]
        2. NK-cell type[A]
    C. Mycosis fungoides, Sezary's syndrome[I]
    D. Peripheral T-cell lymphomas, unspecified[A]
        1. Provisional cytologic categories: medium-sized cell, mixed medium-large cell, large cell, lymphoepithelioid cell
        2. Provisional subtype: hepatosplenic g/d T-cell lymphoma
        3. Provisional subtype: subcutaneous panniculitic T-cell lymphoma
    E. Angioimmunoblastic T-cell lymphoma (AILD)[A]
    F. Angiocentric lymphoma[A]
    G. Intestinal T-cell lymphoma, leukemia with or without enteropathy[A]

continued

Table 1A.12.   Revised European-American Classification of Lymphoid Neoplasms *continued*

T-cell and Putative NK-cell Neoplasms

  H. Adult T-cell lymphoma, leukemia (ATL/L)[A]
  I. Anaplastic large cell lymphoma (ALCL) (CD 30+, T-cell, and null-cell types[A])
  J. Provisional entity: Anaplastic large-cell lymphoma, Hodgkin's-like[A]

[I], indolent; [A], aggressive; [C], controversial.

Table 1A.13.   The Ann Arbor Staging System for Non-Hodgkin's Lymphoma

Stage	Substage
Stage I	
Involvement of a single lymph node region	I
Localized involvement of a single extralymphatic site or organ	I$_E$
Stage II	
Two or more nodal regions on the same side of diaphragm	II
Localized involvement of a single associated extralymphatic site or organ and its regional nodes with or without other lymph node regions on the same side of the diaphragm	IIE
Stage III	
Nodal regions on both sides of diaphragm	III
Nodal regions on both sides of diaphragm in addition to localized involvement of an extralymphatic site or organ	IIIE
Including the spleen	III^S
Or both the spleen and an extralymphatic site	IIIE^S
Stage IV	
Disseminated (multifocal) involvement of one or more extralymphatic sites or organs with or without lymph node involvement or isolated extralymphatic organ involvement with distant lymph node involvement	IV

Sites may be identified by the following: N, nodes; H, liver; P, pleura; O, bone; D, skin; S, spleen.
The number of lymph node groups involved may be indicated by a subscript (e.g., II$_3$). Patients may be further subclassified as A (absence) or B (presence) of systemic symptoms (weight loss > 10% in 6 months, fevers, drenching night sweats).

a favorable prognosis, with median survival as long as 10 years. These lymphomas often respond well to either radiation therapy or chemotherapy. Unfortunately, the indolent lymphomas are characterized by recurrence and eventual resistance to therapy or transformation to an aggressive histology. As the name suggests, the aggressive NHLs have a shorter natural history. Up to 60% of patients with aggressive NHL can be cured with current therapy.

LOCALIZED DISEASE

NHL is considered to be localized if it is confined to one or two immediately adjacent sites (stages I, IE, II, IIE), no tumor mass is larger than 10 cm, and if the patient has no systemic symptoms of lymphoma (fevers, night sweats, weight loss).

Localized Indolent non-Hodgkin's Lymphomas

Some 10 to 20% of patients with indolent lymphomas are determined to have localized (stage I, II) disease on intensive staging. These patients should be considered for involved or extended-field radiation therapy. Long-term disease-free survival of more than 50% is common, and a small number of patients may be cured with this approach. Chemotherapy provides no additional benefit to radiation in patients with favorable prognostic features but may be appropriate if radiation is contraindicated or other adverse prognostic features are present. Asymptomatic patients with poor performance status and localized indolent NHL can be observed clinically.

Localized Aggressive Non-Hodgkin's Lymphoma

In accordance with the results of randomized trials comparing cyclophosphamide plus doxorubicin, vincristine, and prednisone (CHOP) plus radiation therapy with radiation alone and with chemotherapy alone in patients with localized aggressive NHLs, the recommended treatment for patients with localized aggressive disease is CHOP plus involved-field or extended-field radiation therapy. The 5-year overall survival was 87% with 3 cycles of CHOP plus radiation in a Southwestern Oncology Group (SWOG) randomized trial. For patients with adverse prognostic features (e.g., bulky disease), more than three cycles of CHOP should be considered.

Advanced Disease

Advanced Indolent Non-Hodgkin's Lymphomas

With today's therapy, the vast majority of patients with disseminated indolent non-Hodgkin's lymphomas cannot be cured. As the goal of therapy is palliative for most patients, it is appropriate to observe asymptomatic patients until symptoms demand treatment. As always, decisions on treatment should be individualized. Younger patients with good performance status should be considered for aggressive investigational approaches such as high-dose therapy with stem cell transplantation.

Palliative approaches include radiation therapy, single-agent chemotherapy, interferon, monoclonal antibodies (Rituximab), or a combination of these modalities. Active chemotherapeutic agents include the purine analogues (fludarabine, 2-chlorodeoxyadenosine), alkylating agents (chlorambucil, cyclophosphamide), and corticosteroids. Combination regimens include CVP (cyclophosphamide, vincristine, and prednisone), CHOP, and FND (fludarabine, mitoxantrone, and decadron). Durable complete or partial remissions can be achieved in most patients with disseminated low-grade NHL.

Salvage for disseminated recurrent indolent lymphomas may be achieved with similar treatments in 40 to 50% of patients. In moderate doses, the interferons have achieved results similar to those of standard chemotherapy agents, but the side effect profile may not be acceptable to some patients. A promising new monoclonal antibody (Rituximab) directed against the B-cell marker CD-20 has recently been released and has reported response rates of 50% in previously treated patients. For patients with indolent lymphomas the role of high-dose chemotherapy with stem cell rescue remains investigational.

Advanced Aggressive Non-Hodgkin's Lymphomas

In contrast to most patients with indolent lymphomas, a large percentage of patients with aggressive lymphomas are curable with combination chemotherapy. The treatment of most disseminated aggressive non-Hodgkin's lymphomas, anthracycline-based combination regimens, produces long-term disease-free survival in 35 to 45% of all patients. An important randomized trial comparing CHOP with newer combinations (ProMACE CytaBOM [cyclophosphamide, doxorubicin, etoposide, Prednisone, cytarabine, bleomycin, vincristine, methotrexate, and leucovorin], m-BACOD [Methotrexate, leucovorin, bleomycin, doxorubicin, vincristine, and dexamethasone], MACOP-B [methotrexate, leucovorin, doxorubicin, cyclophosphamide, vincristine, bleomycin, and prednisone]) showed no advantage to the newer regimens over CHOP. For patients over 60 years of age the combination of CNOP (cyclophosphamide, mitoxantrone, vincristine, and prednisone) was shown to be inferior to CHOP in a randomized trial.

Low and low-to-intermediate risk (International Prognostic Index) patients younger than 60 should be offered 6 to 8 cycles of CHOP. Younger patients who have high intermediate or high-risk features should be considered for more aggressive approaches such as high-dose chemotherapy and stem cell rescue. The treatment of patients older than 60 is often complicated by intolerance of standard regimens and comorbid medical conditions. Hence, treatments must be individualized, and alternative regimens and/or growth factors may be required to maintain adequate dose intensity.

Relapsed Aggressive Non-Hodgkin's Lymphoma

Retreatment with standard chemotherapy regimens is seldom curative for patients with relapsed aggressive NHL; bone marrow transplantation (BMT) is the treatment of choice for appropriate patients with relapsed aggressive NHL. In a prospective trial, 109 patients below age 60 with relapsed NHL and chemosensitive disease were randomized to receive further chemotherapy or BMT. At 5-year median follow-up, those receiving BMT had an overall survival of 53% versus 32% for those continuing chemotherapy.

CENTRAL NERVOUS SYSTEM THERAPY

Patients who are at high risk for CNS involvement require modified approaches. The risk of spread to the CNS is greatest in patients with lymphoblastic lymphoma, Burkitt's and Burkitt's-like lymphoma, and the HTLV-1-associated NHL. Patients with other aggressive histologic subtypes and with involvement of certain extranodal sites (bone marrow, testicles, and/or the central facial sinuses) also have an increased incidence of CNS disease. CNS therapy entails intrathecal administration of chemotherapy (methotrexate, cytosine arabinoside, hydrocortisone). Craniospinal radiation therapy is also incorporated into many protocols for the treatment of high-grade NHLs.

UNCOMMON NON-HODGKIN'S LYMPHOMA SUBTYPES

MALT Lymphomas

This subtype of indolent NHL often manifests as localized disease, often involving the stomach. This subtype of NHL is associated with *Helicobacter pylori* infections. Effective treatment of the underlying infection with bismuth, omeprazole, metronidazole, and amoxacillin may result in complete regression of the disease.

Cutaneous T-Cell Lymphoma

Cutaneous T-cell lymphoma (CTCL), or mycosis fungoides, is a rare indolent T-cell lymphoma characterized by cutaneous involvement (erythematous patches and plaques) that may gradually progress to generalized skin, lymph node, and visceral involvement. Patients with localized skin disease may be effectively treated with topical alkylating agents (carmustine [BCNU], mechlorethamine). Psoralen with ultraviolet light (PUVA) is also frequently used to control cutaneous disease. For patients with more advanced skin involvement, photopheresis is another effective modality. Electron beam radiation therapy can effectively palliate refractory skin lesions. Systemic chemotherapy, which is palliative, is usually reserved for advanced refractory or visceral disease. Active systemic agents include the alkylating agents, purine analogues, interferon, and the retinoids.

Mantle Cell Lymphoma

Once considered an indolent lymphoma, mantle cell lymphoma is now considered to be an aggressive B-cell malignancy with a median survival of only 3 years with standard treatments. This lymphoma resembles follicular small cleaved cell lymphoma and is associated with the t(11;14), *bcl-1* gene rearrangement. Bone marrow and extranodal involvement is common. Appropriate patients should be considered for intensive treatments such as consolidative BMT.

Lymphoblastic Lymphoma

Lymphoblastic lymphoma is an aggressive T-cell lymphoma often afflicting young patients. Clinical manifestations may include a mediastinal mass, leukemic phase, disseminated disease, hypercalcemia, and increased risk (20 to 30%) of CNS involvement. Treatment approaches are similar to those for acute lymphocytic leukemia involving CNS therapy (intrathecal chemotherapy with or without radiation), aggressive alternating multidrug chemotherapy, and maintenance therapy. Approximately 45% of these patients have long-term disease-free survival with this approach. Patients with adverse features should be considered for high-dose therapy and stem cell rescue.

Diffuse Small Non–Cleaved Cell Lymphoma

Diffuse small non–cleaved cell (Burkitt's) lymphoma is an extremely aggressive disseminated lymphoma that often presents with an acute onset of systemic symptoms and an abdominal mass. Advanced disease, systemic symptoms, and extranodal involvement are common at presentation. Treatment with aggressive CHOP-like regimens with additional methotrexate, CNS treatment, and maintenance therapy can achieve long-term disease-free survival. Approaches similar to the treatment of acute lymphocytic leukemia involving aggressive alternating systemic therapy and CNS prophylaxis have been investigated. Consolidative bone marrow transplantation may be appropriate for certain high-risk patients.

BIBLIOGRAPHY

Aisenberg AC. Coherent view of non-Hodgkin's lymphoma. J Clin Oncol 1995;13:2656–2675.

Armitage JO. Treatment of non-Hodgkin's lymphoma. N Engl J Med 1993;328:1023–1030.

Armitage JO. The changing classification of non-Hodgkin's lymphomas. CA Cancer J Clin 1997;47:323–325.

Cannellos GP. CHOP may have been part of the beginning but certainly not the end: issues in risk-related therapy for large-cell lymphoma. J Clin Oncol 1997;15:1713–1716.

Fisher RI, Gaynor ER, Dahlberg S, et al. Comparison of a standard regimen (CHOP) with three intensive chemotherapy regimens for advanced non-Hodgkin's lymphoma. N Engl J Med 1993;328:1002–1006.

Gianni AM, Bregni M, Siena S, et al. High-dose chemotherapy and autologous bone marrow transplantation compared with MACOP-B in aggressive B-cell lymphoma. N Engl J Med 1997;336:1290–1297.

Harris NL, Jaffe ES, Stein H, et al. A revised European-American classification of lymphoid neoplasms: a proposal from the International Lymphoma Study Group. Blood 1994;84:1361–1392.

Skarin AT, Dorfman DM. Non-Hodgkin's lymphomas: current classification and management. CA Cancer J Clin 1997;47:327–350.

The International Non-Hodgkin's Lymphoma Prognostic Factors Project. A predictive model for aggressive non-Hodgkin's lymphoma. N Engl J Med 1993;329:987–994.

Part B

Solid Tumors

Malignant Melanoma

Clay M. Anderson and John D. Wilkes

BACKGROUND

Malignant melanoma is becoming an increasingly important clinical problem in the Unites States and other temperate regions of the world. Fortunately, despite the increasing incidence of melanoma, the curability of the disease is also increasing, because of better education and screening. Currently, 80% of persons diagnosed with melanoma in the United States will be cured of their disease by appropriate surgical management. Unfortunately, 20% of patients, some of whom had low-risk primary melanomas treated with adequate surgical therapy, eventually die of metastatic disease. This brief review primarily focuses on the various approaches to systemic therapy for advanced melanoma, including chemotherapy, immunotherapy, and combination strategies for both the adjuvant and the stage IV clinical settings.

EPIDEMIOLOGY

Melanoma is the seventh most common malignancy diagnosed in the United States, where in 1998 there will be approximately 41,600 new cases of melanoma and 7,000 deaths. The incidence of melanoma is increasing rapidly; by the year 2000, 1 in 75 Americans will be diagnosed with melanoma at some time in their life. Men are affected 1.2 times as frequently as women.

ETIOLOGY

The increase in melanoma incidence appears to be due in large part to ultraviolet radiation exposure, with highest incidence occurring in Australia, Israel, Hawaii, and Arizona. Polygenetic factors also play a role, as patients with congenital nevi, the dysplastic nevus syndrome, fair complexion, light-colored hair and eyes, and those who sunburn easily have increased risk. It is estimated that 9% of melanomas are familial.

CLINICAL MANIFESTATIONS

Most melanomas begin as a pigmented macular skin lesion that with time enlarges and may form patches, plaques, ulcers, or nodules. Clinical findings that suggest the diagnosis of melanoma include (*a*) asymmetry, (*b*) borders that are irregular, (*c*) color or pigment variation, and/or (*d*) diameter larger than 6 mm.

There are four common clinical types of melanoma: superficial spreading melanoma (70%), nodular melanoma (10 to 15%), lentigo maligna melanoma (10 to 15%), and acral lentiginous melanoma (less than 10%). Rarely, melanomas arise from non-cutaneous sites, including the retina, gastrointestinal tract, or genitourinary tract.

STAGING EVALUATION

After a careful history with attention to risk factors and physical examination with documentation of the primary lesion and any potential metastatic sites (lymph nodes, satellite lesions), patients should be evaluated by an experienced physician for excisional or punch biopsy (Table 1B.1). Lymph node involvement may be determined with sentinel lymph node biopsy. In most cases clinical staging is not possible, and pathologic staging is performed on the completely resected primary lesion and lymph nodes. Chest radiograph and blood chemistry may give some indication of occult metastases.

PROGNOSIS

For primary melanomas, the depth of penetration (pT stage, Breslow's thickness) is the most significant prognostic factor. Superficial spreading melanomas lack a vertical growth phase and have a more favorable prognosis than nodular melanomas, which rapidly enter a vertical growth phase and are more predisposed to metastasize. However, when corrected for thickness, all subtypes of melanoma have similar prognoses. Stage for stage, women tend to have a more favorable prognosis than men.

TREATMENTS

Until recently medical therapy, designed either to prevent recurrence after surgery or to treat regional or distant metastases, has been largely ineffective. In the past several years, however, more promising clinical results have been recorded for both adjuvant therapy and therapy for stage IV disease. We now have a standard adjuvant therapy for resected nodal (stage III) metastasis in the form of high-dose interferon-α, and encouraging clinical responses have been documented in stage IV patients receiving biochemotherapy regimens. In addition, interleukin 2 (IL-2) therapy continues to produce durable remissions in a significant minority of stage IV patients, and vaccine therapy and gene therapy hold hope as future strategies against this difficult disease.

Table 1B.1A. TNM Staging System for Cutaneous Malignant Melanoma

Primary tumor

pTX	Primary tumor cannot be assessed.
pT0	No evidence of primary tumor.
pTis	Melanoma in situ (atypical melanocytic hyperplasia, severe melanocytic dysplasia), not an invasive lesion (Clark's level I).
pT1	Tumor 0.75 mm thick or less and invading the papillary dermis (Clark's level II).
pT2	Tumor larger than 0.75 mm but no larger than 1.5 mm thick and/or invades the papillary-reticular dermal interface (Clark's level III).
pT3	Tumor more than 1.5 mm but not more than 4 mm thick and/or invades the reticular dermis (Clark's level IV).
pT3a	Tumor larger than 1.5 mm but no more than 3 mm thick.
pT3b	Tumor larger than 3 mm but no more than 4 mm thick.
pT4	Tumor larger than 4 mm thick and/or invades the subcutaneous tissue (Clark's level V) and/or satellite(s) within 2 cm of the primary tumor.
pT4a	Tumor larger than 4 mm thick and/or invades subcutaneous tissue.
pT4b	Satellite(s) within 2 cm of the primary.

Regional lymph nodes

NX	Regional nodes cannot be assessed.
N0	No regional lymph node metastasis.
N1	Metastasis no more than 3 cm in greatest diameter in any regional lymph node(s).
N2	Metastasis larger than 3 cm in greatest diameter in any regional lymph node(s) and/or in transit metastases.[a]
N2a	Metastasis larger than 3 cm in greatest diameter in any regional lymph node(s).
N2b	In transit metastases.
N2c	Both N2a and N2b.

Distant metastasis

MX	Presence of distant metastasis cannot be assessed.
M0	No distant metastasis.
M1	Distant metastasis.
M1a	Metastasis in skin or subcutaneous tissue or lymph node(s) beyond the regional lymph nodes.
M1b	Visceral metastases.

[a]*In transit metastases involve skin or soft tissue metastases larger than 2 cm from the primary tumor and not beyond the regional lymph nodes.*

Table 1B.1B. Stage Grouping for Cutaneous Malignant Melanoma

Stage	T	Thickness (mm)	N	M	5-Yr Survival (%)
0	pTis		N0	M0	—
I	pT1	≤ 0.75	N0	M0	95
	pT2	0.76–1.5			
II	pT3	1.51–4	N0	M0	80
III	pT4	>4	N0	M0	40
	Any pT	—	N1	M0	
		—	N2	M0	
IV	Any pT	—	Any N	M1	<10

Adapted with permission from American Joint Committee on Cancer. Cancer staging manual. 5th ed. Philadelphia: Lippincott-Raven, 1997.

ADJUVANT THERAPY

Melanoma is an unpredictable neoplasm; even thin primary melanomas sometimes recur in lymph nodes and/or distant sites years after the removal of the primary lesion. In addition, many patients present with intermediate-thickness or deep primary lesions or have clinically evident nodal disease at the outset. These patients have a lifetime risk of recurrence after surgery that varies from 25 to 75%. Once these patients recur, they are likely to die of the disease. Various strategies tried after surgery in these at-risk populations include single-agent chemotherapy, combination chemotherapy, immunotherapy with Bacillus Calmette-Guérin, *Corynebacterium parvum*, various vaccines or levamisole, combinations of chemotherapy and immunotherapy (not including biochemotherapy), and high-dose chemotherapy with bone marrow transplantation. Until recently no approach produced significant reproducible benefits compared with observation.

In 1995, the results of several randomized studies comparing interferon-α with placebo were published. All four trials showed a trend toward improved disease-free and overall survival in the interferon arm. The most significant benefit was seen from the Eastern Cooperative Oncology Group (ECOG) 1684 trial, which used high-dose interferon-α for 1 year in patients with nodal involvement or primaries more than 4 mm thick. This trial, which formed the basis for FDA approval of interferon-α, showed a 10% absolute improvement in overall survival at 5 years with interferon compared with no treatment after surgery (15% absolute improvement in survival in the node-positive patients at 5 years).

Because of the modest benefit, cost, and toxicity of this high-dose interferon strategy, investigators are pursuing newer vaccine strategies and shorter, more intensive biochemotherapy approaches as possible adjuvant therapy for high-risk melanoma.

TREATMENT FOR DISSEMINATED DISEASE

Metastatic melanoma is a difficult clinical problem because the disease exhibits primary resistance to most chemotherapy drugs in a majority of cases. Despite the fact that melanoma responds to immunotherapy approaches better than other solid tumors, only 10% of patients obtain significant clinical benefit from this approach. In the stage IV setting the only FDA-approved therapy is single-agent dacarbazine (DTIC). This alkylating agent has never been proved to prolong survival compared with supportive care alone in stage IV melanoma. At present no other treatment strategy has been proved superior to single-agent DTIC in terms of survival benefit, and there remains no real standard therapy for stage IV disease.

Treatments that have shown some clinical activity include single-agent and combination chemotherapy, biologic response modifiers, other forms of immunotherapy, and strategies incorporating both chemotherapy drugs and immunotherapy agents (biochemotherapy). Vaccines and gene therapy have unproven clinical activity in this setting.

Chemotherapy

Other than single-agent DTIC, chemotherapy drugs that have shown some clinical activity against melanoma include cisplatin; the vinca alkaloids; the nitrosoureas, including lomustine and carmustine; bleomycin; and hydroxyurea. Newer agents, including the taxanes and the nitrosourea fotemustine, are also active. Response rates are in the range of 10 to 20%. Conspicuously lacking in activity are the classic alkylators, intercalating agents, and topoisomerase II inhibitors.

Combinations of the active drugs have consistently produced higher responses in phase II studies (20 to 40%) but no improved survival in phase III studies. The two most popular combination regimens used in the community are CVD (cisplatin, vinblastine, and dacarbazine) and the Dartmouth regimen (cisplatin, carmustine, dacarbazine, and tamoxifen), both of which are fairly well tolerated and showed impressive response rates in phase II studies. The role of tamoxifen, which has little activity as a single agent, is unclear, but the only randomized study showed it did not contribute to the response rate of the Dartmouth regimen. Newer combinations being investigated include fotemustine, temozolamide (a dacarbazinelike compound with oral bioavailability), and tirapazamine (a hypoxic cell sensitizer).

Biologic Therapy

Because of the lack of activity of cytotoxic drugs against melanoma and the interesting early observations of regressing primaries, vitiligo, and spontaneous remissions in melanoma patients, immunotherapy approaches have been an active area of investigation for decades. Two cytokine agents, IL-2 and interferon-α, have led the way in terms of documented durable remissions in stage IV melanoma patients. Interleukin-2, also known as T-cell growth factor, has no antitumor activity on its own but is a potent stimulator of lymphokine-activated killing activity in natural killer (NK) cells and T cells. The exact mechanism by which IL-2 affects melanoma in vivo is still unclear. While at higher doses it has significant toxicity, including hypotension, capillary leak syndrome, and renal insufficiency, it can lead to durable remissions in almost 10% of stage IV patients. IL-2 may have more clinical activity when combined with interferon and/or chemotherapy drugs. The addition of stimulated and expanded immune cells to IL-2 (adoptive immunotherapy) has not produced improved clinical results.

Interferon-α, another cytokine, differs from IL-2 in that it can kill cancer cells or inhibit their growth directly. It is also a potent immunostimulant, and it has both antiangiogenic and differentiating properties. In melanoma interferon-α can produce responses in the range of 15% of stage IV patients, but only 2 to 5% are complete or durable. Interferon-α does potentiate the effects of IL-2 and certain chemotherapy drugs. The combination of IL-2 at more moderate doses and interferon-α may be more effective and less toxic than high-dose IL-2 alone, although randomized trials have yet to confirm this hypothesis.

Biochemotherapy

During the 1980s, numerous investigators began to combine interferons and IL-2 with select chemotherapy drugs to explore possible synergistic clinical activity against melanoma. Until recently these approaches seemed to increase toxicity without significantly improving response rates or survival relative to either approach alone. Dacarbazine plus interferon-α or IL-2 has been shown to be no better than dacarbazine alone. Cisplatin plus IL-2 seems to have slightly better clinical activity than moderate-dose IL-2 alone, but no randomized studies have been done.

More recently, several centers have reported on the combination of cisplatin-based chemotherapy with IL-2 and interferon-α (biochemotherapy regimens). Overall response rates up to 70% and complete response rates of 10 to 20% have been observed, with most of the complete responses being durable. These results are very encouraging, but this form of therapy is more toxic than other regimens, and ongoing randomized studies must be reported before we know whether this is a real advance.

Vaccines

Much like the biologic therapy approach, vaccine therapy for stage IV melanoma has had a fairly long track record, but with less documented success to date because of lack of identification of melanoma antigens and technical obstacles. To a large degree both of these limitations have been overcome in the past several years. Newer vaccines, including anti-idiotypic antibodies, melanoma antigen peptides, and peptide-pulsed dendritic cells, are replacing the older autologous or allogeneic whole-cell vaccines of the 1970s and 1980s. The clinical effectiveness of vaccine therapy is still unknown.

Gene Therapy

With the identification of the genes for some important melanoma antigens and cytokines important in the immune response against melanoma, the stage has been set for the application of gene therapy against this disease. Researchers at the National Cancer Institute (NCI) and other centers are transfecting immune cells or tumor cells ex vivo with cytokine genes or melanoma antigen genes. They are selecting for successfully transfected cells and then reinfusing those cells into the patient to generate a more potent and specific immune response against the patient's own tumor. Whether these approaches will lead to more successful treatments for stage IV patients is uncertain.

FUTURE DIRECTIONS

While historical results for systemic therapy in advanced melanoma have been disappointing, there is reason to be optimistic. First, rapidly emerging new agents, including temozolamide, tirapazamine, and fotemustine, may have unique activity against this difficult disease. Second, newer cytokines, including IL-12 and IL-15, that are emerging from phase I and II trials may be effective in combination with chemotherapy against melanoma. Third, we eagerly await results of randomized studies from the M. D. Anderson Cancer Center, the NCI, an intergroup trial, and the European Organization for Research and Treatment of Cancer (EORTC) that are comparing biochemotherapy with combination chemotherapy. Last, basic research into the phenotypic and molecular determinants of resistance of melanoma cells to cytotoxic drugs and specific immunity will yield important clinical results within a few years.

BIBLIOGRAPHY

Anderson CM, Buzaid AC, Legha SS. Systemic treatments for advanced cutaneous melanoma. Oncology 1995;9:1149–1158.

Atkins MB, O'Boyle KR, Sosman JA, et al. Multiinstitutional phase II trial of intensive combination chemoimmunotherapy for metastatic melanoma. J Clin Oncol 1994;12:1553–1560.

Balch CM, Soong SJ, Bartolucci AA, et al. Efficacy of an elective regional lymph node dissection of 1 to 4 mm thick melanomas for patients 60 years of age or younger. Ann Surg 1996;224:255–266.

Buzaid AC, Legha SS. Combination of chemotherapy with IL-2 and interferon-α for the treatment of advanced melanoma. Semin Oncol 1994;21:23–28.

Cascinelli N, Bufalino R, Morabito A, et al. Results of adjuvant interferon study in WHO melanoma programme. Lancet 1994;343:913–914.

Kirkwood JM, Strawderman MH, Ernstoff MS, et al. Interferon α 2b adjuvant therapy of high-risk resected melanoma: The Eastern Cooperative Oncology Group trial EST 1684. J Clin Oncol 1996;14:7–17.

National Institutes of Health Consensus Development Conference Statement. Diagnosis and treatment of early melanoma. JAMA 1992;268:1314–1319.

Sondak VK, Wolfe JA. Adjuvant therapy of melanoma: Overview of reported studies and studies in progress. Curr Opin Oncol 1997;9:189–204.

Sparano JA, Fisher RI, Sunderland M, et al. Randomized phase III trial of treatment with high-dose IL-2 either alone or in combination with interferon alfa-2a in patients with advanced melanoma. J Clin Oncol 1993;11:1969–1977.

Adult Central Nervous System Tumors

John D. Wilkes

BACKGROUND

Malignant neoplasms may arise from any structure within the cranial vault. Most of these tumors are malignant gliomas that demonstrate high-grade features. These tumors are extremely heterogeneous in their presentation, management approaches, and outcomes. Thus, the multimodality involvement of neurosurgeons, radiation oncologists, medical oncologists, neurologists, and neuroradiologists has paramount importance. Despite intensive investigation of many agents, the role of chemotherapy remains quite limited for all but a few subsets of these patients.

EPIDEMIOLOGY

There were an estimated 17,400 cases of primary CNS neoplasms diagnosed in 1998 in the United States. In adults the incidence of primary CNS malignancy increases with age, as most cases are diagnosed after age 45. Grade III (anaplastic astrocytomas) and IV (glioblastoma multiforme) astrocytomas are the most common primary brain tumors in adults, accounting for 2.3% of all cancer-related deaths. In children, primary central nervous system (CNS) tumors are the most common solid tumor and second most common cause of cancer death. The incidence of CNS tumors appears to be increasing, and there is a slight male predominance.

ETIOLOGY

The cause of primary CNS tumors remains unknown. Genetic factors have been implicated, although fewer than 5% of patients diagnosed have a family history of brain tumors. Inherited disorders also predispose to the development of primary brain tumors (Li-Fraumeni syndrome, von Hippel-Lindau disease, neurofibromatosis, tuberous sclerosis). Implicated environmental factors include radiation, exposure to vinyl chloride or petrochemicals, and head trauma.

CLINICAL MANIFESTATIONS

Patients with CNS tumors may present with signs of increased intracranial pressure such as weakness, headache, or nausea and vomiting. Focal neurologic deficits are seen in approximately 50% of patients, and about 20% present with seizures. CNS hemorrhage is not common with high-grade lesions. Sometimes subtle personality changes may be the only clinical manifestation of the tumor.

DIAGNOSIS AND STAGING

Magnetic resonance imaging with gadolinium contrast is the single most useful test to diagnose a CNS tumor. Although 5% of malignant gliomas are multifocal, most high-grade gliomas present as a single, infiltrating, contrast-enhancing mass with surrounding edema arising from the white matter. Low-grade gliomas are more often nonenhancing infiltrative lesions best appreciated on T2 imaging. Computed tomography (CT) may be useful to identify the calcifications seen in about 50% of oligodendrogliomas but may be false-negative in low-grade gliomas. More recently PET (positron emission tomography) has proven to be extremely useful in differentiating postoperative and postradiation changes from recurrent disease. There is no staging system for primary CNS neoplasms.

PATHOLOGY

Primary CNS malignancies may arise from the astrocytes (astrocytoma), oligodendrocytes (oligodendroglioma), meninges (meningioma), ependymal cells (ependymoma), or germative neuroepithelial cells (medulloblastoma). Astrocytomas constitute 75 to 90% of all malignant brain tumors and based on pathologic findings, may be further classified into low-grade astrocytoma, anaplastic astrocytoma, or glioblastoma multiforme. Oligodendrogliomas are usually low-grade tumors, although transformation to more aggressive anaplastic subtypes may occur. Meningiomas are usually benign. Primary CNS lymphomas are reviewed in the discussion of AIDS-related malignancies at the end of this chapter.

PROGNOSIS

The prognosis of patients with primary CNS tumors is directly related to histologic type. Patients with low-grade astrocytomas and oligodendrogliomas have a median survival of 5 to 10 years with conventional treatment (discussed later). In contrast, patients with anaplastic astrocytomas and glioblastoma multiforme have median survivals of 3 and 1 years, respectively. For high-grade tumors, factors affecting prognosis include age, performance status, duration and type of symptoms, and the extent of surgical resection. The prognosis of low-grade astrocytomas is affected by age, duration of symptoms, postoperative neurologic status, and tumor ploidy.

PRINCIPLES OF MANAGEMENT

The standard treatment of low-grade gliomas (low-grade astrocytomas, oligodendrogliomas) is yet to be defined. The initial management involves surgical intervention for a tissue diagnosis. It remains unclear whether early resection or debulking improves outcome over deferred therapy. Retrospective studies do suggest a benefit to aggressive primary surgical management. Current recommendations are for surgical resection with a focus on debulking and preserving neurologic function. Adjuvant radiation therapy for low-grade gliomas remains controversial, and some defer therapy until signs of clinical progression are present. Patients with limited resections or biopsies alone are more likely to be treated with immediate adjuvant radiation therapy. Two randomized trials to address the issue of early versus delayed radiation therapy for low-grade astrocytomas are under way. The benefit of immediate adjuvant therapy has been established for patients with ependymoma, with 5-year survival rate of 80% compared with 33% in patients undergoing surgery alone.

The initial management of patients with high-grade astrocytomas (anaplastic astrocytoma, glioblastoma) is biopsy, surgical resection, or debulking for diagnosis and relief of symptoms. Extensive initial resection lengthens survival in younger patients with good performance status. Adjuvant radiation therapy improves 1-year survival 3 to 24% over surgery alone. Radiation therapy as primary treatment for unresectable lesions or as adjuvant therapy is extremely important in the management of these malignancies. Various radiation techniques have been evaluated in an attempt to overcome the inherent radioresistance of CNS malignancies and to lessen toxicity to normal brain tissue.

CHEMOTHERAPY

The nitrosoureas (carmustine, lomustine, streptozocin), alkylating agents (procarbazine), and the platinums are the most extensively studied agents for the treatment of primary brain tumors.

ADJUVANT THERAPY

In general, younger patients with relatively good performance status and extensive resections fare better with adjuvant therapy than do older patients, those with poor performance status, and those who receive limited resections. While no adjuvant chemotherapy has proven benefit for patients with low-grade astrocytomas, adjuvant chemotherapy following surgery and radiation has been shown to improve time to treatment failure and survival for adults with anaplastic astrocytoma. Similarly, oligodendrogliomas appear to be chemosensitive and are being studied in the adjuvant setting.

Several randomized trials have evaluated the role of systemic adjuvant BCNU in patients with high-grade astrocytoma, and a marginal improvement in survival has been demonstrated in some trials. A meta-analysis evaluating systemic chemotherapy for patients with high-grade astrocytomas revealed only a 10% improved survival at 1 year. Recent reports from randomized placebo-controlled studies of patients with malignant glioma treated with adjuvant BCNU wafers demonstrated a 2-year survival rate of 31% versus 6% in the control group. Aside from a single study that suggested a benefit to procarbazine, CCNU, and vincristine (PCV) over BCNU in patients with anaplastic astrocytoma, multiagent chemotherapy regimens have shown no superiority over single-agent BCNU. The limited benefits of adjuvant chemotherapy in high-grade astrocytomas make it reasonable to defer therapy until recurrence.

RECURRENT DISEASE

The management of recurrent CNS tumors in adults depends on several factors, including the patient's performance status, age, time to recurrence, initial histology, response to initial treatment, and extent of recurrence. Reresection, radiation, and systemic chemotherapy are all options. Both single-agent nitrosoureas and PCV combinations have been evaluated in the treatment of patients with recurrent glioma. For patients with recurrent low-grade astrocytomas, systemic chemotherapy produces little benefit unless transformation to a higher-grade glioma has occurred. In contrast, oligodendroglioma appears to be quite chemosensitive, with response rates approaching 90%. More recently, BCNU biodegradable polymers (Gliadel wafers) have been implanted in the resection cavity and have demonstrated a significant survival benefit for patients with recurrent malignant gliomas. In a trial of 222 patients, the 6-month survival was 60% compared with 43% in the placebo arm.

MISCELLANEOUS CNS TUMORS

There are few data to support the routine use of chemotherapy as an adjuvant to surgery and/or radiation for patients with less common CNS tumors such as brainstem gliomas, cerebellar astrocytomas, and malignant meningiomas. Ependymomas appear to be more sensitive to a variety of chemotherapeutic agents such as BCNU, platinums, vincristine, and ifosfamide. Response rates for recurrent disease vary from 22 to 80%, with time to progression of 12 to 16 months. Medulloblastomas are also responsive to a variety of chemotherapeutic agents, including the nitrosoureas, vincristine, methotrexate, cyclophosphamide, procarbazine, and the platinums. Single-agent response rates vary between 33 and 80%. Much like primary germ cell tumors, pineal germinomas are also quite sensitive to chemotherapy regimens such as BEP (bleomycin, etoposide, cisplatin).

BIBLIOGRAPHY

Brem H, Pianadosi S, Burger PC, et al. Placebo-controlled trial of safety and efficacy of intraoperative controlled delivery by biodegradable polymers of chemotherapy for recurrent gliomas. The Polymer-Brain Tumor Treatment Group. Lancet 1995;345:1008–1012.

Cairncross G, Macdonald D, Ludwin S, et al. Chemotherapy for anaplastic oligodendroglioma. National Cancer Institute of Canada Clinical Trials Group. J Clin Oncol 1994;12:2013–2021.

Delattre JY, Uchuya M. Radiotherapy and chemotherapy for gliomas. Curr Opin Oncol 1996;8:196–203.

Fine HA, Dear KB, Loeffler JS, et al. Meta-analysis of radiation therapy with or without adjuvant chemotherapy for malignant gliomas in adults. Cancer 1994;71:2585–2597.

Kim L, Hochberg FH, Thornton AF, et al. Procarbazine, lomustine, and vincristine (PCV) chemotherapy for grade III and IV oligoastrocytomas. J Neurosurgery 1996;85:602–607.

Lesser GJ, Grossman S. The chemotherapy of high-grade astrocytomas. Semin Oncol 1994;21:220–235.

Levin VA, Silver P, Hannigan J, et al. Superiority of postradiotherapy chemotherapy with CCNU, procarbazine, and vincristine (PCV) over BCNU for anaplastic gliomas; NCOG 6G61 final report. Int J Radiat Oncol Biol Phys 1990;18:321–324.

Macdonald DR. Low-grade gliomas, mixed gliomas, and oligodendrogliomas. Semin Oncol 1994;21:236–248.

Valtonen S, Timonen U, Toivanen P, et al. Interstitial chemotherapy with carmustine-loaded polymers for high-grade gliomas: a randomized double-blind study. Neurosurg 1997;41:44–49.

Head and Neck Cancer

John D. Wilkes

BACKGROUND

Carcinomas of the head and neck constitute an extremely heterogeneous group of malignancies that as a rule behave aggressively and are often advanced at the time of diagnosis. Patients with head and neck cancers require a coordinated multidisciplinary approach involving head and neck surgeons, radiation oncologists, medical oncologists, and dentists. Chemotherapy was once thought to offer little benefit in head and neck cancers, but with the identification of more effective agents and the refinement of treatment approaches, chemotherapy is playing an increasing role in the management of these challenging patients.

EPIDEMIOLOGY

There were approximately 41,000 cases of head and neck cancer diagnosed (3% of all new cancer diagnoses in the United States) and more than 12,000 deaths in 1998. This disease is more common in men than in women, and the incidence rises with age. More than 95% of these malignancies are squamous cell carcinomas, although rare histologies such as melanoma, sarcoma, adenocarcinomas (usually salivary, parotid), and lymphomas may be seen. Anatomically, larynx cancers are most common, followed by cancers of the tongue, lip, buccal or alveolar mucosa, oropharynx, floor of mouth, hypopharynx, nasopharynx, and salivary glands. Second primary tumors of the upper aerodigestive tract remain a significant concern; they may arise at a rate of 3 to 4% per year.

ETIOLOGY

Overall, the cancers of the head and neck are primarily related to tobacco and alcohol use. The use of both alcohol and tobacco is synergistic for cancers of the oropharynx and oral cavity. Exposure to ultraviolet light is a risk factor for cancer of the lip, while certain occupational exposures and Epstein-Barr virus exposure increase the risk for nasopharyngeal cancer. Poor oral hygiene, mechanical irritation, marijuana use, and the Plummer-Vinson syndrome have been implicated in the causation of head and neck cancers. There is also an inverse relation between the intake of fruits and vegetables and the risk of cancers of the head and neck.

CLINICAL MANIFESTATIONS

The symptoms of head and neck cancers are variable, depending on the site or sites involved. Common subjective complaints include dysphagia, odynophagia, changes in phonation, epistaxis, otalgia, and nasal congestion. Physical examination may reveal halitosis, cranial neuropathies, mucosal ulcerations, nodules, or induration. Palpable lymphadenopathy may also be appreciated.

Clinically, cancers of the head and neck are most often characterized by local or regional recurrences (90%), although distant metastatic disease occurs in up to 40% of cases. Hypercalcemia may be seen with advanced disease (15%).

STAGING EVALUATION

The staging and pretreatment evaluation of a patient with head and neck cancer should begin with a careful history and physical examination, blood counts, chemistry panels, and a chest radiograph (Table 1B.2). General endoscopy under anesthesia with careful identification of the primary lesion and biopsy is mandatory. Esophagoscopy must also be performed, as there is a 10 to 15% incidence of synchronous primary tumors in the upper aerodigestive tract. Bronchoscopy is not mandatory unless there is a suspicious finding on chest radiograph.

Computed tomography (CT) and/or magnetic resonance imaging (MRI) is necessary to provide further information on both primary disease and lymph nodes. Other diagnostic evaluations may include angiography, Panorex films, or pharyngoesophagograms. Bone scans should be performed on patients with symptoms or positive lymph nodes and on asymptomatic patients with an unexplained elevation in serum alkaline phosphatase.

PROGNOSIS

A number of factors affect the prognosis of a patient with cancer of the head and neck. As always, staging affects prognosis, with stage I or II disease having a 5-year survival rate of more than 80%, while those with stage IV disease have 5-year survival rates below 10% regardless of primary treatment modality. For example, T1 (stage I) cancers involving sites such as the glottic larynx and lip have 5-year cure rates as high as 80%. More advanced cancers at the same sites, however, carry a very poor prognosis, with cure rates as low as 10 to 15%.

Anatomic location is also a significant prognostic factor. Generally, the prognosis worsens as one proceeds anatomically from the lips to the hypopharynx. The hypopharynx has extensive lymphatic drainage, and tumors at this site remain clinically silent until late in the disease course. As a result, patients often present with advanced disease (lymph node metastases in 40 to 70%), and survival rates for carcinoma of the hypopharynx are perhaps the lowest of all sites in the head and neck. In contrast,

Table 1B.2A. TNM Staging System for Head and Neck Cancers

Regional lymph nodes

NX	Regional lymph nodes cannot be assessed.
N0	No regional lymph node metastasis.
N1	Metastasis in a single ipsilateral lymph node, less than 3 cm.
N2a	Metastasis in a single ipsilateral lymph node larger than 3 but less than 6 cm.
N2b	Metastasis in multiple ipsilateral lymph nodes, none larger than 6 cm.
N2c	Metastasis in bilateral or contralateral lymph nodes, none larger than 6 cm.
N3	Metastasis in a lymph node larger than 6 cm in greatest dimension.

Distant metastasis

MX	Minimum requirements to assess the presence of distant metastasis cannot be met.
M0	No known distant metastasis.
M1	Distant metastasis present.

T-staging for cancers of the head and neck is complex, varying significantly with the anatomic location of the primary lesion. For most sites in the head and neck, these N-stage, M-stage, and stage groupings are uniform. Nasopharyngeal, thyroid, and salivary gland tumors do not adhere to these nodal and stage groupings. In clinical evaluation, the actual size of the nodal mass should be measured, and allowance should be made for intervening soft tissues. Most masses over 3 cm in diameter are not single nodes but confluent nodes or tumors in soft tissues of the neck. Midline nodes are considered homolateral nodes.

Table 1B.2B. Stage Grouping for Head and Neck Cancers

Stage	Tumor	Nodes	Metastasis
0	Tis	N0	M0
I	T1	N0	M0
II	T2	N0	M0
III	T3	N0	M0
	T1,T2,T3	N1	M0
IVA	T4	N0	M0
	T4	N1	M0
	Any T	N2	M0
IVB	Any T	N3	M0
IVC	Any T	Any N	M1

Adapted with permission from American Joint Committee on Cancer. Cancer staging manual. 5th ed. Philadelphia: Lippincott-Raven, 1997.

cancers of the lip tend to present early and have the best prognosis, with more than 90% survival at 5 years.

TREATMENTS

There are few well-designed controlled prospective studies comparing treatment modalities in patients with head and neck cancer. Therefore, it is difficult to state unequivocally the optimal therapy for a specific site or stage. Also, detailed discussion of clinical subtleties, surgical complexities, and radiation practices is beyond the scope of this chapter. The ultimate therapeutic choice must be individualized to the patient, with the experiences of the members of the multidisciplinary team factoring largely into the management plan.

PRIMARY THERAPY

Surgical resection and radiation therapy remain the primary treatment modalities for most patients with squamous cell carcinomas of the head and neck. The choice of treatment is often a complex decision process incorporating the skills of the treating physicians, the needs of the patient, and the treatment that produces the least functional disability. Whenever possible, patients should be managed in a multidisciplinary fashion.

ADJUVANT CHEMOTHERAPY

Although systemic adjuvant chemotherapy does decrease the incidence of distant metastases, numerous randomized prospective trials have been unable to demonstrate a survival advantage to this approach. Adjuvant chemoradiation therapy is being actively investigated in high-risk patients.

NEOADJUVANT CHEMOTHERAPY

Many chemotherapy drugs and combinations have been used in the neoadjuvant setting. The potential advantages to this approach include improved drug delivery, higher local response rates (75 to 85%), improved tolerance by the patient, diminished chance of drug resistance, and earliest treatment of micrometastatic disease. Although neoadjuvant chemotherapy has not been proved in randomized, prospective trials to improve local or regional control or survival, it is commonly used to treat patients with locally advanced disease. There is significant controversy as to whether preoperative chemotherapy responses can allow for more limited surgical resection or radiation. Although response rates are encouraging, the use of neoadjuvant chemotherapy for most sites in the head and neck remains investigational (discussed later).

Organ Preservation

The use of neoadjuvant (induction) chemotherapy for organ preservation has also been investigated. In a prospective randomized trial, the Veterans Administration compared laryngectomy plus postoperative radiation therapy with induction chemotherapy (cisplatin plus 5-FU) followed by irradiation in responding patients. Two-thirds of patients treated with chemotherapy followed by radiation therapy were able to achieve larynx preservation with no compromise in overall survival. A confirmatory trial is ongoing through the Radiation Therapy Oncology Group (RTOG).

Recent data from the EORTC suggest that a similar organ preservation approach may be feasible for hypopharyngeal primaries. In a prospective randomized trial comparing surgery plus postoperative radiation therapy against induction chemotherapy (cisplatin plus 5-FU) followed by irradiation in responding patients, local and regional failures were similar in the two groups. Although the median survival was statistically better for patients receiving induction chemotherapy followed by radiation, 5-year disease-free and overall survival were the same. Functional larynx preservation was achieved in 42% of patients at 3 years and 35% at 5 years.

CONCURRENT OR ALTERNATING CHEMORADIATION THERAPY

For patients with locally advanced carcinomas of the head and neck, concurrent or alternating chemotherapy and radia-tion approaches have been explored. These investigational schedules employ either standard radiation and concurrent single-agent chemotherapy as a radiation sensitizer or full-strength chemotherapy with concurrent alternative radiation schedules (planned treatment breaks). Another approach that entails alternating chemotherapy and radiation has yielded promising initial results. In general, concurrent or alternating chemoradiation therapy regimens have the potential for significant toxicity. Nonetheless, initial trials of this approach are promising.

METASTATIC DISEASE

Distant metastases occur in up to 60% of patients whose primary tumors do not respond to initial treatment. For reasons previously mentioned, the hypopharynx has the highest incidence of distant metastases, followed by the base of the tongue and anterior tongue.

Systemic chemotherapy is often prescribed for patients with locally advanced, previously irradiated and/or disseminated disease. Response rates from pooled clinical trials are listed in Table 1B.3. The significant variation in these data should be interpreted with some caution, as high response rates may indicate small trial size, select patient populations, and variable response criteria.

In general, combination chemotherapy for head and neck cancer yields responses in 40 to 60% of patients, and cisplatin-containing regimens appear to be more active than nonplatinum regimens. Combination regimens have better response rates than single agents at the expense of increased toxicity. There is as yet no clearly superior approach, and treatments should be individualized. Newer classes of agents such as the taxanes appear to have promising response rates and favorable toxicity profiles.

RECURRENT DISEASE

Most treatment failures occur within the first 2 years following definitive surgery and/or irradiation. Treatment options at the time of recurrence depend on the primary modalities employed. In general, surgery should be considered if feasible. If further radiation can be provided, this may also afford excellent

Table 1B.3. Chemotherapy for Advanced Head and Neck Cancers

Regimen	Response Rates (%)
Single agents	
Methotrexate	10–30
Cisplatin	17–30
Carboplatin	15–25
Bleomycin	18–21
Vinblastine	27
Doxorubicin	25
5-fluorouracil (5-FU)	13–15
Paclitaxel	25–40
Docetaxel	32–44
Gemcitabine	13
Ifosfamide	26
Vinorelbine	20
Combinations	
Cisplatin, 5-FU	20–70
Cisplatin, 5-FU, vinblastine	20
Cisplatin, 5-FU, leucovorin (PFL)	56
Cisplatin, paclitaxel	60–72
Paclitaxel, carboplatin	20–23

palliation. Last, chemotherapy can be offered for palliation, as described previously.

BIBLIOGRAPHY

Bachaud J, David J, Boussin G, et al. Combined postoperative radiotherapy and weekly cisplatin infusion for locally advanced squamous cell carcinoma of the head and neck: preliminary report of a randomized trial. Int J Radiat Oncol Biol Phys 1991;20;243–246.

Harari PM. Why has induction chemotherapy for advanced head and neck cancer become a United States community standard of practice? J Clin Oncol 1997;15:2050–2055.

Lefebvre JL, Chevalier D, Luboinsky B, et al. Larynx preservation in pyriform sinus cancer: preliminary results of a European Organization for Research and Treatment of Cancer phase III trial. J Natl Cancer Inst 1996;88:890–899.

Merlano M, Benasso M, Corvo R, et al. Five-year update of a randomized trial of alternating radiotherapy and chemotherapy compared with radiotherapy alone in treatment of unresectable squamous cell carcinoma of the head and neck. J Natl Cancer Inst 1996;88:583–589.

Shah JP, Lydiatt W. Treatment of cancer of the head and neck. CA Cancer J Clin 1995;45:352–368.

Spaulding MB, Fischer SG, Wolf GT et al. Tumor response, toxicity, and survival after neoadjuvant organ-preserving chemotherapy for advanced laryngeal carcinoma. J Clin Oncol 1994;12;1592–1599.

Spitz MR. Epidemiology and risk factors for head and neck cancer. Semin Oncol 1994;21;281–288.

Taylor SG, Murthy AK, Vannetzel JM, et al. Randomized comparison of neoadjuvant cisplatin and fluorouracil infusion followed by radiation versus concomitant treatment in advanced head and neck cancer. J Clin Oncol 1994;12:385–395.

Vokes EE, Weichselbaum RR, Lippman SM, Hong WK. Head and neck cancer. N Engl J Med 1993;328;184–194.

Thyroid Cancer

Victoria J. Dorr

INCIDENCE

In 1997 in the United States there were about 16,100 cases and 1,230 deaths attributable to cancer of the thyroid. Occult thyroid cancer is identified in up to 6 to 15% of autopsies. These are usually microscopic foci of papillary carcinoma. The incidence of thyroid cancer is higher in areas with an increased level of radiation exposure. The median age of occurrence is the fourth decade.

ETIOLOGY AND RISK FACTORS

Low-dose radiation (up to 2000 rad) is a known risk factor for thyroid cancer. Until the 1950s, radiation was commonly given to the head and neck for benign ailments. With a median interval of 20 years to onset, an increase in occult and clinical thyroid cancer was detected. The risk of subsequent malignancy was highest when the exposure occurred during thyroid development in childhood. Interestingly, high doses of radiation have not been associated with an increased risk of malignancy, presumably because of thyroid tissue ablation with high doses.

Prior to iodination of salt, iodine deficiency was associated with an increased incidence of thyroid malignancy. Follicular pathology is most likely to occur in these circumstances, although anaplastic cell type has also been reported.

Medullary thyroid cancer is associated with familial multiple endocrine neoplasia types 2a and 2b. Both Gardner's syndrome and Cowden's disease have been associated with an increased risk of thyroid neoplasms.

SIGNS AND SYMPTOMS

The classic presentation of thyroid cancer is of a solitary asymptomatic thyroid nodule. Symptoms of a thyroid malignancy may include those associated with hyperthyroidism, hypothyroidism or calcitonin secretion, although thyroid dysfunction is rare in thyroid malignancies. Symptoms of mechanical obstruction (hoarseness, dyspnea, or dysphagia) may occur. Observation of the thyroid gland size is important, as normally the thyroid gland is not visible. On physical examination a solitary palpable hard nodule may be noticeable. Fixation to surroundings tissues may also be noted. Occasionally cervical lymphadenopathy is noted. A primary presentation of thyroid cancer as a lymph node metastasis occurs in up to 25% of cases, particularly in young children.

THYROID NODULE EVALUATION

Thyroid nodules are common, affecting 4 to 7% of adults. Nodularity and size of the thyroid gland increase with age. Overall, there is a 5 to 10% risk of malignancy with a thyroid gland nodule. Women are more likely to develop thyroid nodules, but men are twice as likely as women to have a malignant thyroid nodule. Patients with a history of childhood irradiation and a thyroid nodule are likely to have a malignancy identified (approximately a third of the time). Multiple nodules are less likely to be associated with malignancy than single ones.

Patients with nodules that are rapidly growing; young patients; those with nodules that are firm or fixed or are associated with hoarseness, hemoptysis, or lymphadenopathy; and those who have a history of exposure to radiation should have rapid evaluation. Lesions that are incidentally noted on CT or ultrasound may be cautiously observed if nonpalpable and less than 0.5 cm.

Laboratory testing of thyroid function is not useful in differentiating benign from malignant thyroid conditions. However, thyroid function testing should be performed to assess for underlying thyroid disease. Malignant tumors are rarely found to be functional. Hashimoto's thyroiditis can be associated with hypothyroidism; a low thyroid-stimulating hormone (TSH) in the face of a normal thyroid hormone level may indicate a functional adenoma or multinodular goiter.

Any new thyroid nodule or any that increase in size should be sampled with fine-needle aspiration, which has become the cornerstone of thyroid nodule evaluation, replacing biopsy because of its simplicity, safety, and efficacy. The procedure entails inserting a 22- to 25-gauge needle into the nodule, usually without anesthesia, and aspirating. A 90% success rate is reported, and complications are rare. An aspirate interpreted as definitely benign virtually excludes the possibility of malignancy. A false-negative rate of 1% is expected. An aspirate interpreted as malignant requires surgical removal of the nodule. However, fine-needle aspiration 20 to 40% of the time is interpreted as indeterminate or inadequate. In these cases additional evaluation is required. The best test in these circumstances is probably a repeat aspirate. If the second aspirate is also indeterminate, a third attempt under ultrasound guidance is recommended. Since follicular adenocarcinoma is a diagnosis based on capsular penetrance, cytology patterns of microfollicular pattern, follicular neoplasm, or suspicious cytology should be considered for surgical resection. Approximately 25% of these cases are malignant.

Radioisotope scanning for thyroid cancers may be useful. In general, thyroid cancers, as opposed to normal tissue, pick up less of the radioisotope. These areas are considered cold on thyroid scans. The sensitivity of scanning with iodine is 83% and with a technetium radioisotope, about 93%. However, more than 80% of thyroid nodules are cold, resulting in a high number of false-positive findings. The specificity is low for both radioisotopes: 25% for radioiodine scans and 15% for technetium. Therefore, the clinical utility of radioisotope scanning is useful only if negative; a positive scan does not aid in differentiating benign from malignant nodules.

Ultrasonography can be used to define the size and location of the nodule. If a nodule is cystic on ultrasound, it is unlikely to be malignant. The sensitivity of ultrasonography in detecting malignancy is 95%, but the specificity is only 18%. This is because the vast majority of lesions are noncystic. Aspiration of cystic lesions frequently returns nondiagnostic results. Hemorrhagic cysts or those larger than 4 cm are worrisome, and additional evaluation, including surgical resection based on clinical judgment, may be warranted.

Thyroid suppression as a test for thyroid cancer is based on the assumption that thyroid malignancies are not responsive to TSH, while benign nodules are. Thus, administration of sufficient exogenous thyroid replacement to suppress endogenous production should shrink the nodule. Nodules that remain stable or grow during thyroid replacement have 85% sensitivity and 25% specificity for thyroid cancer.

Patients with benign lesions on cytological evaluation can be treated with thyroxine for 6 to 12 months to see whether the nodules resolve. If the lesions have shrunk after 6 to 12 months, thyroxine should be stopped and the nodule monitored. If the nodule enlarges while the patient is taking thyroxine, repeat aspirate or surgical resection should be performed. MRI or CT to evaluate for resectability is indicated for patients with anaplastic thyroid cancer.

STAGING

The staging system for thyroid cancer is shown in Table 1B.4.

ANAPLASTIC THYROID CANCER

Anaplastic cancer of the thyroid constitutes approximately 5% of thyroid cancers. Anaplastic thyroid cancer is a rapidly growing, hard, fixed mass, occasionally with overlying skin breakdown. A mean survival of 6 months is reported. Because of the rapid growth most patients develop tracheal compression,

Table 1B.4. Staging Systems for Thyroid Cancer

Primary Tumor

TX	Tumor size cannot be assessed.
T0	No evidence of primary tumor.
T1	Tumor less than 1cm and limited to the thyroid.
T2	Tumor larger than 1 cm and less than 4 cm and limited to the thyroid.
T3	Tumor larger than 4 cm limited to the thyroid.
T4	Tumor of any size extending beyond the thyroid capsule.

Nodes

NX	Nodes cannot be assessed.
N0	No regional lymph node metastasis.
N1a	Metastasis in ipsilateral cervical lymph node(s).
N1b	Metastasis in bilateral, midline, or contralateral cervical or mediastinal adenopathy.

Distant Metastasis

MX	Presence of distant metastasis cannot be assessed.
M0	No distant metastasis.
M1	Distant metastasis.

Papillary or Follicular

Stage	Under Age 45	Over 45 years
I	Any T, any N, M0	T1, N0, M0
II	Any T, any N, M1	T2 or T3, N0, M0
III	T4, N0, M0, or any T, N1, M0	
IV	Any T, any N, M1	

Medullary (all ages)

Stage	
I	T1, N0, M0
II	T2 or T3 or T4, N0, M0
III	Any T, N1, M0
IV	Any T, Any N, M1

All undifferentiated cases are stage IV.

and tracheostomy may be required for airway protection. Aggressive surgical debulking generally offers limited benefit and does not prolong survival. The treatment of choice is en bloc resection if technically feasible.

PAPILLARY THYROID CARCINOMA

While papillary thyroid cancer is clinically infrequent (fewer than 30 cases per million population worldwide), it is a common incidental finding at autopsy (up to 15%). The peak incidence is in the fourth and fifth decades of life. Papillary carcinoma accounts for up to 75% of thyroid cancers. Papillary cancer presents as a solitary thyroid nodule 75% of the time, but it can present as a solitary ipsilateral lymph node enlargement. Multifocal disease is common, occurring in 30 to 50% of cases. Lymph node metastases occur in up to 40 to 80% of cases, but lymph node involvement does not predict long-term outcome. Patients with aneuploid tumors appear to have the worst prognosis. Poor prognostic characteristics include age over 50 years, large tumor, extensive extrathyroidal invasion, distant metastasis, and poorly differentiated tumors.

The disease-specific mortality rates for papillary thyroid cancer are 2% at 10 years, 3% at 20 years, and 5% at 30 years. Patients with tumor limited to the thyroid had 2% 20-year mortality, and patients with locally invasive tumors had 26% mortality at 20 years. Patients with distant metastatic disease had 69% mortality at 10 years.

Surgical resection for thyroid cancer is the cornerstone of therapy. Conflicting studies argue the relative merits of total thyroidectomy versus lobectomy and isthmectomy. The benefit of total thyroidectomy includes a theoretic advantage in the ability to use total body radioiodine scanning after surgical resection to assess for recurrence. Serum thyroglobulin levels can also be used for follow-up. Risks include an increased risk of laryngeal nerve damage and an 8% risk of hypoparathyroidism. Total thyroidectomy should be performed in patients with prior neck irradiation and in patients with locally advanced or metastatic disease. Lymph nodes should be resected conservatively. Thyroxine should be given postoperatively with the intent of suppressing TSH to undetectable levels.

Thyroid scanning with radioactive iodine (RAI) 4 to 6 weeks after surgery is indicated for high-risk patients. If uptake is noted, a prophylactic dose of RAI (30 mCi) should be considered. False-positives may occur with periodontal surgery, esophageal stricture, hiatal hernia, Zencker's diverticulum, ectopic kidney, or lung cancer. Prior to RAI, patients must not take thyroxine for 4 to 6 weeks; hypothyroid symptoms may be blunted by the use of 50 to 75 µg triiodothyronine for 4 weeks, with discontinuation 2 to 4 weeks prior to scan. Thyroglobulin should be used postoperatively to monitor for thyroid cancer recurrences, although up to 15% of women have antithyroglobulin antibodies, which makes this screening test useless for them.

Follow-up with thyroglobulin and TSH measurement and physical examination should take place twice a year for three years and annually thereafter. Annual chest radiography is recommended.

RAI 100 to 200 mCi should be the first-line therapy for metastatic disease and for cervical node involvement. Repeat dosing is done approximately every 6 months. A maximum of 500 mCi for children and 800 to 1000 mCi for adults is recommended. A tumor with lower thyroid uptake may still be successfully treated with RAI. Cervical and lung lesions tend to respond better than bone or brain lesions. Side effects of RAI therapy may include radiation thyroiditis, sialoadenitis, pulmonary fibrosis, radiation sickness (malaise, nausea, and headache), brain edema if metastases are present, and sterility at doses larger than 800 mCi. External beam radiation therapy can be used for unresectable or recurrent neck disease and for palliation as indicated.

FOLLICULAR CARCINOMA

Follicular thyroid cancer accounts for up to 10% of thyroid cancer. It is most common in areas with iodine deficiency. Women are more likely to be affected than are men. Median age of onset is the sixth decade. Poor prognostic features include size larger than 3 cm, age over 50, and extrathyroidal spread. Pseudocapsules are common. The definition of malignancy as opposed to fibroadenoma is based on penetrance of the pseudocapsule or blood vessel invasion. Thus, needle aspiration is not useful for diagnostic purposes in this lesion. Nodal metastases are uncommon. Patients with minor capsular invasion have a good prognosis, with survival similar to that of age-matched controls; patients with major penetrance of capsule, however, are at significant risk for metastatic disease. Lung and bone are the most frequent sites of metastases.

The treatment of choice is surgical resection by total thyroidectomy. RAI ablation should be considered in high-risk patients. Lifelong suppression of TSH with thyroxine is desirable. The 5-year survival is 80%.

HURTHLE CELL CARCINOMA

Hurthle cell carcinoma, which is considered a variant of follicular carcinoma, occurs more commonly in women than in men. Treatment is total thyroidectomy. RAI ablation is rarely useful in this tumor type. The 5-year survival rate is 60 to 70%.

UNDIFFERENTIATED CANCER: SPINDLE OR GIANT CELL ANAPLASTIC VARIETY

Undifferentiated cancers are aggressive tumors, with survival less than 6 months in general. These tumors are directly invasive and may destroy the trachea. Unless complete resection is feasible, palliative therapy is generally recommended. Palliation can be obtained with external beam radiation therapy or with doxorubicin-based chemotherapy. Responses to these modalities are temporary.

MEDULLARY THYROID CANCER

Medullary thyroid cancer accounts for 5 to 10% of thyroid cancer. It arises from parafollicular C cells. These tumors can secrete calcitonin, carcinoembryonic antigen (CEA), adrenocorticotropic hormone (ACTH), serotonin, histaminase, prostaglandins, neuron-specific enolase, or calcitonin gene–related peptide. Most cases (70%) occur sporadically. A familial predisposition is seen in patients with multiple endocrine neoplasia (MEN) type 2 (tends to be bilateral disease) and in those with familial medullary thyroid carcinoma. Treatment is total thyroidectomy and ipsilateral neck node dissection. Patients with microscopic disease have a 95% 10-year survival. Patients with palpable nodes have a 50% 10-year survival. Calcitonin and CEA should be monitored after surgery. Imaging can also be done with nuclear medicine scans with thallium, metaiodobenzylguanidine (MIBG), or octreotide. These scans lack sensitivity, however. RAI therapy is not indicated. External beam radiation therapy can be used for palliation. Doxorubicin chemotherapy may produce a response.

BIBLIOGRAPHY

Candy B, Rolla AR. Neoplasms of the thyroid. In: Holland JF, Frei E, Bast RC, et al, eds. Cancer medicine. 4th ed. Baltimore: Williams & Wilkins, 1997;1551–1562.

Fraker DL, Skarulis M, Livolsi V. Thyroid tumors. In: DeVita VT, Hellman S, Rosenberg SA, eds. Cancer: principles & practice of oncology. 5th ed. Philadelphia: Lippincott-Raven, 1997;1617–1729.

Landis SH, Murray T, Bolden S, Wingo PA. Cancer statistics 1998. CA Cancer J Clin 1998;48:6–29.

McKittrick RJ, Stephens RL. Chemotherapy of endocrine tumors. In: Perry MC, ed. The chemotherapy source book. 2nd ed. Baltimore: Williams & Wilkins, 1997;1201–1214.

Thyroid cancer. PDQ treatment for health professionals. National Cancer Institute. http://cancernet.nci.nih.gov/clinpdq/soa/Thyroid_cancer_Physician. html; 1/18/98.

Breast Cancer

Victoria J. Dorr

INCIDENCE

Breast cancer is the most frequently diagnosed cancer in women and the second most frequent cause of cancer death in women. The incidence of breast cancer has been increasing steadily over the past several decades. Fortunately, the annual death rate from breast cancer is relatively stable, suggesting that while more women are diagnosed with breast cancer, fewer are dying from it. In 1997 an estimated 180,200 cases of breast cancer occurred in women, with 43,900 deaths secondary to breast cancer. The lifetime risk of developing breast cancer is 12.2%, or 1 in 8 women. The lifetime risk of dying of breast cancer is 3.6%, or 1 in 28 women.

ETIOLOGY AND RISK FACTORS

Many risk factors for the development of breast cancer have been identified.

GENETIC AND FAMILIAL FACTORS

The Romans as early as the first century A.D. reported that certain families were at high risk for breast cancer. Today, about a third of women with breast cancer relate a family history of one or more first-degree relatives with breast cancer; of these 4 to 9% have hereditary breast cancer (autosomal dominant transmission with a high frequency of breast and other cancers). Hereditary breast cancer is, however, believed to be responsible for up to 25% of breast malignancies that occur prior to age 30. Breast cancer in a first-degree relative is associated with a twofold increased risk of breast cancer. Table 1B.5 summarizes the risks of having a hereditary breast cancer.

Two recently discovered genes, BRCA1 and BRCA2, are believed to account for 90% of hereditary breast cancer. BRCA1, which is on chromosome 17q21, is believed to regulate transcription. The penetrance, or cumulative risk, of developing a malignancy with BRCA1 is 59% at age 50 and 82% at age 70. BRCA1 is associated with an 85% lifetime risk of developing breast cancer, a 40% lifetime risk of developing ovarian cancer, a 7% lifetime risk of developing prostate cancer, and a 4% lifetime risk of developing colon cancer. BRCA2, on chromosome 13q12–13, is associated with an 85% lifetime risk of developing beast cancer, a 17% lifetime risk of ovarian cancer, a 7% risk of head and neck cancer, and a 28% lifetime risk of prostate can-

Table 1B.5. What Is the Risk of Having Hereditary Breast Cancer?

If ovarian cancer occurs prior to age 50	7%
If breast cancer occurs prior to age 30	12
If 2 first-degree relatives have breast cancer before age 40	40
If 3 family members have breast cancer before age 50	40
If 1 breast and 1 ovarian cancer before age 50 in family	46
If 2 breast and 1 ovarian cancer before age 50 in family	82
If 2 breast and 2 ovarian cancer before age 50 in family	91

cer. Genetic testing for both BRCA1 and BRCA2 is available. Because of the large number of mutations identified, screening a person for BRCA1 or BRCA2 first requires screening of a family member with a known malignancy to identify the mutation specific for that family. The false-positive and false-negative rates of genetic testing are unknown. Few states have safeguards to protect against employment or insurance discrimination based on genetic testing. Thus, genetic testing is recommended only after counseling by professionals familiar with all of the implications of testing. Patients with more than two relatives with breast, ovarian, or other cancers; those with two or more generations of family members affected by cancer; and those with bilateral cancer, multiple primary tumors, or early-onset breast cancer possibly should be considered for genetic counseling.

Li-Fraumeni syndrome is an autosomal dominant syndrome associated with an increased incidence of breast, brain, and adrenal neoplasms, as well as sarcomas, lymphomas, and leukemias. The cause of this syndrome is believed to be the transmission of one abnormal p53 gene. The p53 gene is a tumor suppressor gene; thus it requires only one additional mutation or deletion of p53 to induce cancer. This syndrome is believed to account for up to 1% of breast cancers.

DEMOGRAPHIC FACTORS

The United States is 13th of 48 countries in frequency of deaths from breast cancer (the United Kingdom is the highest). The highest rates of breast cancer are in urban areas of the midwestern and northeastern United States; the lowest rates are in the southern and mountain states. Native Hawaiian women have the highest age-adjusted rate of breast cancer, followed by the white, African-American, Hispanic, Asian, and Native American populations in order of descending frequency. Breast cancer is more frequent among women of higher socioeconomic social class. Marriage is associated with a lower incidence of breast cancer. Table 1B.6 summarizes the relative risks for a variety of risk factors associated with breast cancer and puts them in perspective in relation to each other.

PREVENTION

Women at high risk for breast cancer should be followed with close surveillance or may be considered for prophylactic surgery. Prophylactic mastectomy has decreased the incidence of breast cancer in women at high risk but is not entirely protective. For women with a high risk of breast cancer, monthly breast self-examination should be taught, and a clinical breast examination should be performed every 4 to 6 months. Mammography should be performed annually. Mammography surveillance in women with a first-degree relative with breast cancer is generally recommended to begin 10 years earlier than the youngest family member developed cancer. Screening for ovarian cancer in women suspected of having hereditary breast cancer should include an annual pelvic examination, CA-125, and consideration to pelvic ultrasound evaluation. Patients at high risk should be considered candidates for ongoing prevention studies. Tamoxifen, raloxifene, and retinoid therapy are being evaluated in this role.

Table 1B.6 Relative Risk of Developing Breast Cancer

Older age (65–69 vs 30–34)	17.0
Breast biopsy of atypical hyperplasia and a first-degree relative with breast cancer	8.9
Resident of North America or Europe	4.5
Atypical hyperplasia on breast biopsy	4.4
Prior breast cancer in the contralateral breast	4.0
Radiation therapy more than 1 Gy	4.0
Family history of first-degree relative with breast cancer	3.0
Nulliparous or first birth after age 40	2.5
Late menopause	2.0
Obesity (more than 200 pounds)	2.0
Early menarche	1.5
Urban, high socioeconomic status	1.5
More than 24 g (2 drinks) of alcohol daily	1.5
Hormone replacement therapy for more than 15 years	1.4
Oral contraceptives for more than 10 years	1.4
Hormone replacement therapy for more than 10 years	1.2
Hormone replacement therapy for more than 5 years	1.1
Daily light to moderate exercise	0.8

SCREENING

Early detection of breast cancer with annual mammography screening has demonstrated a reduction in mortality by 25 to 35% in women over age 50. Screening mammography in women aged 40 to 49 continues to generate controversy. The American Cancer Society and the National Cancer Institute both have endorsed regular screening mammography in this group of women. The National Institute of Health has recommended that the decision be left to the primary physician. Women who are at high risk for breast cancer (a first-degree relative with breast cancer) should be evaluated with mammography annually starting 10 years younger than when the youngest family member developed cancer.

SIGNS AND SYMPTOMS

Most patients with breast cancer present with a nontender mass detected by the patient. Pain, although more frequently associated with breast cysts, is a presenting symptom in up to 10% of patients. Palpable breast cancer is usually well defined, a dominant mass, whereas diffuse fibrotic changes, especially in the upper outer quadrants of the breast, are characteristic of benign breast disease. Lobular carcinoma of the breast may present as a diffuse thickening of the breast and thus is more difficult to detect. Diffuse inflammation of the breast should always raise the concern of inflammatory breast cancer. The peau d'orange change is characteristic of inflammatory breast cancer. Crusting and scaling of the nipple should be recognized as possible Paget's disease, which is associated with a diagnosis of ductal carcinoma in situ within 2 years in most patients.

Cysts are the most common benign condition occurring in the breast. Ultrasound can be used to distinguish a cyst from a solid tumor; however, most clinicians prefer to aspirate these lesions. Aspiration should also relieve the patient of any symptoms associated with the cyst. Concern of a malignancy should be raised if the aspirate is bloody, if a palpable mass remains after aspirate, if the cyst rapidly reaccumulates, or if an abnormality persists on mammography after aspirate. Nipple discharge is associated with malignancy in about 11% of cases, but patients who are postmenopausal are more likely to have a malignancy (36% risk of malignancy) when a nipple discharge is noted.

DIAGNOSIS

A careful history and physical examination are always the cornerstone of any evaluation. Bilateral mammography should also be performed. Malignancies may be bilateral in up to 1% of cases. Signs of malignancy on mammography include a dominant mass associated with distortion of the breast architecture or spiculated and crablike appearance. Microcalcifications may also be identified. Malignant microcalcifications tend to occur in clusters of more than three and are smaller than benign calcifications. If a suspicious mass is noted on physical examination but the mammogram is negative, a fine-needle aspirate or biopsy should **AL-WAYS** be undertaken. A false-negative rate of up to 15% can occur on mammography.

Abnormalities that are detected on mammography may require additional evaluation. This can include magnification views of the breast, ultrasonography, and mammography or ultrasound-directed biopsy of the breast.

Fine-needle aspiration can be performed in the office to evaluate suspicious lesions. Benefits include speed, relative painlessness, and low cost. The drawbacks include lack of detailed histology, inability to differentiate in situ from invasive cancer, and the need for an experienced cytopathologist. Most important, care should be taken in patients with a mass, an equivocal mammogram, and a "negative" fine-needle aspiration cytology report. Up to 10% of these patients are found to have cancer. False positives occur in fewer than 1% of cases. A core-cutting needle biopsy can also be performed rapidly, painlessly and inexpensively in an office. The accuracy of a core-cutting needle biopsy is better than fine-needle aspiration, but false negatives still occur in up to 6% of cases.

Excisional biopsy has the advantage of allowing complete evaluation of the tumor size and its characteristics prior to definitive local therapy. It does require two separate procedures and is thus more expensive. Additionally, it creates an incision that must be incorporated into the definitive surgery.

Nonpalpable lesions have in the past been approached with needle-localized excisional biopsy. Specimen radiography after biopsy is essential to confirm that the abnormality has been removed. Failure to remove the mammography abnormality occurs in up to 5% of cases. More recently stereotactic core needle biopsies have been advocated. These may be mammography or ultrasound guided. Sensitivity to this technique ranges from 71 to 100%.

STAGING

A careful history and physical examination are the cornerstones of staging evaluation (Table 1B.7). Careful attention should be paid to areas where breast cancer commonly spreads, including skin, lymph nodes, bone, lung, and liver. A complete blood count and chemistry profile including liver functions should be performed. A chest radiograph is routine.

In patients with early-stage breast cancer who are free of pain

Table 1B.7A. TNM Staging System for Breast Cancer

TNM System

Primary tumor

TX   Primary tumor cannot be assessed.

T0   No evidence of primary tumor.

Tis   Carcinoma in situ; intraductal carcinoma, lobular carcinoma in situ, or Paget's disease of the nipple with no associated tumor mass.

T1   Tumor 2 cm or less in greatest dimension.[a]

T1a   0.5 cm or less in greatest dimension.

T1b   More than 0.5 cm but not more than 1 cm in greatest dimension.

T1c   More than 1 cm but not more than 2 cm in greatest dimension.

T2   Tumor more than 2 cm but not more than 5 cm in greatest dimension.[a]

T3   Tumor more than 5 cm in greatest dimension.[a]

T4   Tumor of any size with direct extension to chest wall or skin (chest wall includes ribs, intercostal muscles, and serratus anterior muscle but not pectoral muscle).

T4a   Extension to chest wall.

T4b   Edema (including peau d'orange), ulceration of the skin of the breast, or satellite skin nodules confined to the same breast.

T4c   Both T4a and T4b.

T4d   Inflammatory carcinoma.

Regional lymph nodes

NX   Regional lymph nodes cannot be assessed (e.g., previously removed).

N0   No regional lymph node metastasis.

N1   Metastasis to movable ipsilateral axillary lymph node(s).

N2   Metastasis to ipsilateral lymph node(s) fixed to one another or to other structures.

N3   Metastasis to ipsilateral internal mammary lymph node(s).

Distant metastasis

MX   Presence of distant metastasis cannot be assessed.

M0   No distant metastasis.

M1   Distant metastasis (includes metastasis to ipsilateral supraclavicular lymph nodes).

Inflammatory carcinoma is a clinicopathologic entity characterized by diffuse brawny induration of the skin of the breast with an erysipeloid edge, usually without an underlying palpable mass. Radiologically there may be a detectable mass and characteristic thickening of the skin over the breast. The clinical presentation is due to tumor embolization of dermal lymphatics or to capillary congestion. Inflammatory carcinoma is classified T4d.

Dimpling of the skin, nipple retraction, or other skin changes may occur in T1, T2, or T3 without changing the classification.

[a]Paget's disease associated with tumor mass is classified according to the size of the tumor.

Table 1B.7B. Stage Grouping for Breast Cancer

Stage	Tumor	Nodes	Metastasis
0 (in situ)	Tis	N0	M0
I	T1	N0	M0
IIA	T0	N1	M0
	T1	N1	M0
	T2	N0	M0
IIB	T2	N1	M0
	T3	N0	M0
IIIA	T0	N2	M0
	T1	N2	M0
	T2	N2	M0
	T3	N1	M0
	T3	N2	M0
IIIB	T4	Any N	M0
	Any T	N3	M0
IV	Any T	Any N	M1

and have a normal alkaline phosphatase, a bone scan is positive in fewer than 1% of cases and is generally not recommended. Some physicians routinely obtain a baseline bone scan at the time of diagnosis for later comparison. Patients with bone pain or abnormal alkaline phosphatase should be considered for a bone scan. As tumor size and lymph node involvement increase, so does the risk of occult bone metastasis, and a bone scan may be warranted in patients with more advanced malignancy.

Routine CT or liver imaging is usually reserved for patients who are symptomatic or who have abnormal liver function tests. As with bone scans, routine CT in asymptomatic patients with early breast cancer has an extremely low yield. Patients with locally advanced tumors do have an increased risk of occult metastasis. Careful staging in this population has resulted in upstaging of approximately 25% of patients with locally advanced breast cancer. MRI is reserved for evaluation of symptomatic processes.

PROGNOSIS

Overall 50% of women diagnosed with breast cancer are expected to remain disease free for the remainder of their lives. Approximately a third of women diagnosed with breast cancer will die of it. Staging is important because of its correlation with survival; this is demonstrated in Table 1B.8.

Approximately 80% of cancers are ductal, 10% lobular, and 5% medullary, with the remaining 5% composed of well-differentiated breast cancers with a better than average progno-

Table 1B.8. Ten-Year Survival of Breast Cancer

Stage at Diagnosis	Description	10 year survival (%)
Stage 0	In situ	95–99
Stage I	Occult invasive (<1 cm)	90–95
Stage I	Overt invasive	70–75
Stage II	Positive 2x nodes	40–45
Stage III	Locally advanced	10–15
Stage IV	Metastatic	Rare

sis (tubular, papillary, colloid, adenoid cystic). Ductal and lobular cancers have about the same prognosis. Lobular cancer is more likely to be bilateral and have a mirror image occurrence in the contralateral breast. Patients with medullary carcinoma are less likely to have nodal involvement, but the prognosis is similar to that of node positive ductal or lobular carcinoma.

Early National Surgical Adjuvant Breast Project (NSABP) studies demonstrate the importance of lymph node involvement. These studies confirm that lymph node involvement is the single most important prognostic factor for breast cancer. Patients with lymph node–negative tumors generally have recurrence rates up to 30%; patients with node-positive tumors have recurrence rates of 50 to 75%. The number of nodes involved is also a prognostic factor. Recurrence rate and lymph node involvement are presented in Table 1B.9.

Tumor size is an independent predictor of disease recurrence. Table 1B.10 presents the 5-year survival of women with axillary node–negative breast cancer based on tumor size.

Hormone receptors (ER [estrogen receptor] and PR [progesterone receptor]) have also been noted to be independent prognostic factors. Receptor status correlates with nuclear grade, histologic differentiation, and cell turnover. Receptor status is an independent predictor of disease-free survival. Hormone receptors also predict response to hormone therapy. This is demonstrated in Table 1B.11.

DNA flow cytometry measurements of ploidy and the number of cells in the synthesis phase (S phase) of the cell cycle have also been evaluated as prognostic factors. Patients with aneuploid stage I and II breast cancers have a recurrence rate twice that of diploid tumors. In prospective studies no data yet available confirm the importance of these items for correlation to disease-free or overall survival.

Epidermal growth factor receptor is the gene product of the HER-2-neu oncogene. Preliminary data suggest that patients with higher levels of her-2-neu protein had a poorer prognosis

Table 1B.9. Recurrence Rate of Breast Cancer in Patients with Lymph Node Involvement

Number of Positive Lymph Nodes	Recurrence Rate (%)
0	19
1	23
2	40
3	43
4	44
5	54
6–10	63
11–15	72
16–20	75
>21	82

Table 1B.10. Ten-Year Survival in Axillary Node–Negative Breast Cancer

Tumor Size (cm)	Patients	5-Year Survival (%)
<0.5	269	99.2
0.5–0.9	791	94.1
1.0–1.9	4668	92.3
2.0–2.9	4010	90.6
3.0–3.9	2072	86.2
4.0–4.9	845	84.6
>5.0	809	82.2

Table 1B.11. Prediction of Breast Cancer Response to Hormonal Therapy

ER+	PR+	77%
ER−	PR+	46
ER+	PR−	27
ER−	PR−	11

than patients with lower levels. HER-2-neu expression may predict tumor sensitivity to individual chemotherapeutic agents.

Independent prognostic factors should be thought of as major and minor. Major prognostic factors include lymph node states, proliferative activity, histologic grade, and ploidy. Minor factors include hormone receptor status, blood or lymph vessel invasion, and all others. Almost all patients have one bad prognostic factor if enough factors are assessed. Extremes in tumor size may modify the importance of other factors. An assessment of each patient's risk must be made before she can make an informed decision about the potential benefits of additional therapy.

TREATMENT

LOCAL THERAPY

After the malignancy is confirmed, it is appropriate to discuss all local treatment options with the patient. Surgical options include mastectomy, mastectomy with reconstruction, and conservative surgery (lumpectomy) with radiation therapy. Axillary node dissection remains the standard of care in all patients. Approximately a third of women with clinically node-negative disease are found to have axillary metastasis at the time of surgery. In an effort to decrease the morbidity of lymphedema after an axillary node dissection, research is focusing on sentinel lymph node biopsy rather than complete axillary dissection. Estrogen and progesterone receptors should be measured on the specimen.

An NSABP study demonstrated that in women with tumors smaller than 4 cm treated with lumpectomy, axillary node dissection and radiation, both overall and disease-free survival were equivalent to results of a modified radical mastectomy. Absolute contraindications to breast-conserving surgery include first- or second-trimester pregnancy, multifocal disease, diffuse microcalcifications, and prior breast radiation therapy. Precautions include a high ratio of mass to breast size, a history of collagen vascular disease, large breast, and tumor beneath the nipple. In patients who choose a complete mastectomy, both delayed and immediate reconstruction are reasonable alternatives to the use of an external prosthesis.

Postoperative radiation therapy is required after a partial mastectomy. If adjuvant chemotherapy is planned, delaying radiation therapy until after completion of the chemotherapy appears safe and may be preferable in patients with a high risk of distant dissemination.

The Early Breast Cancer Trialists' Collaborative Group presented in a meta-analysis an evaluation of the addition of radiation therapy to all breast surgeries. The addition of radiation therapy to all surgeries resulted in a rate of recurrence that was a third that of surgery alone; but there was no significant difference in 10-year survival (59.7% with and 58.6% without radiation therapy). However, an increased non–breast cancer death rate was seen in women who underwent irradiation. Breast conservation surgery was associated with a statistically insignificant increased risk of recurrence in the remaining breast tissue but no significant difference in 10-year overall survival. Recent studies once again challenge whether postmastectomy radiation therapy should be performed routinely. Postmastectomy chest wall radiation therapy is not given routinely but should be considered for patients who have a known residual tumor or who are in the high-risk group of patients with more than four involved axillary nodes or tumors larger than 5 cm.

ADJUVANT THERAPY

The Early Breast Cancer Trialists' Collaborative Group reviewed 133 prospectively randomized trials of systemic adjuvant therapy in stage I and II breast cancer. These trials included 75,000 women treated with chemotherapy, hormonal therapy, or immune therapy. In the Early Breast Cancer Trialists' Collaborative Group, 30,000 women were enrolled on tamoxifen trials. An overall 25% reduction in recurrence and a 17% reduction in death was noted in the tamoxifen treated groups ($p < .00001$). For patients who were ER positive, the reduction in recurrence was 32% and the reduction in death was 21%; for those who were ER negative, the figures were 13 and 11%, respectively. No significant differences were noted with varying dosages of tamoxifen, but a duration of tamoxifen use of 2 to 5 years was significantly more effective than less than 2 years. Additionally, a 39% reduction in the risk of a new breast cancer arising was seen in tamoxifen-treated patients.

Cytotoxic chemotherapy consisted primarily of CMF (cyclophosphamide, methotrexate, and 5-fluorouracil) given for 6 to 12 months. Chemotherapy was demonstrated to decrease recurrence and increase survival in both premenopausal and postmenopausal women with stage I and II disease. A 30% reduction in the risk of recurrence and a 20% reduction in the risk of death was observed at 10 years with chemotherapy. Polychemotherapy was found to be superior to single-agent chemotherapy. No added benefit was seen in maintenance chemotherapy of 2 years versus 6 months. The combination of chemotherapy with hormone therapy in the women over age 50 demonstrates an additive benefit. There was a 45% reduction in risk of recurrence, and a 30% reduction in the risk of death occurred at 10 years with the combination.

The role of ovarian ablation in premenopausal women was evaluated and found to have benefits similar to that of chemotherapy for premenopausal women. An additive benefit of ovarian ablation and chemotherapy was the reduction of the risk of recurrence by an additional 9% and the risk of death by 11% over chemotherapy alone.

Stage I

Up to 30% of women with stage I breast cancer have a recurrence. Patients with tumors smaller than 1 cm have a 10-year disease free survival of 92%; for 1 to 1.9 cm the disease-free survival is 78%, and in tumors larger than 2 cm the disease-free survival is 69%. Patients with excellent prognostic factors (tumor smaller than 1 cm, ER positive, nuclear grade 1, diploid, and more than 35 years old) can probably be observed or considered for hormone therapy.

For patients with ER-negative tumors, adjuvant chemotherapy with a proven effective regimen should be considered (see adjuvant therapy regimens listed later in this chapter). For premenopausal patients with high-risk prognostic factors that are ER positive (tumor larger than 2 cm, aneuploid, or high nuclear grade) adjuvant chemotherapy with consideration of additional hormone manipulation (ovarian ablation and/or tamoxifen or other effective hormone agent) can be recommended. For patients with postmenopausal ER-positive breast cancer, hormone therapy can be recommended, with discussion of additional chemotherapy particularly in patients with poorer prognostic factors (tumors larger than 2 cm or high nuclear grade).

Stage II

Overall, 50 to 75% of patients with stage II disease have a recurrence. Premenopausal and postmenopausal patients should be considered for adjuvant chemotherapy. Patients with hormone receptor–positive tumors should also receive a hormone regimen. Ovarian ablation in premenopausal women may be a consideration as well.

Elderly patients and those with a poor performance status secondary to competing comorbidities may be considered for hormone therapy alone. In patients with more than four nodes positive, dose-intensive chemotherapy with stem cell support remains investigational at this writing.

Stage III

A multimodality approach to the management of local or regional advanced breast cancer is warranted.

1. Confirm diagnosis of breast cancer by obtaining fine-needle aspiration or core biopsy of the breast. Evaluation for hormone receptors should be performed on this tissue.
2. A chest radiograph, bone scan, liver imaging, chemistry, and complete blood count should be performed to evaluate for metastatic disease.
3. Initiate systemic doxorubicin (Adriamycin)-based chemotherapy (doxorubicin, cyclophosphamide, or AC; CAF; 5-FU, doxorubicin, cyclophosphamide, or FAC; see chemotherapy section for details) unless there is a medical contraindica-tion. If cardiac dysfunction is present, chemotherapy with cyclophosphamide, methotrexate, 5-FU (CMF), CMFVP (cyclophos-

phamide, methotrexate, fluorouracil, vincristine, and prednisone), or mitoxantrone-based chemotherapy should be given.
4. Treatment should continue until maximal tumor response (3 to 5 cycles) is seen.
5. Evaluate operability.
    a. If minimal or no residual tumor in surgical specimen, postoperative radiation therapy may be withheld.
    b. If T3 and feasible, breast-conserving surgery can be performed. Marking or tattooing around the area of primary tumor helps to ensure complete resection should a complete response occur.
    c. If inoperable after 3 to 5 cycles, consider additional chemotherapy or radiation therapy.
6. Postoperatively, complete three to five additional cycles of chemotherapy for a total of eight cycles.
7. Hormonal therapy is given in postmenopausal and hormone receptor–positive women.

Stage IV

Most stage IV disease is responsive to therapy. Durable complete remissions may occur in up to 10 to 20% of patients, although long-term disease-free survival indicative of a cure is rare. Surgical procedures are generally limited to those that permit diagnosis and determination of hormone receptor status. Control of local disease can be achieved with either surgery or radiation therapy.

External beam irradiation plays a major role in the palliation of symptomatic disease. Bone disease may also be palliated with the use of strontium or samarium nuclear medicine injections. Some degree of myelosuppression after treatment with these agents is expected. Recent studies suggest also a role for pamidronate, both in ameliorating pain from bone metastasis and in preventing new bone metastasis.

If visceral disease is absent and hormone receptors are positive, hormone therapy with effective agents is an excellent first treatment. Ovarian ablation may be used in premenopausal women. Patients with an initial response to hormone therapy who later relapse may be effectively salvaged with additional hormonal intervention. Responses have occurred with withdrawals from tamoxifen as well as diethylstilbestrol (DES).

If visceral disease is present or hormone receptors are negative, chemotherapy with effective agents is recommended. Multiple regimens are available, and the choice of chemotherapy remains the subject of multiple ongoing investigational protocols.

Dose-intensive chemotherapy with stem cell support remains investigational. A single randomized trial of dose-intensive versus standard chemotherapy has shown a substantial benefit in disease-free and overall survival with the use of dose-intensive therapy. However, this study has been strongly criticized for the use of what is believed to be relatively ineffective standard chemotherapy. Other studies have reported long-term survivors (up to 15 to 25%) who received dose-intensive therapy.

Recurrent Disease

Recurrent breast cancer is often responsive to therapy, although treatment is rarely curative. Radiation is indicated for local or symptomatic disease. Surgery may be indicated as well for local disease. Patients with a prior response to hormone therapy should be considered for other forms of hormonal therapy. Some patients have a response to hormonal therapy withdrawal, lasting on average 10 months.

If patients fail to respond to hormone therapy, salvage chemotherapy may be indicated. Generally therapy with anthracyclines or taxanes may be considered for patients with a failure after methotrexate-based chemotherapy. Failure to respond to anthracycline-based chemotherapy generally is followed by taxane therapy. Hyperthermia with radiation can be considered for patients with a localized chest wall recurrence who have received radiation therapy. Dose-intensive chemotherapy with stem cell support may be a consideration in a select population as well.

MONOCLONAL ANTIBODY THERAPY

Herceptin, the first monoclonal antibody for the treatment of metastatic breast cancer, has been recently approved by the FDA. Herceptin targets the HER-2/*neu* gene; this is a growth factor that is "over-expressed" in 25 to 30% of women with breast cancer. In the first phase III study, 222 women with metastatic breast cancer received Herceptin at a loading dose of 4 mg/kg intravenously, then 2 mg/kg weekly thereafter. The side effects were minimal, consisting of fever and chills in 40% of patients, primarily with the first dose. A reduction in cardiac function was seen in 9 patients, of whom 6 were symptomatic. All of these patients had prior anthracycline therapy or a cardiac history. The overall response was 21% (4% CR and 17% PR). The median duration of response was 8.4 months. The second phase III study compared chemotherapy with or without Herceptin in 469 patients. Overall, the response rate improved from 36.2% with chemotherapy alone to 62% with chemotherapy and Herceptin therapy. The time to progression was also significantly improved from 5.5 months to 8.6 months with the combination of chemotherapy and Herceptin. This was seen in patients who were stratified to receive doxorubicin and cyclophosphamide and those who received paclitaxel. Patients who received doxorubicin and cyclophosphamide had an 18% incidence of myocardial dysfunction versus 3% with chemotherapy alone. Herceptin therapy is indicated for patients with metastatic breast cancer and an overexpression of HER-2/*neu*. Concurrent administration of doxorubicin is not recommended.

HORMONE THERAPY

In 1895 Beatson demonstrated the efficacy of oophorectomy in treating a patient with premenopausal breast cancer. In the early 1900s 30% rates of response to oophorectomy were noted in premenopausal women, with responses lasting 6 to 12 months. Responsiveness to hormone therapy is directly related to the amount of ER or PR on cells. Responses to hormonal therapy generally require 6 to 8 weeks.

Tamoxifen

Tamoxifen binds reversibly to the estrogen receptor. Tamoxifen is considered cytostatic; it is a cell cycle inhibitor that arrests cells in the G0 and in G1 cell cycle phase. In patients with metastatic breast cancer, a 76% response rate to tamoxifen is seen in patients who are ER positive and PR positive; and a response rate of 10% in patients who are ER negative and PR negative was seen. Tamoxifen, which is weakly estrogenic, protects postmenopausal women against osteoporosis but may promote bone loss in premenopausal women. It also exerts a favorable effect on lipids and cholesterol, improving cardiovascular risk factors similarly to estrogen.

Side effects of tamoxifen include headaches, hot flashes, decreased levels of antithrombin 3 with a slightly increased risk of thromboembolism, and a recent report of earlier onset of cataracts. Clonidine, Bellergal-S, vitamin E, or megestrol acetate (Megace) may be used for symptomatic hot flashes. Tamoxifen exerts an estrogenic effect on the uterus and has been associated with endometrial hyperplasia as well as an increased risk of endometrial cancer. An annual pelvic examination and rapid evaluation of any extramenstrual bleeding is recommended. The recommended dose in postmenopausal women is 20 mg daily. There is controversy regarding dose for premenopausal women. Doses of 40 to 120 mg/day have been recommended in premenopausal women. These doses have been associated with a tendency to suppress menses but no demonstrated increased antitumor response.

A tamoxifen flare is reported to occur in 10% of cases of patients with active breast cancer. This occurs in the first few weeks of therapy. Effects include increased pain or hypercalcemia. A tumor flare generally heralds a response to treatment.

A study by the NSABP demonstrated no benefit to 10 years versus 5 years of tamoxifen administration in node-negative estrogen receptor–positive breast cancer. The optimal duration of tamoxifen administration in node-positive patients is unknown. Tamoxifen has been investigated as primary breast therapy in the elderly; a 27% complete remission (CR) and a 61% overall response rate were noted. An increased risk of local recurrence has been reported, although overall survival is the same.

Torimefene

Toremifene (Fareston) is a pure antiestrogen; thus no tumor flare and no increase in endometrial cancer theoretically should occur. It also could theoretically accelerate osteoporosis. Cross-resistance between tamoxifen and toremifene is reported. The recommended dose of toremifene is 60 mg daily.

Progestational Agents

Megestrol and methoxyprogesterone (Provera) have responses equivalent to that of tamoxifen but slightly shorter in duration. A response rate of 14 to 22% with megestrol occurs in tamoxifen failures. A major disadvantage to progestational agents is weight gain. The recommended dose is megestrol 160 mg daily or medroxyprogesterone 500 mg three times weekly.

Aromatase Inhibitors

Aminoglutethimide is equivalent to surgical adrenalectomy, and hydrocortisone replacement is required. Side effects include lethargy in 48%, rash, hypotension, ataxia, fever, and myelosuppression. The recommended dose is aminoglutethimide 250 mg twice a day for 2 weeks, then four times a day with hydrocortisone 20 to 30 mg every morning.

Several newer selective aromatase inhibitors have been investigated. Steroid replacement is not required with these agents. Side effects of these agents include hot flashes, nausea, vomiting, and anorexia. The recommended doses are letrozole (Femara) 2.5 mg daily and anastrazole (Arimidex) 1 mg daily.

Diethylstilbestrol

DES has a 63% response rate in ER-positive tumors. Side effects include nausea, increased nipple pigmentation, fluid retention, congestive heart failure, thromboembolism, and in 40% of women, uterine breakthrough bleeding. The recommended dose is 5 mg three times a day. Withdrawal responses have been seen with DES.

Androgens

Halotestin's side effects include virilization, acne, increased libido, cholestatic jaundice, and peliosis hepatis. The recommended dose of halotestin is 20 to 30 mg daily.

Luteinizing Hormone-Releasing Hormone Agonists

Chemical ovarian ablation can be induced by goserelin acetate (Zoladex) or leuprolide acetate (Lupron). Goserelin has a reported 45% response rate in premenopausal women; leuprolide is similar. An 11% response rate in ER-positive postmenopausal women has also been seen. The recommended dose of goserelin is 3.6 mg subcutaneously monthly. Leuprolide is dosed at 7.5 mg subcutaneously monthly.

CHEMOTHERAPY

In 1969 Cooper reported an amazing 88% response rate in hormone-resistant breast cancer. Follow-up studies found Cooper's regimen had response rates of 60%, with a 10 to 15% CR seen. Doxorubicin has for some time been the most active single agent in breast cancer. Recently, however, the taxanes, docetaxel and paclitaxel, have demonstrated similar or superior results to those of doxorubicin in metastatic breast cancer. Additionally, the taxanes have produced significant responses in patients with doxorubicin-resistant breast cancer. In the adjuvant setting most investigators prefer to use doxorubicin-based regimens (AC, CAF, FAC) rather than methotrexate-based regimens (CMF, CMFVP). Clear superiority of the doxorubicin-based regimens has not yet been proved, although several studies demonstrate a trend toward better response rates. In patients with metastatic disease, there is a slight advantage in response to doxorubicin regimens as compared with methotrexate regimens, but this has not translated into a significant improvement in overall survival. Table 1B.12 summarizes responses seen in metastatic breast cancer with a variety of agents in the first and second line.

FOLLOW-UP

The peak time to recurrence of breast cancer is 2 to 5 years. The risk of recurrence steadily decreases after the fifth year but never reaches zero. Only 20 to 30% of recurrences are asymptomatic, and symptoms suggesting recurrence were caused by cancer only approximately a third of the time.

Table 1B.13 offers three options for following the woman with breast cancer. Intensive follow-up may be indicated for women participating in clinical research protocols or in women at high risk for recurrent disease. Patients with symptomatic lesions should be evaluated with radiologic tests as symptoms dictate. Patients with progressively rising tumor markers or worsening liver function should be considered for reevaluation with CT and bone scan if diagnosis of recurrent disease would affect the therapy plan. Positron emission tomography may be

Table 1B.12. Efficacy of Chemotherapy in Advanced Breast Cancer (CR + PR)

Agent	First Line Response Rate (%)	Second Line Response Rate (%)
Doxorubicin 60–75 mg/m^2	43–54	28
Docetaxel 75–100 mg/m^2	48–68	35–51
Paclitaxel 175–300 mg/m^2/3–24 hr	29–63	6–38
Paclitaxel 140 mg/m^2/96 hr		48
Vinorelbine	30–41	16
Edatrexate	34–41	
Gemcitabine	25–37	
Cyclophosphamide	36	
Mitomycin C	32	
5-FU	28	
Methotrexate	26	
Melphalan	25	9
FAC (5-FU, doxorubicin, cyclophosphamide)	52	
CMF (cyclophosphamide, methotrexate, 5-FU)	44	
MVAC (methotrexate, vincristine, doxorubicin, cisplatin)	25–83	
Cisplatin + 5-FU		40
Mitomycin + vinblastine		14–30
NFL (mitoxantrone, 5-FU, leucovorin)		45–65
VATH (vinblastine, doxorubicin, thiotepa, halotestin)		49
DVM (doxorubicin, vincristine, mitomycin C)		24

useful in distinguishing benign from malignant questionable lesions. It is recommended that apparent initial recurrence be confirmed by pathologic diagnosis if clinically feasible, particularly in patients with a long disease-free interval.

DUCTAL CARCINOMA IN SITU

Ductal carcinoma in situ (DCIS) refers to the presumably malignant proliferation of cells within the mammary ducts and lobules of the breast but without invasion of the basement membrane. The increased identification of this lesion is thought to be due to the widespread use of screening mammography. DCIS can present as a palpable mass, nipple discharge, or Paget's disease of the nipple. On mammography DCIS frequently appears as clus-

Table 1B.13. Follow-up of the Woman with Breast Cancer

	Minimal	Moderate	Intense
Physical examination q 3–4 mo years 1–3; q 6 mo years 4, 5; annually thereafter	•	•	•
Mammography annually	•	•	•
Pap smear annually	•	•	•
Flexible sigmoidoscopy or colonoscopy every 3–5 years	•	•	•
Complete blood count biannually years 1–5; annually thereafter		•	•
Chemistry profile, liver panel with each physical examination		•	•
Tumor marker (CEA, CA 15–3, or CA 27–29) with each physical examination		•	•
Bone scan annually			•
Chest radiograph annually			•
5-year cost of follow-up	$1725	$3875	$6630

tered microcalcifications, although a spiculated mass may also be DCIS. DCIS is divided into comedo and noncomedo subtypes (cribriform, micropapillary, solid, or clinging). In general, the comedo type has a higher proliferative activity and is more likely to be associated with microinvasion than the other types.

The natural history of DCIS demonstrates that there is an increased risk of approximately 30% at 10 years of the development of invasive cancer. Mastectomy appears to be curative for 98% of patients with DCIS. Because of the increased frequency of detecting smaller areas of DCIS, conservative therapy with local excision has gained favor. An increased risk of local recurrence accompanies this approach. Approximately half of the patients with local recurrence have invasive tumors. The role of postoperative irradiation in this group remains unanswered. Studies have demonstrated that there is a decreased risk of local recurrence with postlumpectomy radiation therapy. Some studies show similar rates of recurrence to radiation when wide (larger than 1 cm) margins were obtained and when the tumor margins were carefully inked and evaluated for local invasiveness. Local recurrences are more frequent with the comedo type of DCIS.

LOBULAR CARCINOMA IN SITU

Lobular carcinoma in situ (LCIS) lacks both mammographic and clinical signs. It consists of a solid proliferation of small uniform round to oval cells with a slow proliferative rate. This lesion is frequently multicentric (60 to 80%) and is frequently bilateral. Studies demonstrate a sevenfold greater risk of developing breast cancer in patients with LCIS than the general population, and the risk of breast cancer is equal in the biopsied and contralateral breast.

Management options include close observation similar to that of a woman in a high-risk category of hereditary familial breast cancer. Alternatively, consideration can be given to bilateral simple mastectomy. Radiation therapy has no known role in the management of LCIS.

Bibliography

Breast cancer. PDQ treatment for health professionals. National Cancer Institute. http://cancernet.nci.nih.gov/clinpdq/soa/Breast_cancer_Physician.html; 1/18/98.

Dickson RB, Lippman ME, Harris J, et al. Cancer of the breast. In: DeVita VT, Hellman S, Rosenberg SA, eds. Cancer: principles & practice of oncology. 5th ed. Philadelphia: Lippincott-Raven, 1997;1541–1616.

Early Breast Cancer Trialists' Collaborative Group. Effects of radiotherapy and surgery in early breast cancer. N Engl J Med 1995:333;1444–1455.

Kardinal CG, Cole JT. Chemotherapy of breast cancer. In: Perry MC, ed. The chemotherapy source book. 2nd ed. Baltimore: Williams & Wilkins, 1997;1125–1185.

Landis SH, Murray T, Bolden S, Wingo PA. Cancer statistics 1998. CA Cancer J Clin 1998:48;6–29.

Lung Cancer

Mohammed A. Raheem and Victoria J. Dorr

BACKGROUND

Lung cancer is the most common cause of cancer death in both men and women. In the United States alone, 178,000 new lung cancer cases were expected in 1998 (98,300 in men and 79,800 in women) and 160,400 deaths (94,400 in men and 64,300 in women). Only 14% of lung cancer patients are alive 5 years after diagnosis.

ETIOLOGY

Known causes of lung cancer include the following:

1. Tobacco use: carcinogenic effects of tobacco are caused by polycyclic aromatic hydrocarbons from tars produced during combustion. Nicotine can form nitrosamines such as 4-(N-methyl-N-nitrosamino)-1-(3-pyridyl)-butanone (NNK), which is a strong carcinogen in rodents.
2. Environment: arsenic, asbestos, beryllium, chloromethylethers, chromium, hydrocarbons, mustard gas, nickel, and radiation are carcinogens.
3. Familial predisposition is also a factor.

CANCER SCREENING

Chest radiography and sputum cytology have been tested, but to date no early screening effort has demonstrated a reduction in the lung cancer mortality rate.

PATHOLOGY

NON-SMALL CELL LUNG CANCER

Non-small cell lung cancer (NSCLC) includes squamous cell, adenocarcinoma, and large cell histologies. Squamous cell carcinoma accounts for almost a third of lung cancers. Usually these cancers originate in the central bronchus. Adenocarcinoma accounts for about 30 to 45% of lung cancers. Usually these tumors demonstrate peripheral growth. Adenocarcinoma is more common in women than in men. Large cell carcinoma accounts for about 9% of lung cancers and is characterized by large cells with large nuclei and prominent nucleoli. Adenosquamous carcinoma accounts for about 1 to 2% of lung cancers.

SMALL CELL LUNG CANCER: OAT CELL CARCINOMA

Small cell lung cancer (SCLC) accounts for about 20 to 25% of lung cancers. Typically small cell cancers are peribronchial.

Early and wide metastases are common, making complete surgical resection rarely possible.

CLINICAL PRESENTATION

Signs and symptoms are due to local tumor growth and intrathoracic spread. These may include, in descending order of frequency, cough, dyspnea, chest pain, hemoptysis, pneumonitis, vocal cord paralysis, superior vena cava syndrome, pleural effusion, Pancoast's syndrome, and pericardial effusion. Signs and symptoms due to systematic involvement may include anorexia, weight loss, fatigue, fever, and anemia.

Important paraneoplastic syndromes include the following:

Syndrome of inappropriate antidiuretic hormone (ADH) secretion (SIADH). Autonomous secretion of ADH is hallmarked by hyponatremia. Most commonly this occurs with small cell lung cancer.

Syndrome of ectopic adrenocorticotropic hormone (ACTH) secretion. Hyperadrenocorticalism due to ectopic ACTH production is characterized by cushingoid features, severe weakness, weight loss, edema, and hypertension.

The humoral hypercalcemia of malignancy, which is due to ectopic parathyroid hormone (PTH) secretion.

The ectopic production of human chorionic gonadotrophin (HCG).

Other paraneoplastic syndromes:

Eaton-Lambert syndrome, which is characterized by proximal limb muscle weakness that improves with repeat contraction; it is most commonly associated with SCLC.

Subacute sensory neuropathy, a peripheral neuropathy characterized by progressive impairment of all sensory modalities with areflexia and sensory ataxia and associated with SCLC.

Clubbing.

Hypertrophic pulmonary osteoarthropathy (HPO).

Nonbacterial thrombotic endocarditis (NBTE), in which the mitral valve is usually involved. NBTE may result in emboli to central nervous system, kidneys, and coronary arteries. It is usually associated with adenocarcinoma and bronchoalveolar cell carcinoma.

Migratory thrombophlebitis.

Hypercoagulable state.

DIAGNOSIS AND STAGING

For diagnosis and staging one needs a good patient history and physical examination, including performance status evaluation and evaluation for weight loss; chest radiograph; and chest computed tomography (CT), including adrenals, CBC, and SMA 12 (Table 1B.14). Diagnostic tests that may yield a diagnosis of lung cancer include sputum cytology, fiberoptic bronchoscopy, CT-guided transthoracic needle biopsy, and surgical biopsy. Pulmonary function testing should be done prior to lung resection. Mediastinoscopy should also be performed if resection is contemplated. For small cell cancer, CT of the brain and bone marrow aspirate and bilateral biopsy should be done to complete staging.

Table 1B.14A. TNM Staging System for Lung Cancer

Primary Tumor

TX   Tumor proved by the presence of malignant cells in sputum or bronchial washing but not visualized by bronchoscopy.

T0   No evidence of primary tumor.

Tis   Carcinoma in situ.

T1   Tumor 3 cm or less in greatest dimension, surrounded by lung or visceral pleura without bronchoscopic evidence of invasion more proximal than lobar bronchus (i.e., not the main bronchus).

T2   Tumor with any of the following features of size or extent.
         More than 3 cm in greatest dimension.
         Involving main bronchus 2 cm or more distal to the carina.
         Invading the visceral pleura.
         Associated with atelectasis or obstructive pneumonitis that extends to the hilar region but does not involve the entire lung.

T3   Tumor of any size that directly invades the chest wall (including superior sulcus tumors), diaphragm, mediastinal pleura, or parietal pericardium; or tumors in the main bronchus less than 2 cm distal to carina but without involvement of the carina; or associated atelectasis or obstructive pneumonitis of the entire lung.

T4   Tumor of any size that invades mediastinum, heart, great vessels, trachea, esophagus, vertebral body, or carina; or tumor with a malignant pleural effusion.

Nodal Involvement

N0   Regional lymph nodes cannot be assessed.

N1   Metastasis to lymph nodes in the peribronchial or the ipsilateral hilar region or both, including direct extension.

N2   Metastasis in ipsilateral mediastinal and/or subcarinal lymph node(s).

N3   Metastasis in contralateral mediastinal, contralateral hilar, ipsilateral or contralateral scalene, or supraclavicular lymph nodes.

Distant Metastasis

M0   No distant metastasis.

M1   Distant metastasis.

Table 1B.14B. Stage Grouping for Lung Cancer

Stage	TNM Description		
	Tumor	Nodes	Metastasis
IA	T1	N0	M0
IB	T2	N0	M0
IIA	T1	N1	M0
IIB	T2	N1	M0
	T3	N0	M0
IIIA	T3	N1	M0
	T1–3	N2	M0
IIIB	Any T4	Any N	M0
	T1–4	N3	
IV	Any T	Any N	M1

STAGING FOR SCLC

Limited Stage

Limited-stage small cell lung cancer means tumor confined to the hemithorax of origin, the mediastinum, and the supraclavicular nodes, which can be encompassed within a "tolerable" radiation therapy port. There is no universally accepted definition of limited stage, and patients with pleural effusion, massive pulmonary tumor, and contralateral supraclavicular nodes have been both included in and excluded from limited stage by various groups.

Extensive Stage

Extensive-stage SCLC means tumor that is too widespread to fit the definition of limited stage disease.

THERAPY OF NSCLC

Surgery is the major potentially curative therapeutic option for NSCLC. Radiation therapy can produce cure in a small minority and palliation in most patients. In advanced-stage disease, chemotherapy offers modest improvements in median survival, primarily in patients with good performance status and minimal weight loss, although overall survival is poor. Where studied, chemotherapy has been reported to produce short-term improvement in disease-related symptoms. The effect of chemotherapy on quality of life requires more study.

OCCULT OR IN SITU CARCINOMA

Primary surgical resection remains the mainstay of therapy for occult or in situ carcinoma. Endoscopic phototherapy with a hematoporphyrin derivative has been described as an alternative to surgical resection in carefully selected patients. This investigational treatment seems to be most effective for very early central tumors that extend less than 1 cm within the bronchus.

STAGE I DISEASE

Surgery (lobectomy or pneumonectomy if feasible) is the standard treatment for stage I disease. Careful evaluation of lung function and assessment of evidence of metastatic disease should be completed before surgery. Limited surgery may be required in some patients with minimal lung reserve. Patients with unsatisfactory pulmonary function should be considered for differential testing to assess the function of the anticipated remaining lung. Careful evaluation for metastasis should be performed. Patients with lymphadenopathy on CT should undergo mediastinoscopy to confirm disease involvement, as false positives are frequent. Patients with adrenal masses should also undergo CT-guided biopsy if it will change the treatment plan, again because of a high frequency of false-positives on CT (see Adrenal Tumors).

Limited resection has been compared with lobectomy in patients with tumors that are amenable to this approach. Local recurrence was greater in patients treated with local resection, but overall survival was not affected in patients with disease smaller than 3 cm. Overall, survival was worse in patients treated with local resection and tumor size larger than 3 cm.

Inoperable patients with stage I disease and with sufficient pulmonary reserve may be considered for radiation therapy with curative intent. Some 5-year survival rates of 10 to 27% have been seen; however, patients with T1, N0 tumors had better outcomes, with 5-year survival rates of 32 to 60%.

Clinical trials to date have not demonstrated a clear benefit to adjuvant radiation therapy or chemotherapy. Consideration of enrollment of patients in clinical trials is important, as recurrence rates remain unacceptably high. Patients with incomplete resection (positive margins) should be considered for adjuvant radiation.

STAGE II

Surgery is the treatment of choice for patients with stage II NSCLC. Careful evaluation of lung function and assessment for metastatic disease should be completed before surgery. Limited surgery may be required in patients with minimal lung reserve. Patients with unsatisfactory pulmonary function should be considered for differential testing to assess the function of the anticipated remaining lung. Careful evaluation for suspected metastasis should be performed. Patients with lymphadenopathy on CT should undergo mediastinoscopy to confirm disease involvement, as false-positives are common. Patients with adrenal masses should also undergo CT-guided biopsy, again because of a high frequency of false-positives on CT (see Adrenal Tumors).

In patients who are deemed inoperable or who are not candidates for surgery, radiation therapy with curative intent has a 3-year survival of 20%. Radiation therapy is usually considered in an adjuvant role after surgical resection, although a clear benefit has not been demonstrated in randomized trials. An improvement in local disease-free events is seen.

Adjuvant chemotherapy in this population holds considerable promise, although no survival benefit has been seen with adjuvant chemotherapy to date. This may change with the advent of more tolerable and more effective agents. Enrollment in clinical trials is encouraged.

STAGE IIIA

For clinically evident N2 disease the 5-year survival is only 2%; chemotherapy followed by radiation therapy is usually the initial approach. Of patients treated with preoperative cisplatin-based chemotherapy, approximately 65 to 75% will be operable, and the 3-year survival is 27 to 28%.

Patients with completely resected stage III disease and postoperative radiation therapy show an improvement in local control but not in overall survival. Two small trials demonstrate a significant benefit in disease-free survival and a trend in favor of an improvement in overall survival with adjuvant chemotherapy with CAP (cisplatin, doxorubicin, and cyclophosphamide).

Patients with localized superior sulcus tumors have a favorable prognosis, with 20% survival at 5 years. Patients may be treated with surgery alone, surgery and radiation, or radiation alone. Adjuvant chemotherapy may also be considered. Patients with locally advanced disease that directly invades the chest wall may be curable with surgical resection if feasible.

For patients deemed unresectable, radiation therapy is effective in palliation, with a very small percentage of patients alive at 5 years. A meta-analysis of patients with stage III disease has shown a 10% reduction in the risk of death when combination chemotherapy and radiation therapy was compared with radiation therapy alone.

STAGE IIIB

Patients with stage IIIB disease are not considered operable in general. These patients should be approached with consideration of radiation or radiation and chemotherapy. As with stage

IIIA, a meta-analysis has shown a 10% survival advantage with combination chemotherapy and radiation therapy over radiation alone. Radiation therapy is effective palliation in patients with poor performance status. Patients with malignant pleural effusions are rarely treatable with radiation therapy. Rarely patients with supraclavicular involvement may be alive at 3 years when treated with radiation therapy with curative intent. Adjuvant chemotherapy is believed to add a small survival benefit.

STAGE IV

Combination chemotherapy with cisplatin- or carboplatin-based chemotherapy is usually considered an option. Response rates of 20 to 40% are seen, but long-term survival is rare. A prospective randomized comparison of vinorelbine plus cisplatin versus vindesine plus cisplatin versus single-agent vinorelbine has reported improved response rate (30%) and median survival (40 weeks) with the vinorelbine plus cisplatin regimen. Vinorelbine by itself has a response rate of 29 to 35%. Paclitaxel and docetaxel have demonstrated activity in NSCLC. Response rates of 21 to 24% have been seen with paclitaxel and 28 to 33% with docetaxel. Paclitaxel plus carboplatin has a reported response rate of 27 to 53%, with a 1-year survival rate of 32 to 54%. Cisplatin plus paclitaxel has demonstrated a higher response rate and better 1-year survival rate than cisplatin plus etoposide. Gemcitabine has response rates of 20 to 70% reported, and CPT-11 (Irinotecan) response rates of 20 to 32%. Topotecan has response rates of 0 to 47%. Meta-analyses have shown that chemotherapy produces modest improvements in short-term survival over supportive care alone in patients with inoperable stages IIIB and IV disease. While a slight improvement in response rates and survival have been seen with newer combinations of chemotherapy, survival is still dismal, and participation in clinical trials is appropriate. Radiation therapy may be used for palliation of symptoms. Endobronchial laser therapy or brachytherapy may be considered for obstructing bronchial lesions.

RECURRENT DISEASE

Patients who have a solitary cerebral metastasis after initial resection of a primary NSCLC lesion and who have no evidence of extracranial tumor may achieve prolonged disease-free survival with surgical excision of the brain metastasis and postoperative whole-brain irradiation. Patients who have multiple lesions or who are not candidates for surgery may be candidates for radiation.

Patients with solitary recurrence of a pulmonary lesion and with no other evidence of metastatic disease may be candidates for local resection. In most cases this is a new primary lung lesion. For recurrent disease with multiple sites of involvement, treatment options include chemotherapy, radiation therapy, and palliative measures only. For patients with limited disease and a good performance status, chemotherapy may offer a small survival advantage.

THERAPY OF SCLC

Few patients present with localized disease because of the propensity for early metastases. Thus, local therapy with surgery or radiation therapy alone is rarely indicated. Chemotherapy is the primary treatment.

LIMITED-STAGE DISEASE

Approximately 30 to 40% of patients have disease localized to one hemithorax. The median survival for this group of patients is 18 to 24 months. Combination chemotherapy has proved superior to single-agent therapy. Response rates of 60 to 95% are reported, with complete response rates of 45 to 75%. The addition of radiation to chemotherapy yields a small benefit in survival at 3 years. Multiple studies have assessed the efficacy of cisplatin and etoposide in combination with radiation therapy in limited-stage small cell lung cancer. These studies have consistently achieved median survivals of 18 to 24 months and 2-year survivals of 40 to 50% with less than 3% treatment-related mortality. Patients with SCLC have a high incidence (60%) of cranial metastasis. Therefore, patients who achieve a complete remission with therapy may be candidates for prophylactic cranial irradiation (PCI). PCI results in a 50% reduction in the risk of cranial metastasis. Unfortunately, PCI may be associated with a decline in neuropsychologic function.

EXTENSIVE DISEASE

More than 60 to 70% of patients present with disease that has spread beyond one hemithorax. These patients have a median survival of 6 to 12 months with therapy. Combination chemotherapy is appropriate. Radiation therapy may be used for palliation. The combination of chemotherapy and radiation has not improved survival in randomized studies of patients with extensive-stage SCLC.

RELAPSED OR RECURRENT SCLC

The median survival for this group of patients is poor, with a median survival of 2 to 3 months. Patients with recurrence beyond 6 months of initial treatment may be candidates for chemotherapy. Patients who fail to respond to therapy or who relapse within 6 months have little chance of benefit from additional therapeutic agents.

BIBLIOGRAPHY

Demetri G. Small cell lung cancer. Oncology 1996;179–201.

Ettinger D. Nonsmall-cell lung cancer. Oncology 1996;81–129.

Handbook for staging of cancer. 4th ed. Philadelphia: Lippincott, 1993;129–136.

Jahanzeb M, Ihde DC. Chemotherapy of lung cancer. In: Perry MC, ed. The chemotherapy source book. ed 2. Baltimore: Williams & Wilkins, 1997;1103–1123.

Landis SH, Murray T, Bolden S, Wingo PA. Cancer statistics 1998. CA Cancer J Clin 1998; 48:6–29.

Mountain CF. Revisions in the international system for staging lung cancer. Chest 1997;111:1711–1717.

Nesbitt JC, Lee JS, Komaki R, Roth JA. Cancer of the lung. In: Cancer medicine. 4th ed. Baltimore: Williams & Wilkins, 1997;1723–1805.

Nonsmall cell lung cancer. PDQ treatment for health professionals. National Cancer Institute. http://cancernet.nci.nih.gov/clinpdq/soa/A:\Nonsmall_cell_lung_cancer_Physician.html; 1/18/98.

Small cell lung cancer. PDQ treatment for health professionals. National Cancer Institute. http://cancernet.nci.nih.gov/clinpdq/soa/A:\Small_cell_lung_cancer_Physician.html; 1/18/98.

Esophageal Cancer

John D. Wilkes

BACKGROUND

Unfortunately, the diagnosis of esophageal cancer is often made late in the disease course, with more than half of patients presenting with advanced and incurable disease. Thus the survival rates remain disappointing; fewer than 10% of patients are at 5 years. Standard approaches are surgery or chemoradiation therapy. Trimodality approaches are considered investigational. New and more effective strategies are clearly needed for patients with this challenging disease.

EPIDEMIOLOGY

About 12,300 cases of esophageal cancer were diagnosed in 1998 in the United States. These cases were approximately equally divided between squamous cancers and adenocarcinomas, although in Western countries a remarkable and worrisome increase in the incidence of adenocarcinomas of the distal esophagus has been seen. This increase, which has been most notable in middle-aged white men, appears to be associated with Barrett's epithelium.

ETIOLOGY

Tobacco and alcohol use are the most common factors related to the development of squamous cell carcinomas of the esophagus. Less commonly, tylosis, lye strictures, achalasia, and Plummer-Vinson syndrome are implicated. Risk factors for adenocarcinoma remain uncertain, although a strong association with Barrett's epithelial metaplasia is probably significant.

CLINICAL MANIFESTATIONS

At presentation, 90% of patients have dysphagia and weight loss, which has usually been progressive over 3 to 6 months. Odynophagia and retrosternal discomfort are common. Vomiting, regurgitation, aspiration, pneumonia, bleeding, Horner's syndrome, and recurrent laryngeal nerve paralysis are most frequently noted in patients with locally advanced disease.

STAGING EVALUATION

A complete history, physical examination, and chest radiograph are needed for all patients suspected of having esophageal cancer (Table 1B.15). Esophagoscopy with biopsies is the diagnostic test of choice. If available, endoscopic ultrasound is the

Table 1B.15A. TNM Staging System for Esophageal Cancer

Primary Tumor

TX	Primary tumor cannot be assessed.
T0	No evidence of primary tumor.
Tis	Carcinoma in situ.
T1	Tumor invades the lamina propria or submucosa.
T2	Tumor invades the muscularis propria.
T3	Tumor invades adventitia.
T4	Tumor invades adjacent structures.

Regional Lymph Nodes

NX	Regional lymph nodes cannot be assessed.
N0	No demonstrable metastasis to regional lymph nodes.
N1	Metastasis to regional lymph nodes.

Distant Metastases

M0	No known distant metastasis.
M1	Distant metastasis present; specific site(s).
M1a	Metastasis to celiac or cervical lymph nodes.
M1b	Non–regional lymph node and/or other distant metastases.

Table 1B.15B. AJCC Stage Grouping for Esophageal Cancer

Stage	Tumor	Nodes	Metastasis	5-Year Survival (%)
0	Tis	N0	M0	—
I	T1	N0	M0	40–50
IIA	T2	N0	M0	20–30
	T3	N0	M0	
IIB	T1	N1	M0	
	T2	N1	M0	
III	T3	N1	M0	10–20
	T4	Any N	M0	
IVA	Any T	Any N	M1a	0–5%
IVB			M1b	

Adapted with permission from American Joint Committee on Cancer. Cancer staging manual. 5th ed. Philadelphia: Lippincott-Raven, 1997.

most reliable method of assessing T and N stage. Once diagnosed, a barium swallow is useful to determine the length of the lesion and degree of stenosis. CT of chest and upper abdomen is most useful to assess for mediastinal involvement and/or metastases. Bronchoscopy should be performed if the tumor involves the upper or middle third of the esophagus. Pulmonary function tests and cardiac evaluation are appropriate for any candidate for surgery.

PROGNOSIS

Adverse prognostic factors for esophageal cancer include length of tumor, depth of penetration, presence of nodal metastases, and pretreatment weight loss of more than 10%. Survival by stage groupings can be found in Table 1B.15.

TREATMENTS

SURGERY

Surgery alone is likely to be curative only for patients with select T1 lesions and possibly for those with Barrett's epithelium with high-grade dysplastic changes. Complications are not insignificant. The cure rate as a single modality is approximately 5 to 20%, and only about 50% of patients are operable. Median survival is less than 1 year, and symptomatic patients are unlikely to be cured with surgery alone. Nonetheless, surgical resection remains an effective form of palliation in selected patients.

RADIATION THERAPY

Radiation therapy for esophageal cancer may be either palliative or curative. Palliation is achieved in 60 to 85% of patients. Radiation tends to be used as single-modality therapy in the palliative setting or in patients who are unfit for more aggressive approaches. When it is offered for curative intent, patients receiving radiation alone achieve 18% survival at 1 year and 6% at 5 years. Both preoperative and postoperative radiation have been evaluated in clinical trials, and neither appears to have any significant effect on the natural course of the disease.

CHEMOTHERAPY

Despite numerous agents with moderate activity, chemotherapy alone is ineffective for controlling localized esophageal cancer. Similarly, neither preoperative nor adjuvant chemotherapy has been demonstrated to be effective. Chemotherapy has been employed for palliation of metastatic disease. Active agents and commonly used regimens with response rates for locally advanced and metastatic disease are listed in Table 1B.16.

CHEMOTHERAPY PLUS RADIATION THERAPY

The natural history of esophageal cancer is characterized by distant recurrence following locally directed therapies. As a result, systemic chemotherapy is thought to be an extremely important component of effective treatment. The combination of

Table 1B.16. Chemotherapy for Unresectable or Metastatic Esophageal Cancer

Regimen	Overall Response Rates (%) (Pooled data)
Single Agent	
Cisplatin	24–55
Paclitaxel	32
5-FU	10–36
Mitomycin	26–33
Navelbine	25
Bleomycin	18–30
Doxorubicin	18
Methotrexate	36
Combination	
Infusional 5-FU, cisplatin	35–61
Cisplatin, methotrexate	76
Cisplatin, 5-FU, etoposide	50–65
Cisplatin, doxorubicin, etoposide	50
5-FU, doxorubicin, cisplatin	33
Methotrexate, bleomycin, cisplatin	32
Cisplatin, bleomycin	25

chemotherapy and radiation has been evaluated as both a preoperative strategy and as definitive therapy.

A number of trials suggest a potential benefit of intensive preoperative chemoradiation therapy followed by esophagectomy (Table 1B.17). Forastiere and coworkers recently reported a 40% pathologic complete response rate and median survival of 31.3 months using a 30-day infusional 5-FU plus cisplatin regimen and concurrent radiation therapy. Similar resectability rates, pathologic response rates, and survival rates have been achieved by investigators in both single-arm and randomized trials. At this point many investigators think intensive trimodality therapy should be considered only for select patients with excellent performance status or in the context of a clinical trial.

Nonrandomized data from various institutions suggest the combination of radiation and chemotherapy without surgical intervention may be as effective. In 1991 Coia and associates reported the results of chemoradiation therapy from Fox Chase Cancer Institute. Patients with stage I and II lesions treated with 5-FU, mitomycin, and radiation therapy achieved 70% local control and 29% overall survival at 3 years. A randomized intergroup trial compared 5-FU plus cisplatin given weeks 1, 5, 8, and 11 plus radiation therapy against radiation therapy alone. The combined regimen resulted in better survival (12.5 versus 8.9

Table 1B.17. Concurrent Chemoradiotherapy Regimens

Chemotherapy Regimen	Radiation	Results
Johns Hopkins		
Cisplatin 26 mg/m² days 1–5, 26–30; 5-FU 300 mg/m² days 1–30	2Gy/day; 44 Gy total	90% resectability, 40% pathologic CR, 31.3-month median survival, 58% 2-year survival
University of North Carolina		
5-FU 1 g/m²/day CIVI × 96 hr (days 1–4), 29–32; cisplatin 100 mg/m² day 1 only	1.8 Gy/day; 45 Gy total	94% resectability, 51% pathologic CR, 26-month median survival, 53% 2-year survival
University of Michigan		
Vinblastine 1 mg/m²/days 1–4,17–21; cisplatin 20 mg/m² CIVI days 1–5, 17–21; 5-FU 300 mg/m² CIVI days 1–21	1.5 Gy bid 45 Gy total	91% resectability, 24% pathologic CR, 29-month median survival, 59% 2-year survival
Ireland		
5-FU 15 mg/kg over 16 hr days 1–5; cisplatin 75 mg/m² day 7; repeat cycle at week 6	267 cGy/day; 40 Gy total	88% resectability, 25% pathologic response, 16-month median survival, 37% 2-year survival

CIVI, continuous intravenous infusion.

months) than radiation therapy alone. There was a 36% survival reported at 2 years. Enthusiasm for this approach has been tempered by the high local recurrence rate and toxicity seen with the combined approach.

BIBLIOGRAPHY

Ajani J. Contributions of chemotherapy in the treatment of carcinoma of the esophagus: results and commentary. Semin Oncol 1994;21:474–482.

Bates BA, Detterbeck FC, Bernard SA, et al. Concurrent radiation therapy and chemotherapy followed by esophagectomy for localized esophageal cancer. J Clin Oncol 1996;14:156–163.

Forastiere AA, Heitmiller RF, Lee DJ, et al. Intensive chemoradiation followed by esophagectomy for squamous cell and adenocarcinoma of the esophagus. Cancer J Sci Am 1997;3:144–152.

Herskovic A, Martz K, Al-Sarraf M, et al. Combined chemotherapy and radiation therapy compared with radiation therapy alone in patients with carcinoma of the esophagus. N Engl J Med 1992;329:1593–1598.

Walsh TN, Noonan N, Hollywood D, et al. A comparison of multimodal therapy and surgery for esophageal adenocarcinoma. N Engl J Med 1996;335:462–467.

Gastric Cancer

John D. Wilkes

BACKGROUND

While the overall incidence of cancer in the United States appears to have peaked in 1993, the incidence of adenocarcinoma of the distal stomach has steadily been decreasing since the 1930s. However, the incidence of proximal gastric cancers, especially in patients under 40 years of age, has been increasing dramatically. Despite the overall decline in incidence, the survival rate for patients with gastric cancer remains unchanged over the same period, and this malignancy remains the eighth most common cause of cancer death.

EPIDEMIOLOGY

In 1998 there were an estimated 22,600 new cases of gastric cancer diagnosed in the United States, with approximately 13,700 deaths. Worldwide, gastric cancer has a strong geographic variation, being 7 to 10 times as common in Japan and Chile as in the United States. Movement from a high-incidence area to a lower-incidence area results in an eventual reduction in risk for subsequent generations. There is also an increased incidence of gastric cancer in African-American men and in persons of lower socioeconomic status. The peak incidence is in the seventh decade.

ETIOLOGY

Dietary and environmental factors are thought to play a role in the pathogenesis of gastric cancer. Diets low in fruits and vegetables or high in nitrates and salt predispose to gastric cancer. Environmental factors include smoking, lack of food refrigeration, and poor water quality. Occupational exposures may play a minor role. Pernicious anemia, atrophic gastritis, blood type A, and prior gastric resection also appear to increase the risk of gastric cancer. The potential role of *Helicobacter pylori* infection remains to be determined.

CLINICAL MANIFESTATIONS

As is too frequently the case with gastrointestinal neoplasms, the signs and symptoms of gastric cancer are often nonspecific, resulting in significant delays in diagnosis. Symptoms may include fatigue, pain, anorexia, vomiting, or weight loss. Metastatic disease to the liver, lymph nodes (Virchow's node, Sister Mary Joseph's periumbilical node), or peritoneum (Blumer's rectal shelf, ascites) may be identifiable on physical examination.

STAGING EVALUATION

Upper endoscopy with biopsy is the most useful diagnostic procedure (Table 1B.18). If available, endoscopic ultrasound may provide the most accurate means of assessing both T stage and local nodal involvement. Barium studies may provide complementary information. CT of the chest, abdomen, and pelvis must be performed to evaluate for both local disease extension and distant metastases. Bone scans should be obtained in any patient with bone pain or an elevated alkaline phosphatase.

PROGNOSIS

The minority (17%) of patients with gastric cancer present with localized disease and have a relatively favorable prognosis. Patients with pretreatment weight loss of more than 10% or with proximal tumors have a worse prognosis. The extent of disease by TNM stage is the strongest predictor of survival (Table 1B.18).

TREATMENTS

SURGERY

Resection of the primary tumor, when feasible, is the only known curative therapy for gastric cancer. Procedures include total gastrectomy and partial distal gastrectomy with either Billroth I (gastroduodenostomy) or Billroth II (gastrojejunostomy) anastomoses. Surgical resection or bypass may be performed for palliation of advanced stage IV disease. Regional lymphadenectomy is recommended with all of these procedures, but splenectomy is not routine. In select patients with extensive or metastatic gastric cancer, palliative gastric resection may be indicated to control bleeding, obstruction, or pain.

ADJUVANT THERAPY

Distant and/or local failure following primary resection occurs in 60 to 70% of patients with resected gastric cancer. There is no evidence as yet that postoperative adjuvant chemotherapy offers any benefit following curative resection. A meta-analysis of 11 published randomized trials confirms the lack of benefit in this approach.

Small randomized clinical trials show that adjuvant radiation therapy decreases local failure but does not appear to affect survival. A large intergroup randomized trial evaluating the role of adjuvant radiation therapy and chemotherapy is under way.

RADIATION THERAPY

Radiation therapy may provide palliation of bleeding or obstruction for patients with unresectable primary tumors.

Table 1B.18A. TNM Staging System for Gastric Cancer

Primary tumor

TX   Primary tumor cannot be assessed.

T0   No evidence of primary tumor.

Tis   Carcinoma in situ.

T1   Tumor invades the lamina propria or submucosa.

T2   Tumor invades the muscularis propria or the subserosa.

T3   Tumor penetrates the serosa without invasion of adjacent structures.

T4   Tumor invades adjacent structures.

Regional lymph nodes

NX   Regional lymph nodes cannot be assessed.

N0   No regional lymph node metastasis.

N1   Metastasis in 1–6 regional lymph nodes.

N2   Metastasis in 7–15 regional lymph nodes.

N3   Metastasis in more than 15 regional lymph nodes.

Distant metastases

MX   Presence of distant metastases cannot be assessed.

M0   No distant metastasis.

M1   Distant metastasis present.

Table 1B.18B. Stage Grouping for Gastric Cancer

Stage	Tumor	Nodes	Metastasis	5-Year Survival (%)
0	Tis	N0	M0	>90
IA	T1	N0	M0	60
IB	T1	N1	M0	43
	T2	N0	M0	
II	T1	N2	M0	30
	T2	N1	M0	
	T3	N0	M0	
IIIA	T2	N2	M0	18
	T3	N1	M0	
	T4	N0	M0	
IIIB	T2	N2	M0	9
IV	T4	N1	M0	<5
	T1–4	N3	M0	
	T4	N2	M0	
	Any T	Any N	M1	

Adapted with permission from American Joint Committee on Cancer. Cancer staging manual. 5th ed. Philadelphia: Lippincott-Raven, 1997.

Table 1B.19. Chemotherapy for Unresectable or Metastatic Gastric Cancer

Regimen	Overall Response Rates (%)(Pooled data)
Single Agents	
Mitomycin	30
5-FU	21
Cisplatin	19–25
Carmustine	19
Hydroxyurea	19
Doxorubicin	17
Chlorambucil	17
Etoposide	12
Methotrexate	11
Combinations	
5-FU, doxorubicin (FA)	19
5-FU, doxorubicin, mitomycin (FAM)	9–42
Etoposide, leucovorin, 5-FU (ELF)	17–53
Etoposide, doxorubicin, cisplatin (EAP)	20–64
5-FU, doxorubicin, cisplatin (FAP)	19–38
5-FU, doxorubicin, Mtx (FAMTX)	21–59

CHEMOTHERAPY

Various chemotherapeutic agents have been evaluated in locally advanced and metastatic gastric cancer. Most single agents have only modest activity (Table 1B.19). Responses from single agents are usually partial and brief. Combinations have demonstrated better response rates than single agents but have not as yet been shown to improve patient survival, and they are associated with more toxicity.

BIBLIOGRAPHY

Herman J, Bonenkamp JJ, Boon MC, et al. Adjuvant therapy after curative resection for gastric cancer: a meta-analysis of randomized trials. J Clin Oncol 1993;11:1441–1447.

Kelson D. The use of chemotherapy in the treatment of advanced gastric and pancreas cancer. Semin Oncol 1994;21:58–66.

Kelson D, Atiq OT, Saltz L, et al. FAMTX versus etoposide, doxorubicin, and cisplatin: a random assignment trial in gastric cancer. J Clin Oncol 1992;10:541–548.

O'Brien ME, Cunningham D. The role of chemotherapy for metastatic gastric cancer. J Inf Chemother 1995;5:112–116.

Schipper DL, Wagener DJ. Chemotherapy of gastric cancer. Anti-Cancer Drugs 1996;7:137–149.

Pancreatic Cancer

John D. Wilkes

BACKGROUND

Carcinoma of the pancreas is the fifth leading cause of cancer deaths in the United States, and despite significant improvements in imaging modalities and perioperative capabilities, overall treatment results remain disappointing. The median survival for all patients is a dismal 3 to 6 months, and the 5-year survival is only 4%. Unfortunately, there is no effective means of early detection, including the use of the tumor marker CA-19–9. Thus, 80% of patients have unresectable or metastatic disease at diagnosis. Approximately 95% of pancreatic neoplasms are adenocarcinomas arising from the exocrine pancreas. Endocrine tumors of the pancreas are covered in the following subchapter, Neuroendocrine Tumors of the Gastrointestinal Tract.

EPIDEMIOLOGY

Approximately 29,000 new cases of pancreatic cancer were diagnosed in 1998, with a nearly equal number of deaths. The peak incidence occurs in the seventh and eighth decades, and African-Americans have one of the highest incidences worldwide.

ETIOLOGY

Although the causes of pancreatic cancer remain uncertain, there appears to be a genetic predisposition in a minority of cases (5%), with a mutation in the tumor-suppressor gene (CDKN2, p16) identified in patients with familial pancreatic cancer. There is also a doubled incidence of pancreas cancer in smokers. Dietary factors may also contribute to risk, as animal studies suggest a possible increased risk related to excessive fat intake and N-nitroso compounds. Other dietary factors, such as caffeine and alcohol use, have not been conclusively demonstrated as causal factors. Patients who have undergone gastrectomy or have diabetes or chronic pancreatitis also may be at increased risk for pancreas cancer.

CLINICAL MANIFESTATIONS

The vague nature of symptoms of pancreatic neoplasms is largely responsible for the fact that 80 to 85% of patients have advanced and incurable disease at diagnosis. The most common symptoms include anorexia, weight loss (70 to 100% of patients), back or abdominal pain (70 to 90%), jaundice, steatorrhea, glucose intolerance, and depression (50%). Physical findings may include jaundice, a palpable gallbladder (Courvoisier's sign), venous thrombosis, and migratory superficial thrombophlebitis (Trousseau's syndrome). Metastatic disease to the liver, lymph nodes (Virchow's node, Sister Mary Joseph's periumbilical node), or peritoneum (Blumer's rectal shelf, ascites) may be also identifiable on physical examination.

STAGING EVALUATION

A diagnosis of small, localized pancreatic cancer is often difficult to obtain (Table 1B.20). CT-guided biopsy and endoscopic retrograde cholangiopancreatography (ERCP) are the least invasive means. Laparoscopy or surgical exploration may be required to obtain a tissue diagnosis. Following diagnosis, the best imaging study to stage patients and evaluate resectability is dynamic CT. This improvement over conventional CT can identify unresectability (nodal or vascular structure involvement, occlusion, local organ invasion, and/or distant metastases) in up to 85% of patients. Some institutions still recommend angiography, although the improved vascular resolution provided by dynamic CT may make this less important. Endoscopic ultrasonography may help identify metastatic disease in lymph nodes but is not yet routine. As always, a careful history and physical examination are key components to any staging workup. A chest radiograph, hematologic profile, and routine chemistries may help identify occult metastatic disease and assist in determining the patient's tolerance of planned treatments.

PROGNOSIS

The prognosis of patients with pancreas cancer is highly dependent on resectability. Tumor invasion of adjacent structures and lymph node involvement are adverse prognostic signs. For patients who are completely resected, pathologic involvement of lymph nodes is the most significant predictor of survival. Patients with involved lymph nodes following resection have a median survival of only 6 to 8 months.

TREATMENTS

SURGERY

Surgical resection remains the only curative approach for adenocarcinomas of the pancreas, and it is appropriate only for carefully staged patients with disease confined to the pancreas (stage I). Standard procedures include total pancreatectomy and partial pancreaticoduodenectomy (Whipple procedure). One advantage of the latter procedure is the ability of the residual pancreas to perform endocrine functions. Patient selection and improved op-

Table 1B.20A. TNM Staging System for Pancreatic Cancer

Primary Tumor

TX	Primary tumor cannot be assessed.
T0	No evidence of primary tumor.
Tis	In situ carcinoma.
T1	Tumor limited to the pancreas 2 cm or less in greatest diameter.
T2	Tumor limited to the pancreas more than 2 cm in greatest diameter.
T3	Tumor extends directly to duodenum, bile duct, or peripancreatic tissues.
T4	Tumor extends directly to stomach, spleen, colon, or adjacent large vessels.

Regional Lymph Nodes

NX	Regional lymph nodes cannot be assessed.
N0	No regional lymph node metastasis.
N1	Regional lymph node metastases.
pN1a	Metastasis in a single regional lymph node.
pN1b	Metastases to multiple regional lymph nodes.

Distant Metastases

MX	Presence of distant metastases cannot be assessed.
M0	No distant metastasis.
M1	Distant metastasis present.

Table 1B.20B. Stage Grouping for Pancreatic Cancer

Stage	Tumor	Nodes	Metastasis	Median Survival (mo)
0	Tis	N0	M0	–
I	T1	N0	M0	12–18
	T2	N0	M0	
II	T3	N0	M0	7–10
III	T1–3	N1	M0	6–8
IVA	T4	Any N	M0	3–4
IVB	Any T	Any N	M1	

Adapted with permission from American Joint Committee on Cancer. Cancer staging manual. 5th ed. Philadelphia: Lippincott-Raven, 1997.

erative and perioperative techniques have resulted in an increase in 5-year survival (25%) following curative resection. For patients with unresectable disease, surgical bypass may provide palliation of obstruction, jaundice, pain, and/or bleeding.

The importance of effective biliary decompression for patients with carcinoma of the pancreatic head cannot be overstated. This can be achieved through internal or external stents.

Surgical decompression is preferred for patients with favorable performance status in whom long-term stents may become occluded or infected.

RADIATION THERAPY

As a single modality, radiation therapy can palliate symptoms of locally advanced pancreatic cancer and may yield limited prolongation of life in some patients. The median survival of patients treated with radiation therapy alone is 8 to 10 months.

The combination of chemotherapy and radiation has been evaluated in the neoadjuvant, adjuvant, and palliative settings. Data from some investigators suggest an ability to improve resectability with preoperative 5-FU and radiation; however, this approach remains investigational. For palliation, many institutions offer combinations of 5-FU and concurrent radiation therapy. In an older randomized trial, this approach has been demonstrated to increase the proportion of 1-year survivors from 10% with radiation therapy alone to 40%. Similarly, the median survivals for the combination were reported to be 35 weeks versus 18 weeks in the radiation therapy alone arm. There are a variety of approaches employing either bolus or continuous 5-FU as a radiation enhancer.

In the postoperative adjuvant setting, the Gastrointestinal Oncology Study Group (GITSG) demonstrated improved median survival (21 versus 11 months) with 5-FU plus split-course radiation therapy compared with no adjuvant therapy. Results from a confirmatory trial being conducted in Europe are pending. At present, based on the results of the GITSG study, many clinicians offer adjuvant chemoradiation therapy to appropriate patients without either a split radiation course or 2 years of weekly 5-FU (as originally reported by GITSG).

CHEMOTHERAPY

There is no role for adjuvant chemotherapy alone for patients with resected pancreatic cancer outside of well-designed clinical trials. In the setting of advanced or metastatic disease, very few chemotherapeutic agents have demonstrated significant activity. The evaluation of active agents is complicated by both patient-related and tumor-related factors, including poor performance status, impaired nutrition, and absence of bidimensional measurable disease.

Nevertheless, several chemotherapeutic agents do have some clinical activity in adenocarcinoma of the pancreas (Table 1B.21), although their effect on survival, ability to provide palliation, and overall quality of life remain to be determined. As yet there is no strong evidence that systemic chemotherapy provides a

Table 1B.21. Chemotherapy for Unresectable or Metastatic Pancreas Cancer

Regimen	Overall Response Rates (%)(Pooled data)
Single Agents	
Gemcitabine	6–11
5-FU	7–12
Ifosfamide	7–22
Mitomycin	10–27
Doxorubicin	8–13
Streptozotocin	11
Combinations	
5-FU, doxorubicin, mitomycin	13–14
Streptozotocin, mitomycin, 5-FU	4–14
5-FU, doxorubicin, cisplatin	15
5-FU, leucovorin, mitomycin-C, dipyridamole (UCLA regimen)	41
Chemoradiotherapy	
Fox Chase ECOG (preop)	31 (minimal/partial)
5-FU 1 g/m^2 CIVI days 2–5 and 29–32; mitomycin C 10 mg/m^2 day 2 only; 180 cGy fx in 28 days (50.4 Gy)	
MD Anderson (preop)	N/A
5-FU 300 mg/m^2/d CIVI 5 days/week; 180 cGy fx (45–50.4 Gy)	
GITSG (adjuvant)	N/A
5-FU 500 mg/m^2 days 1–3 of each RT course, then weekly for 2 years; 200 cGy fx for 2 weeks repeated after 2-week break (split course, 40 Gy total)	

CIVI, continuous intravenous infusion; RT, radiation therapy.

survival benefit for patients with metastatic pancreatic cancer. Despite higher response rates over single agents in some series, the superiority of combination regimens has not been demonstrated, and the toxicity profiles are often intolerable in this patient population. Patients with poor performance status are exceedingly unlikely to derive any benefit from chemotherapy, and efforts to find alternative means of symptom palliation should be aggressively pursued.

BIBLIOGRAPHY

Ahlgren JD. Chemotherapy for pancreas cancer. Cancer 1996;78:654–663.
Burris HA, Moore MJ, Anderson J, et al. Improvements in survival and clinical

benefit with gemcitabine as first-line therapy for patients with advanced pancreas cancer: a randomized trial. J Clin Oncol 1997;15:2403–2413.

Gastrointestinal Study Group. Comparative therapeutic trial of radiation with or without chemotherapy in pancreatic carcinoma. Int J Radiat Oncol Biol Phys 1979;5:1643–1647.

Kaiser MH, Ellenberg SS. Pancreatic cancer: adjuvant combined radiation and chemotherapy following curative resection. Arch Surg 1985;120:899–903.

Spitz FR, Abbruzzese JL, Lee JE, et al. Preoperative and postoperative chemoradiation strategies in patients treated with pancreaticoduodenectomy for adenocarcinoma of the pancreas. J Clin Oncol 1997;15:928–937.

Wanebo HJ, Vezeridis MP. Pancreatic carcinoma in perspective. Cancer 1996; 78:580–591.

Neuroendocrine Tumors of the Gastrointestinal Tract

John D. Wilkes

BACKGROUND

Neuroendocrine tumors of the gastrointestinal tract are an extremely interesting and rare group of malignancies characterized by the secretion of various hormones. Symptoms of these malignancies may result from local tumor growth, metastatic lesions, or hormonal excess. While surgical resection may be curative in patients with localized disease, most therapeutic strategies are aimed at reduction of tumor burden for palliative purposes in patients with advanced disease. As a general rule, neuroendocrine tumors of the gastrointestinal tract have a relatively indolent clinical course.

EPIDEMIOLOGY

It is estimated that fewer than 2000 cases of gastrointestinal neuroendocrine malignancies are diagnosed each year in the United States. Collectively, these tumors account for only 2% of all gastrointestinal malignancies. Nearly two carcinoid tumors are diagnosed for every islet cell tumor. Insulinomas and gastrinomas are the most common islet cell tumors. Glucagonomas, somatostatinomas, and VIPomas (affecting the vasoactive intestinal peptide) are exceedingly rare.

ETIOLOGY

The causation of gastrointestinal neuroendocrine tumors remains unknown. The association of pancreatic islet cell tumors with the multiple endocrine neoplasia (MEN) type 1 syndrome suggests autosomal dominant transmission. More recent linkage studies identified the MEN-1 gene locus on chromosome 11q13. This provides little information, however, as to the causation of most neuroendocrine tumors of the gastrointestinal tract that are not associated with MEN-1.

CARCINOID TUMORS

CLINICAL MANIFESTATIONS

Carcinoid tumors, the most common neuroendocrine tumors of the gastrointestinal tract, are classified as amine precursor uptake and decarboxylation (APUD) tumors. The appendix (45%), small intestine (30%), and rectum (15%) account for more than 90% of cases. Approximately 60% of carcinoid tumors are asymptomatic at diagnosis. Clinical manifestations of the primary tumor may include obstruction or intussusception. More often the symptoms are related to hormone secretion. Except for those originating in the rectum, carcinoid tumors produce a variety of endocrine substances, including serotonin, histamine, bradykinin, substance P, and kallikrein. The carcinoid syndrome (paroxysmal flushing, diarrhea, abdominal cramping, bronchoconstriction, cardiac valvular lesions, arthropathy, and telangiectasia) results from the release of various endocrine substances, though precisely which substance or substances remains unclear. The carcinoid syndrome rarely occurs in the absence of hepatic metastases, as the liver is extremely efficient in metabolizing the vasoactive amines. The severity of symptoms appears to be directly related to tumor volume. Rarely, the blood supply of a large carcinoid will bypass the liver and drain directly into the systemic circulation, leading to carcinoid syndrome.

Although the demonstration of elevated 24-hour urinary 5-hydroxyindoleacetic acid (5-HIAA) levels is useful in diagnosing metastatic carcinoid, this test cannot help diagnose carcinoids at a curable stage or rectal carcinoids at any stage. Routine imaging studies such as CT and MRI may help identify tumors. Octreotide scans may identify metastatic deposits not visualized on conventional imaging studies.

TREATMENT

Surgical resection is the standard curative modality for localized carcinoids, producing 5-year survival rates of 70 to 90%. As a very general statement, localized carcinoids of the appendix, small bowel, and rectum can be effectively managed with relatively minor interventions (i.e. appendectomy, local excisions). Larger tumors require more aggressive surgery. Carcinoid tumors with gross regional lymphatic metastasis or local extension should be treated with aggressive surgical resection. If all visible malignant disease can be removed, long-term survival rates are excellent, although late recurrences are possible. Aggressive subtotal resections may also provide excellent long-term palliation. There is no proven role for adjuvant chemotherapy.

For patients with metastatic carcinoid, the clinical course is usually quite indolent, with median survivals in excess of 2 years. For such patients, excellent palliation may be achieved through debulking procedures such as resection of large hepatic metastases, hepatic arterial ligation, or chemoembolization. Such procedures may significantly reduce the symptoms related to hormonal excesses.

Octreotide is a long-acting somatostatin analogue that has demonstrated significant utility in the management of neuroendocrine tumors of the gastrointestinal tract. Most patients' carcinoid symptoms can be effectively palliated with subcutaneous injections of this agent two or three times a day. The initial dosing is 50 μg subcutaneously three times daily, and the dose is gradually escalated to 150 μg three times a day. The median duration of symptom control with octreotide is approximately a year.

Combination chemotherapy has been evaluated to some degree for patients with metastatic carcinoid. It should not be offered to asymptomatic patients, who have the potential for significant long-term symptom-free-survival by virtue of the indolent nature of this disease. For symptomatic patients, chemotherapy may provide palliation for more than a year. A variety of single agents and combinations with response rates less than 30% have been reported. Responses are rarely complete and usually brief. The most extensively studied drugs include 5-FU, doxorubicin, dacarbazine, cyclophosphamide, and 5-FU plus streptozocin. Single-agent response rates are 10 to 25%, and 5-FU plus streptozocin produces responses in fewer than 35% of patients. Rarely, patients may obtain transient benefit from the use of interferon-α, but the toxicity profile appears to be unfavorable relative to the clinical benefit.

Adjunctive treatments for carcinoid syndrome include dietary modifications, antidiarrheals, antihistamines (H1 and H2 blockers), and avoidance of certain medications (monoamine oxidase inhibitors).

PANCREATIC ISLET CELL TUMORS

Cancers of the endocrine pancreas are extremely uncommon malignancies, with only 200 to 1000 new cases diagnosed annually. Most islet cell tumors are nonfunctional and malignant. Symptoms result from either tumor bulk or metastases. The functioning endocrine tumors of the pancreas may be benign, producing symptoms through the production of hormones. The term islet cell carcinoma refers to a number of distinct cancers that when functional, have unique metabolic and clinical characteristics (Table 1B.22).

DIAGNOSIS

An extremely high index of suspicion is required to diagnose pancreatic islet cell tumors. Functional tumors may be too small to be detected by conventional imaging techniques, and there are frequently significant delays between initial symptoms and diagnosis. The diagnosis of gastrinoma requires both an elevated serum gastrin and elevated gastric acid levels. Insulinoma

Table 1B.22. Functional Islet Cell Tumors and Clinical Manifestations

Tumor	Clinical Characteristics
Glucagonoma	70% malignant, diabetes, dermatitis (necrolytic erythema migrans), venous thrombosis
Insulinoma	90% benign, solitary, hypoglycemia, 5% MEN-I
Somatostatinoma	90% malignant, adult onset mild diabetes, cholelithiasis
Gastrinoma	60% malignant, peptic ulcer disease, jejunal ulcerations, diarrhea, 20% MEN-I
VIPoma	80% malignant, watery diarrhea, hypokalemia, achlorhydria
Carcinoid	Carcinoid syndrome
Polypeptidoma	Multiple hormonal syndromes

is diagnosed when fasting hypoglycemia accompanies elevated serum insulin and C-peptide levels. Localization of these tumors often poses a significant challenge. Nuclear medicine imaging (Octreotide, FDG/PET), CT and MRI, angiography, and intraoperative imaging with venous sampling for hormones may be required.

TREATMENT

Surgery is the only curative modality for islet cell tumors of the pancreas. The extent of surgical resection is based on both the preoperative tumor localization studies and intraoperative findings. Patients with unresectable disease may have significant long-term palliation of hormonal excess because of the slow-growing nature of most of these tumors. Symptomatic patients with hepatic-dominant disease may benefit from either hepatic arterial occlusion with embolization or chemoembolization.

Combination chemotherapy may provide effective palliation as well as increased survival in selected patients. However, for patients with indolent, slow-growing metastatic islet cell carcinomas, the best therapy may be careful observation and no treatment until palliation is required. If systemic chemotherapy is indicated for symptoms of uncontrollable hormonal excess or tumor growth, combination regimens such as doxorubicin plus streptozocin or 5-FU plus streptozocin may be employed. In a randomized multicenter trial comparing doxorubicin plus streptozocin against 5-FU plus streptozocin, the anthracycline-containing regimen achieved a higher response rate (69 versus 45%), better time to progression (20 versus 7 months), and improved median survival (2.2 versus 1.4 years).

Somatostatin, as described earlier under treatments for carcinoid syndrome, may also provide significant palliation of symptoms related to hormonal excess as a result of advanced islet cell tumors except insulinomas. Diazoxide 300 to 500 mg/day may be helpful in preventing hypoglycemia associated with insulinoma. Omeprazole is extremely effective in reducing the gastric hypersecretion associated with the Zollinger-Ellison syndrome (gastrinoma). Prophylactic anticoagulation therapy should also be considered for patients with glucagonoma. Antidiarrheals such as loperamide can ameliorate the diarrhea associated with VIPomas.

BIBLIOGRAPHY

Delcore R, Friesen SR. Gastrointestinal neuroendocrine tumors. J Am Coll Surg 1994;178:187–211.

Evans DB, Skibber JM, Lee JE, et al. Nonfunctioning islet cell carcinoma of the pancreas. Surgery 1993;114:1175–1182.

Kvols LK, Moertel CG, O'Connell MJ, et al. Treatment of the malignant carcinoid syndrome: evaluation of a long-acting somatostatin analogue. N Engl J Med 1986;315:663–666.

Modlin IM, Lewis JJ, Ahlman H, et al. Management of unresectable malignant endocrine tumors of the pancreas. Surg Gynecol Obstet 1993;176:507–518.

Moertel CG, Johnson CM, McKusick MA, et al. The management of patients with advanced carcinoid tumors and islet cell carcinomas. Ann Intern Med 1994;120:302–309.

Moertel CG, Lefkopoulo M, Lipsitz S, et al. Streptozocin-doxorubicin, streptozocin-fluorouracil, or chlorozotocin in the treatment of advanced islet-cell carcinoma. N Engl J Med 1992;326:519–523.

Hepatobiliary Cancer
John D. Wilkes

HEPATOCELLULAR CARCINOMA
BACKGROUND

Hepatocellular carcinoma (HCC) is possibly the most common solid tumor worldwide, resulting in an estimated 1.25 million deaths annually. Most primary liver tumors are adenocarcinomas (HCC, cholangiocarcinoma). Occasionally mixed hepatocellular cholangiocarcinomas and undifferentiated tumors are diagnosed.

EPIDEMIOLOGY

HCC is a relatively uncommon cancer in the United States, where only about 5000 cases are diagnosed annually. However, this malignancy is the most common cancer in other parts of the world, such as China, Southeast Asia, and Africa. In addition to the geographic variation, there is a strong male predilection, with three men affected for each woman.

ETIOLOGY

HCC is almost always associated with some form of chronic liver disease. In the United States HCC is associated with alcoholic cirrhosis in 50 to 80% of patients, and 5% of cirrhotic patients eventually develop HCC. Worldwide, hepatitis B and C appear to be the most significant causes of HCC, particularly in patients with chronic active hepatitis. Less common causative factors include exposure to aflatoxin or vinyl chloride (sarcomas, angiosarcomas).

CLINICAL MANIFESTATIONS

The primary clinical manifestations of HCC, which relate to the primary mass, may include pain, weight loss, ascites, fatigue, weakness, nausea, and unexplained fever. Physical findings may include hepatomegaly, stigmata of cirrhosis, ascites, and/or splenomegaly. Less commonly, patients may have paraneoplastic manifestations of HCC, including polycythemia, hypoglycemia, hypercalcemia, dysfibrinogenemia, and porphyria cutanea tarda. In patients with underlying cirrhosis, a progressive increase in α-fetoprotein (AFP) or alkaline phosphatase or a rapid deterioration in hepatic function may indicate this neoplasm. The screening of high-risk individuals with serum AFP measurements is recommended. In the United States AFP is elevated in 50 to 70% of patients with HCC.

STAGING EVALUATION

Once the diagnosis of HCC is established, all patients should be assessed for possible surgical resection with angiography, CT portography, or dynamic CT and MRI (Table 1B.23). Information on the arterial anatomy is helpful for the operating surgeon and may eliminate some patients from consideration for resection. Dynamic CT and MRI can document the relation of the tumor to the hepatic and portal veins.

PROGNOSIS

The prognosis of patients with HCC depends on a variety of patient- and disease-related factors including performance status, underlying liver dysfunction, and extent of local tumor replacement. It is important to distinguish the fibrolamellar variant of HCC because an increased proportion of these patients may be cured with resection. AFP levels have also been shown to have prognostic significance, with the median survival of AFP-negative patients being significantly longer than that of AFP-positive patients.

TREATMENTS

The only potential curative therapy for HCC is surgical resection, which depends on tumor size, location, and status of residual liver. Very few patients present with localized resectable disease (T1 to T3, and selected T4; N0; M0) in a portion of the liver that allows complete surgical removal of the tumor with a margin of normal liver. Patients with chronic hepatitis and/or cirrhosis are at high risk when surgical resection is performed. Depending on the patient's and tumor's characteristics, procedures may vary from segmental resection to trisegmental resection. In series of carefully selected patients, partial hepatectomy has resulted in 5-year survival of 10 to 30%. Many of these patients have the fibrolamellar variant. The role of adjuvant therapy following complete resection remains under investigation.

Certain patients with localized but unresectable HCC (select T2 to T4; N0; M0) may be candidates for orthotopic liver transplantation (OLT). The usual contraindications to major hepatic resections may not preclude hepatic transplantation. In a large series, survival rates for OLT vary with clinical and histologic characteristics. Reported 5-year survival was 11% (nonfibrolamellar), 36% (incidental finding), and 41% (fibrolamellar). A series of 20 patients treated with adjuvant doxorubicin following OLT reported a 3-year survival rate of 53%.

Many clinical trials have evaluated the effect of systemic chemotherapy, regional chemotherapy, external beam radia-

Table 1B.23A. TNM Staging System for Hepatocellular Carcinoma

Primary Tumor

TX	Primary tumor cannot be assessed.
T0	No evidence of primary tumor.
T1	Solitary tumor no larger than 2 cm without vascular invasion.
T2	Solitary tumor no larger than 2 cm with vascular invasion or multiple tumors limited to one lobe, none larger than 2 cm without vascular invasion; or a solitary tumor larger than 2 cm without vascular invasion.
T3	Solitary tumor larger than 2 cm with vascular invasion; or multiple tumors limited to one lobe, none larger than 2 cm, with vascular invasion; or multiple tumors limited to one lobe, any larger than 2 cm, with or without vascular invasion.
T4	Multiple tumors in more than one lobe or tumor(s) involving a major branch of portal or hepatic vein(s) or invasion of adjacent organs other than the gallbladder or perforation of the visceral peritoneum.

Regional Lymph Nodes[a]

NX	Regional lymph nodes cannot be assessed.
N0	No regional lymph node metastasis.
N1	Regional lymph node metastases.

Distant Metastases

MX	Presence of distant metastases cannot be assessed.
M0	No distant metastasis.
M1	Distant metastasis present.

[a]*The regional lymph nodes include the hilar (i.e., those in the hepatoduodenal ligament, hepatic and periportal nodes) and those along the inferior vena cava, hepatic artery, and portal vein. Any lymph node involvement beyond these nodes is considered distant metastasis and should be staged as M1.*

1B.23B. Stage Grouping for Hepatocellular Carcinoma

Stage	Tumor	Nodes	Metastasis
I	T1	N0	M0
II	T2	N0	M0
IIIA	T3	N0	M0
IIIB	T1–3	N1	M0
IVA	T4	Any N	M0
IVB	Any T	Any N	M0

Adapted with permission from American Joint Committee on Cancer. Cancer staging manual. 5th ed. Philadelphia: Lippincott-Raven, 1997.

tion plus chemotherapy, and/or radiolabeled antibodies. In general, the response rates and clinical effect of these efforts has been disappointing. Responses are usually limited and brief. Response rates for single-agent systemic chemotherapy have been disappointing. Doxorubicin has produced objective tumor reduction in 15 to 19% of patients, while other agents (5-FU, etoposide, mitoxantrone) have even more limited responses (less than 10%). Combination regimens are not superior to single agents. Recent trials of interferon have suggested some antitumor activity.

Other approaches under evaluation include hepatic artery ligation, chemoembolization of the hepatic artery, cryosurgical ablation, and injection of alcohol. There remains no standard therapy for unresectable HCC, and clinical trials should be considered.

Patients with advanced HCC (any T, N1 or M1) have a dismal prognosis, with median survival of only 3 to 4 months. As previously mentioned, there is no standard therapy for such patients, and clinical trials, such as phase I trials, may be considered.

EXTRAHEPATIC BILE DUCT CANCER

BACKGROUND

Cancer arising in the extrahepatic bile ducts is an uncommon disease in the United States, accounting for approximately 4000 deaths a year. More than 90% of these tumors are adenocarcinomas (papillary, intestinal, mucinous, clear cell, signet ring, adenosquamous). Rare histologies include squamous, small cell, or mesenchymal tumors (embryonal rhabdomyosarcoma, leiomyosarcoma, malignant fibrous histiocytoma).

ETIOLOGY

Bile duct cancer occurs most frequently in patients with a history of chronic inflammatory processes involving the biliary system, such as liver fluke infestation, inflammatory bowel disease, sclerosing cholangitis, and congenital anomalies of the biliary system.

CLINICAL MANIFESTATIONS

The most common symptoms caused by extrahepatic bile duct cancer are jaundice, pain, fever, and pruritus. During diagnostic evaluation many of these tumors are found to be multifocal. Direct hepatic parenchymal invasion or extension along the common bile duct and spread to adjacent lymph nodes are also common. Distant metastases are quite uncommon, although peritoneal seeding does occur.

STAGING EVALUATION

The TNM system should be used to stage extrahepatic bile duct cancer (Table 1B.24). Staging depends on both diagnostic imaging (clinical staging) and when appropriate, surgical exploration with pathologic examination of the resected specimen (pathologic staging). Stages defined by the TNM classification shown in Table 1B.24 apply to all primary carcinomas arising in the extrahepatic bile duct or in the cystic duct but do *not* apply to intrahepatic cholangiocarcinomas, sarcomas, or carcinoid tumors.

PROGNOSIS

In general the prognosis for patients with extrahepatic bile duct tumors is poor, with a median survival of only a year. Prognosis depends significantly on the tumor's anatomic location (proximal versus distal) and resectability. Both perineural invasion and lymph node metastases reduce survival.

TREATMENTS

Complete resection is possible in 25 to 30% of tumors that originate in the distal bile duct. These patients have a 5-year survival rate of 25%, which is a significantly better prognosis than can be expected for proximal tumors. The optimum surgical procedure varies with tumor location, extent of hepatic involvement, and relation of the tumor to major vascular structures. Overall, fewer than 10% of cases of extrahepatic bile duct tumors can be cured surgically.

Most patients with extrahepatic bile duct tumors are incurable at presentation. For palliation, establishment of effective biliary drainage is essential. It may be achieved surgically or by either endoscopic or percutaneous stents. Palliative irradiation (e.g., brachytherapy or external beam radiation therapy) may benefit selected patients. Attempts to improve the effects of radiation (hyperthermia, radiation sensitizers) are under investigation.

The experience with chemotherapy in advanced extrahepatic biliary tumors is limited by the small size of clinical trials, in which favorable response rates probably reflect patient selection. Fluorouracil, doxorubicin, and mitomycin have been reported to produce transient partial remissions in 10 to 20% of patients. A combination regimen, FAM (5-FU, doxorubicin, mitomycin), produced a response rate of 29% in a single trial. Pooled data of regional chemotherapy suggests higher response rates than seen with systemic treatments. An ECOG trial of 5-FU and external beam radiation in patients with unresectable pancreaticobiliary tumors reported a median survival of 1 year, with 19% of patients alive at 2 years. Whenever possible, patients

Table 1B.24A. TNM Staging System for Carcinoma of the Extrahepatic Bile Ducts

Primary Tumor

TX	Primary tumor cannot be assessed.
T0	No evidence of primary tumor.
Tis	Carcinoma in situ.
T1	Tumor invades the subepithelial connective tissue or fibromuscular layer.
T1a	Tumor invades the subepithelial connective tissue.
T1b	Tumor invades the fibromuscular layer.
T2	Tumor invades perifibromuscular connective tissue.
T3	Tumor invades adjacent structures: liver, pancreas, duodenum, gallbladder, colon, stomach.

Regional lymph nodes

NX	Regional lymph nodes cannot be assessed.
N0	No regional lymph node metastasis.
N1	Metastasis in cystic duct, pericholedochal and/or hilar lymph nodes (i.e., in the hepatoduodenal ligament).
N2	Metastasis in peripancreatic (head only), periduodenal, periportal, celiac, and/or superior mesenteric lymph nodes, and/or posterior pancreaticoduodenal lymph nodes.

Distant metastasis

MX	Presence of distant metastasis cannot be assessed.
M0	No distant metastasis.
M1	Distant metastasis.

Table 1B.24B. Stage Grouping for Carcinoma of the Extrahepatic Bile Ducts

Stage	Tumor	Nodes	Metastasis
0	Tis	N0	M0
I	T1	N0	M0
II	T2	N0	M0
III	T1	N1	M0
	T1	N2	M0
	T2	N1	M0
	T2	N2	M0
IVA	T3	Any N	M0
IVB	Any T	Any N	M1

Adapted with permission from American Joint Committee on Cancer. Cancer staging manual. 5th ed. Philadelphia: Lippincott-Raven, 1997.

with unresectable extrahepatic biliary tumors should be considered for inclusion in clinical trials.

CANCER OF THE GALLBLADDER

BACKGROUND

Cancer of the gallbladder is an extremely aggressive disease characterized by absence of early symptoms, advanced stage at presentation, and a grim prognosis. Histologically, 85% of gallbladder tumors are adenocarcinomas (papillary, intestinal type, mucinous, clear cell, signet ring, or adenosquamous), although squamous cell, small cell, and undifferentiated carcinomas have been reported.

EPIDEMIOLOGY AND ETIOLOGY

In most series, the median age at diagnosis is in the seventh decade, and there is a 3.5:1 female to male predominance. The increased risk among Mexicans, Native Americans, and Native Alaskans suggests a genetic susceptibility. Cholelithiasis is an associated finding in 66 to 86% of cases, but fewer than 1% of patients with cholelithiasis develop this cancer. In addition, acute and chronic cholecystitis and ulcerative colitis have been reported as risk factors.

CLINICAL MANIFESTATIONS

Many primary gallbladder tumors are not identified clinically and are unexpected pathologic findings following a cholecystectomy for presumed benign disease. More commonly, however, gallbladder cancer is diagnosed in advanced stages, when the most common symptoms are jaundice, pain, weight loss, nausea, vomiting, and fever.

STAGING EVALUATION

The clinical staging of a patient with gallbladder carcinoma centers on CT of the upper abdomen with attention to regional lymph nodes and parenchymal liver invasion (Table 1B.25). In select cases, ultrasonography, angiography, cholangiography, or ERCP (endoscopic retrograde cholangiopancreatography) may be helpful in determining resectability.

PROGNOSIS

Most symptomatic patients are not diagnosed preoperatively, and most are inoperable (incurable). When unsuspected gallbladder cancer is discovered in the mucosa (Tis, T1a) of the gallbladder at pathologic examination, it is curable in more than

80% of patients. However, symptomatic gallbladder cancer suspected preoperatively has usually penetrated the muscularis and serosa and is curable in fewer than 5% of patients. Some histologic types have a better prognosis than others. Papillary carcinomas have the best prognosis, while undifferentiated carcinomas have an inferior prognosis, with an estimated median survival of only 3 months.

TREATMENTS

Superficial cancers (Tis, T1) discovered incidentally on pathologic examination of a gallbladder removed for presumed benign disease are often cured without further therapy. Patients with localized carcinomas with muscular invasion or beyond (T1b, T2) have a survival of less than 15%. Reexploration to re-

Table 1B.25A. TNM Staging System for Carcinoma of the Gallbladder

Primary tumor

TX	Primary tumor cannot be assessed.
T0	No evidence of primary tumor.
Tis	Carcinoma in situ.
T1	Tumor invades lamina propria or muscle layer.
T1a	Tumor invades the lamina propria.
T1b	Tumor invades the muscle layer.
T2	Tumor invades the perimuscular connective tissue; no extension beyond the serosa or into the liver.
T3	Tumor perforates the serosa (visceral peritoneum) or directly invades one adjacent organ or both (extension 2 cm or less into the liver).
T4	Tumor extends more than 2 cm into liver and/or into two or more adjacent organs (stomach, duodenum, colon, pancreas, omentum, extrahepatic bile ducts, any involvement of liver).

Regional lymph nodes

NX	Regional lymph nodes cannot be assessed.
N0	No regional lymph node metastasis.
N1	Metastasis in cystic duct, pericholedochal, and/or hilar lymph nodes.
N2	Metastasis in peripancreatic (head only), periduodenal, periportal, celiac, and/or superior mesenteric lymph nodes.

Distant metastasis

MX	Presence of distant metastasis cannot be assessed.
M0	No distant metastasis.
M1	Distant metastasis.

Table 1B.25B. Stage Grouping for Carcinoma of the Gallbladder

Stage	Tumor	Nodes	Metastasis
0	Tis	N0	M0
I	T1	N0	M0
II	T2	N0	M0
III	T1	N1	M0
	T2	N1	M0
	T3	N0	M0
	T3	N1	M0
IVA	T4	N0	M0
	T4	N0	M0
IVB	Any T	N2	M0
	Any T	Any N	M1

Adapted with permission from American Joint Committee on Cancer. Cancer staging manual. 5th ed. Philadelphia: Lippincott-Raven, 1997.

sect liver near the gallbladder bed and portal lymphadenectomy may prevent or delay recurrences in selected patients with stage I or II gallbladder cancer. External beam irradiation has been employed for both the primary and adjuvant treatment of gallbladder carcinoma with reported improvement in short-term disease control.

Most patients have unresectable disease as a result of gross direct hepatic invasion, clinical nodal involvement, or peritoneal seeding. Significant palliation can often be achieved with relief of biliary obstruction either surgically, through stenting, or occasionally with external beam radiation therapy.

The benefit, if any, of chemotherapy in patients with advanced gallbladder cancer is extremely limited. The ECOG experience suggests response rates of 7% for N1 disease and only 1% for those with liver involvement. Referral to appropriate clinical trials evaluating new drugs or radiation techniques should be considered.

BIBLIOGRAPHY

Hepatocellular Cancer

Choi BI, Kim HC, Han JK, et al. Therapeutic effect of transcatheter oily chemoembolization therapy for encapsulated nodular hepatocellular carcinoma: CT and pathologic findings. Radiol 1992;182:709–713.

Epstein B, Ettinger D, Leichner PK, et al. Multimodality cisplatin treatment in nonresectable α-fetoprotein-positive hepatoma. Cancer 1991;67:896–900.

Farmer DG, Rosove MH, Shaked A, et al. Current treatment modalities for hepatocellular carcinoma. Ann Surg 1994;219:236–247.

Haug CE, Jenkins RL, Rohrer RJ, et al. Liver transplantation for primary hepatic cancer. Transplant 1992;53:376–382.

Iwatsuki S, Starzl TE, Sheahan DG, et al. Hepatic resection versus transplantation for hepatocellular carcinoma. Ann Surg 1991;214:221–229.

Stillwagon GB, Order SE, Guse C, et al. Prognostic factors in unresectable hepatocellular cancer: Radiation Therapy Oncology Group study 83–01. Int J Radiat Oncol Biol Phys 1991;20:65–71.

Tsukuma H, Hiyama T, Tanaka S, et al. Risk factors for hepatocellular carcinoma among patients with chronic liver disease. N Engl J Med 1993;328:1797–1801.

Venook AP. Treatment of hepatocellular carcinoma: too many options? J Clin Oncol 1994;12:1323–1334.

Yamashita Y, Takahashi M, Koga Y, et al. Prognostic factors in the treatment of hepatocellular carcinoma with transcatheter arterial embolization and arterial infusion. Cancer 1991;67:385–391.

Carcinoma of the Extrahepatic Bile Ducts

Bismuth H, Nakache R, Diamond T. Management strategies in resection for hilar cholangiocarcinoma. Ann Surg 1992;215:31–38.

Henson DE, Albores-Saavedra J, Corle D. Carcinoma of the extrahepatic bile ducts: histologic types, stage of disease, grade, and survival rates. Cancer 1992;70:1498–1501.

Nordback IH, Pitt HA, Coleman J, et al. Unresectable hilar cholangiocarcinoma: percutaneous versus operative palliation. Surgery 1994;115:597–603.

Stain SC, Baer HU, Dennison AR, et al. Current management of hilar cholangiocarcinoma. Surg Gynecol Obstet 1992;175:579–588.

Gallbladder Cancer

Chao T, Greager JA. Primary carcinoma of the gallbladder. J Surg Oncol 1991;46:215–221.

Chijiiwa K, Tanaka M. Carcinoma of the gallbladder: an appraisal of surgical resection. Surgery 1994;115:751–756.

Shirai Y, Yoshida K, Tsukada K, et al. Inapparent carcinoma of the gallbladder: an appraisal of a radical second operation after simple cholecystectomy. Ann Surg 1992;215; 326–331.

Colorectal Cancer

John D. Wilkes

BACKGROUND

Despite recent declines in mortality from colorectal cancer, this malignancy remains the second most common cause of cancer death in the United States. If diagnosed early, more than half of all patients can be cured with current therapy. Screening for colorectal cancer should be a routine component of health care for adults at least 40 years of age, especially for those who have first-degree relatives with colorectal cancer. It is hoped that a better understanding of the genetics and molecular events resulting in the transformation of normal colorectal mucosa to malignancy will yield improved diagnostic and therapeutic strategies for the future.

EPIDEMIOLOGY

It is estimated that colorectal cancer accounted for more than 131,000 new diagnoses of cancer and more than 56,000 deaths in 1998. The mean age at diagnosis is 60 to 65 years, and there is an equal incidence in men and women. Perhaps as a result of sigmoidoscopies and polypectomies, right-sided malignancies are now more common than left colon tumors. The significant worldwide variation in the incidence of colorectal cancer may be a result of genetic or dietary factors (discussed later).

ETIOLOGY

The minority of colorectal cancers appear to be the result of genetic, dietary, and/or inflammatory factors. The genetic predisposition has been well characterized, yet hereditary syndromes, such as familial polyposis and hereditary nonpolyposis colon cancer (HNPCC), account for fewer than 15% of cases. Other high-risk groups include patients with a personal or first-degree family history of colorectal cancer or adenomas or a personal history of breast, ovarian, or endometrial cancer. These high-risk persons account for only 23% of diagnoses. Individuals with diets high in fat and low in fruit and vegetable intake have a higher risk of colorectal cancer, although the pathophysiology remains unclear. Patients with inflammatory bowel disease also have an increased risk of colorectal cancer.

CLINICAL MANIFESTATIONS

The symptoms of colorectal cancer vary with the location of the primary tumor. Carcinomas of the right colon may be asymptomatic for long periods, eventually manifesting as weight loss, vague abdominal pain, or signs of anemia. Left colon lesions often produce a subtle change in bowel movements with constipation and/or diarrhea (may be alternating). Progressive decrease in stool thickness or symptoms of obstruction may occur with more extensive left colon tumors. Rectal tumors often cause gross bleeding, change in bowel movements, pain with defecation, and/or pelvic pain.

STAGING EVALUATION

Once a diagnosis of colorectal cancer has been obtained, a formal staging workup should include blood work (complete blood count, liver and renal function, carcinoembryonic antigen, or CEA), chest radiograph, and CT of the abdomen and pelvis (Table 1B.26). Colonoscopy to the ileocecal valve should be performed on all patients to rule out synchronous primaries. For rectal tumors, endoscopic ultrasonography can provide useful information on tumor depth of penetration and local nodal involvement. Nuclear medicine imaging may provide additional staging information for select patients with questionable extrahepatic disease.

PROGNOSIS

The prognosis for patients with colorectal cancer is related to a variety of clinical, laboratory, and pathologic factors. Clinical manifestations such as bowel obstruction or perforation are indicators of a poor prognosis. Paradoxically, asymptomatic patients appear to have a worse prognosis, often presenting with more advanced disease. Rectal tumors have a poorer prognosis than colon primaries. Elevated pretreatment serum CEA levels appear to be associated with a poor prognosis. The degree of tumor penetration into the bowel wall (T stage) and the presence or absence of lymph node metastases (N stage) are the most significant prognostic features, and they form the basis for the staging system. Tumors with mucinous or neuroendocrine differentiation typically also have a poor prognosis.

TREATMENTS

Appropriately managed, cancers of the colon and rectum are treatable and often curable diseases. Treatment recommendations for cancers of the colon and rectum are based on the American Joint Committee on Cancer (AJCC) staging system.

Table 1B.26A. TNM Staging System for Colorectal Cancer

Primary tumor

TX	Primary tumor cannot be assessed.
T0	No evidence of primary tumor.
Tis	Carcinoma in situ: intraepithelial or invasion of the lamina propria.[a]
T1	Tumor invades submucosa.
T2	Tumor invades muscularis propria.
T3	Tumor invades through the muscularis propria into the subserous or into the nonperitonealized pericolic or perirectal tissues.
T4	Tumor directly invades other organs or structures and/or perforates the visceral peritoneum.[b]

Regional lymph nodes

NX	Regional nodes cannot be assessed.
N0	No regional lymph node metastasis.
N1	Metastasis in one to three regional lymph nodes.
N2	Metastasis in four or more regional lymph nodes.

Distant metastasis

MX	Presence of distant metastasis cannot be assessed.
M0	No distant metastasis.
M1	Distant metastasis.

[a]*This includes cancer cells confined within the glandular basement membrane (intraepithelial) or lamina propria (intramucosal) with no extension through the muscularis mucosae into the submucosa.*
[b]*Direct invasion of other organs or structures includes invasion of other segments of colorectum by way of serosa (e.g., invasion of the sigmoid colon by a carcinoma of the cecum).*

Table 1B.26B. Stage Grouping for Colorectal Cancer

AJCC	Duke's	Tumor	Nodes	Metastasis	5-Year Survival (%)
0	N/A	Tis	N0	M0	—
I	A	T1, T2	N0	M0	>90
II	B	T3, T4	N0	M0	70–85
III	C	Any T	Any N M0	45–60%	
IV	N/A	Any T	Any N	M1	<5

Adapted with permission from American Joint Committee on Cancer. Cancer staging manual. 5th ed. Philadelphia: Lippincott-Raven, 1997.

COLON CANCER

Primary Management

The initial treatment of colon cancer is resection of the bowel segment containing the primary tumor in addition to the mesentery and regional lymph nodes. The procedure, which depends on the anatomic location of the primary, is curative in approximately 50% of patients.

Adjuvant Therapy

Recurrence of disease is a major cause of death in patients with colon cancer, and intensive research investigating adjuvant strategies has yielded improved survival in certain subsets of patients. Large multi-institutional randomized trials from the NSABP, North Central Cancer Treatment Group (NCCTG), and Intergroup have demonstrated a consistent benefit for systemic adjuvant chemotherapy with 5-FU plus either levamisole or leucovorin. The Intergroup trial of 5-FU plus levamisole versus observation reported prolonged disease-free and overall survival in patients with stage III colon cancer receiving chemotherapy. Similar results were obtained in the NSABP trial for stage II and III patients comparing the methotrexate, Oncovin (vincristine), and 5-FU (MOF) regimen against weekly 5-FU plus high-dose leucovorin. Overall, more than 4000 patients have participated in randomized trials comparing adjuvant chemotherapy with surgery alone. Reduction in mortality of 22 to 33% has been consistently reported for stage III patients, but the potential benefits, if any, for patients with stage II colon cancer remain unclear.

Stage I Colon Cancer

These uncommon tumors have an extremely high rate of cure with resection alone. No adjuvant therapy is indicated.

Stage II Colon Cancer

Resection of the bowel segment containing the primary tumor remains the only standard treatment. As mentioned, the role for adjuvant therapy in these patients remains unproved. However, subsets of patients with stage II disease with high-risk clinical (obstruction, perforation) or pathologic features (aneuploidy, perineural or lymphatic invasion, T4 tumors) may be considered for adjuvant therapy as described for stage III colon cancer. The role of adjuvant radiation therapy for patients with T4 primaries remains under investigation. As always, referral of patients with stage II disease to appropriate clinical trials is recommended.

Stage III Colon Cancer

Following complete resection of the primary tumor, patients with pathologically involved lymph nodes should be offered adjuvant chemotherapy with either 1 year of 5-FU plus levamisole or 6 months of 5-FU plus leucovorin, as previously mentioned. As yet no data suggest superiority of either 5-FU-based adjuvant regimen. Innovative adjuvant strategies employing regional chemotherapy, monoclonal antibodies, autologous tumor vaccines, and radiation therapy are all under clinical evaluation but are not yet considered standard practice.

Stage IV Colon and Rectal Cancer

Certain patients with isolated colorectal metastases may benefit from and in some cases even be cured by locally directed approaches. Local therapies may include hepatic or pulmonary resection, regional chemotherapy, or other local ablative techniques (cryosurgery, embolization, interstitial radiation therapy). For operable patients with no more than three hepatic metastases, resection may result in 5-year survival rates as high as 30%. For patients with unresectable metastases isolated to the liver, hepatic intra-arterial chemotherapy with floxuridine, dexamethasone, and leucovorin has consistently produced higher response rates than systemic chemotherapy. However, concerns related to cost, hepatotoxicity, and unproven survival benefit have led to the initiation of a phase III trial comparing this regional infusion approach with standard 5-FU plus leucovorin.

The care for patients with widely metastatic colon or rectal cancer is palliative and must be individualized. There remains no standard approach and little evidence to support a survival advantage to systemic chemotherapy. However, systemic chemotherapy with 5-FU-based regimens, a common treatment for patients with advanced stage IV disease, achieves palliation in approximately 15 to 20% of patients. There is no added benefit of combination chemotherapy over 5-FU alone. In contrast, modulation of 5-FU with leucovorin has produced increased response rates with varying effects on survival. The Roswell Park regimen entails high-dose leucovorin and 5-FU administered weekly, while the Mayo Clinic regimen incorporates a low-dose leucovorin schedule administered 5 consecutive days on a 28-day schedule. The toxicity profiles of these regimens vary significantly, with the Mayo schedule appearing to have a superior therapeutic index and cost profile. Some investigators have found improved response rates for continuous-infusion 5-FU schedules, although the added cost and complications associated with venous access devices and external pumps remains a concern. The choice of a 5-FU-based chemotherapy regimen for an individual patient should be based on response rates, toxicity profile, and quality-of-life issues.

Irinotecan, a topoisomerase-I inhibitor, has been approved for use in patients with 5-FU-refractory colorectal cancer. Partial re-

sponse rates as high as 20% have been reported in this population. In certain patients, palliation may be achieved with surgical
resection or bypass of obstructing tumors or radiation therapy.

Recurrent Colorectal Cancer

Following primary treatment of colorectal cancer, periodic
evaluations may lead to the earlier identification and more effective management of recurrent disease in select patients. Postoperative monitoring should be reserved for detection of
asymptomatic recurrences that can be resected for cure and for
early detection of metachronous tumors. The use of a serum
CEA in this clinical setting is extremely controversial and should
be restricted to patients who would be candidates for resection
of liver or lung metastases.

The management of recurrent colorectal cancer depends on
the sites and extent of the recurrent disease. Second primaries
and locally recurrent colon cancer (at the prior surgical margin
or suture line) may be resectable. Otherwise, the treatment of patients with recurrent colorectal cancer is no different from that
described for patients with stage IV disease.

RECTAL CANCER

Primary Management

Surgery, the primary treatment, cures approximately 45% of
patients with rectal cancer. However, a major limitation of
surgery is the inability to obtain wide radial margins because of
the pelvic anatomy. Thus, local recurrence and death from disease constitute a more significant risk for patients with rectal
cancer.

Adjuvant Therapy

Patients with stage II or III rectal cancer are at high risk for local and systemic relapse and have been the subject of intensive
adjuvant investigations. Two trials have confirmed the benefits
of 5-FU plus radiation therapy for patients with stage II and III
rectal cancers. The GITSG trial demonstrated an increase in both
disease-free and overall survival when chemotherapy and radiation were administered following surgical resection in stage II
and III patients. A NCCTG trial demonstrated a 10% improvement in overall survival with continuous-infusion fluorouracil
5-FU (versus bolus 5-FU) throughout the course of radiation
therapy. Based on these trials, combined treatment with 5-FU
and pelvic irradiation (45 to 55 Gy) is recommended for patients
with stages II and III rectal cancer. Current research involves
comparisons between various chemoradiation therapy sched-

ules, preoperative versus postoperative adjuvant therapy, and sphincter-preserving approaches.

Stage 0 Rectal Cancer

Limited surgical procedures such as local excision, polypectomy, or full-thickness resection by transanal or transcoccygeal routes are appropriate. No adjuvant therapy is indicated.

Stage I Rectal Cancer

The appropriate primary treatment of stage I rectal cancer is surgical resection. According to characteristics of the patient and tumor, a number of procedures can be performed. These include low anterior resection (LAR) with a conventional anastomosis or coloanal anastomosis, abdominoperineal resection (APR), or local resection with or without perioperative external beam irradiation plus fluorouracil (5-FU). No adjuvant radiation or chemotherapy is indicated following LAR or APR for stage I disease.

Stage II Rectal Cancer

Patients with locally advanced (T3, T4) rectal tumors commonly have subclinical involvement of pelvic structures following surgical resection and remain at high risk for disease recurrence. Following standard surgical resections, these patients should be offered adjuvant chemoradiation therapy as previously outlined.

Stage III Rectal Cancer

Patients with lymph nodes identified pathologically following resection of a primary rectal cancer have more than a 50% chance of both local and distant recurrence. All patients with stage III disease should be offered standard adjuvant therapy as outlined earlier. Preoperative radiation therapy with or without chemotherapy to preserve sphincter function with subsequent adjuvant chemotherapy is under investigation.

Stage IV and Recurrent Rectal Cancer

The management strategies for stage IV and recurrent cancer of the rectum are identical to those of similar patients with colon cancer, outlined earlier. Additionally, in some patients, reresection or radiation therapy may provide palliation for recurrent disease in the pelvis.

BIBLIOGRAPHY

Buroker TR, O'Connell MJ, Wieand HS, et al. Randomized comparison of two schedules of fluorouracil and leucovorin in the treatment of advanced colorectal cancer. J Clin Oncol 1994;12:14–20.

Meta-Analysis Group In Cancer. Reappraisal of hepatic arterial infusion in the treatment of nonresectable liver metastases from colorectal cancer. J Natl Cancer Inst 1996;88:252–258.

Moertel CG. Chemotherapy for colorectal cancer. N Engl J Med 1994;330: 1136–1142.

Moertel CG, Fleming TR, Macdonald JS, et al. An evaluation of the carcinoembryonic antigen (CEA) test for monitoring patients with resected colon cancer. J Am Med Assoc 1993;270:943–947.

Moertel CG, Fleming TR, Macdonald JS, et al. Fluorouracil plus levamisole as effective adjuvant therapy after resection of stage III colon carcinoma: a final report. Ann Intern Med 1995;122:321–326.

O'Connell MJ, Mailliard JA, Kahn MJ, et al. Controlled trial of fluorouracil and low-dose leucovorin given for 6 months as postoperative adjuvant therapy for colon cancer. J Clin Oncol 1997;15:246–250.

O'Connell MJ, Martensen JA, Wieand HS, et al. Improving adjuvant therapy for rectal cancer by combining protracted infusion fluorouracil with radiation therapy after curative surgery. N Engl J Med 1994;331:502–507.

Pedersen IK, Burcharth F, Roikjaer O, et al. Resection of liver metastases from colorectal cancer: indications and results. Dis Colon Rectum 1994;37:1078–1082.

Rustgi AK. Hereditary gastrointestinal polyposis and nonpolyposis syndromes. N Engl J Med 1994;331:1694–1702.

Safi F, Link KH, Beger HG. Is follow-up of colorectal cancer patients worthwhile? Dis Colon Rectum 1993;36:636–644.

Swedish Rectal Cancer Trial. Improved survival with preoperative radiotherapy in resectable rectal cancer. N Engl J Med 1997;336:980–987.

Wolmark N, Rockette H, Fisher B, et al. The benefit of leucovorin-modulated fluorouracil as postoperative adjuvant therapy for primary colon cancer: results from National Surgical Adjuvant Breast and Bowel Project protocol C-03. J Clin Oncol 1993;11:1879–1887.

Anal Cancer

John D. Wilkes

BACKGROUND

Anal canal cancer is an uncommon malignancy that arises from the squamous mucosa extending from the anal verge to the pectinate line. Anal cancer was once a disease treated with aggressive surgical resection but is now a paradigm for successful multidisciplinary cancer management and organ preservation.

EPIDEMIOLOGY

Although anal cancer is increasing in frequency, it remains a relatively rare disease, accounting for fewer than 2% of all cancers of the lower gastrointestinal tract. There were an estimated 3300 cases and 500 deaths attributed to this disease in 1998. Most cases are diagnosed in patients more than 60 years of age.

ETIOLOGY

There is strong evidence to support a causal relationship between the human papillomavirus (HPV) and anal cancer. The disease is most common in those who practice receptive anal intercourse, male homosexuals, and those having a history of benign anorectal disease (condyloma, fistulas). Overall, women are affected more frequently than men, although there is a strong male predominance in patients less than 35 years old. There is also an increased risk associated with smoking and chronic immunosuppression.

CLINICAL MANIFESTATIONS

The symptoms of anal cancer often mimic those of benign anorectal disease, which may lead to significant delays in diagnosis. Pain, bleeding, and the sensation of a mass are the most common subjective complaints. Physical examination often reveals a firm, ulcerated, circular lesion. Squamous cell carcinomas constitute most primary cancers of the anus. The uncommon cloacogenic tumors arise from the cuboidal epithelium overlying the columns of Morgangni. Cancers of the anal margin are considered skin cancers and should be treated as such.

STAGING EVALUATION

The staging of a patient with anal cancer should include a careful digital rectal examination (under anesthesia if necessary) to evaluate local extension and invasion (Table 1B.27). CT to evaluate pelvic lymph nodes should also be performed.

Table 1B.27A. TNM Staging System for Cancers of the Anal Canal

Primary tumor

TX	Primary tumor cannot be assessed.
T0	No evidence of primary tumor.
Tis	Carcinoma in situ.
T1	Tumor 2 cm or less in greatest dimension.
T2	Tumor more than 2 cm but not more than 5.0 cm in greatest dimension.
T3	Tumor more than 5 cm in greatest dimension.
T4	Tumor of any size that invades adjacent organ(s), e.g., vagina, urethra, bladder (involvement of the sphincter muscle(s) alone is not T4).

Regional lymph nodes

NX	Regional lymph nodes cannot be assessed.
N0	No regional lymph node metastasis.
N1	Metastasis in perirectal lymph node(s).
N2	Metastasis in unilateral internal iliac and/or inguinal lymph node(s).
N3	Metastasis in perirectal and inguinal lymph nodes and/or bilateral internal iliac and/or inguinal lymph nodes.

Distant metastasis

MX	Presence of distant metastasis cannot be assessed.
M0	No distant metastasis.
M1	Distant metastasis.

Tumors of the anal margin (below the anal verge and involving the perianal hair-bearing skin) are classified with skin tumors.

Table 1B.27B. Stage Grouping for Cancers of the Anal Canal

Stage	Tumor	Nodes	Metastasis
0	Tis	N0	M0
I	T1	N0	M0
II	T2, T3	N0	M0
IIIA	T1, T2, T3	N1	M0
	T4	N0	M0
IIIB	T4	N1	M0
	Any T	N2	M0
	Any T	N3	M0
IV	Any T	Any N	M1
IV	Any T	Any N	M1

Adapted with permission from American Joint Committee on Cancer. Cancer staging manual. 5th ed. Philadelphia: Lippincott-Raven, 1997.

Endorectal ultrasound may aid in pretreatment staging. Suspicious inguinal lymph nodes should be sampled for biopsy. Any patient to be considered for chemoradiation therapy must have routine blood counts, chemistry panels, and a chest radiograph.

PROGNOSIS

The major prognostic factors for anal cancer include site (anal margin is more favorable than anal canal), tumor size (primary tumors smaller than 2 cm have a better prognosis), histologic differentiation (well-differentiated tumors are more favorable than poorly differentiated tumors) and lymph node status (presence of involved lymph nodes decreases survival).

TREATMENTS

Frequently anal cancer is a curable disease. In the past aggressive surgical resection was the primary approach, however, since the late 1970s chemoradiation therapy has provided excellent results in most patients while preserving sphincter function, and surgery is no longer the treatment of choice for most patients.

As a result of the experience from Wayne State University, concurrent chemotherapy and radiation therapy have become standard treatment for most patients with anal canal tumors. There are consistent reports of 5-year survival rates greater than 70% with an acceptable toxicity profile and organ preservation. Most regimens employ infusional 5-FU plus mitomycin with radiation doses of 30 to 57 Gy. The addition of mitomycin has been demonstrated to improve results (higher colostomy-free and disease-free survival) over radiation and 5-FU alone. Patients with AIDS and anal cancer often cannot tolerate the standard 5-FU–mitomycin–radiation therapy–radiation therapy approach. Alternative strategies include the use of 5-FU plus cisplatin and lower-dose radiation (30 Gy). Abdominoperineal surgical resection has been relegated to salvage therapy for patients with either gross or microscopic residual disease following chemoradiation therapy. Other salvage approaches include additional chemoradiation therapy with 5-FU plus cisplatin with lower doses of radiation therapy. Treatment recommendations by AJCC staging are as follows:

STAGE 0 ANAL CANCER

Surgical resection alone is indicated for lesions of the perianal area not involving the anal sphincter. The surgical approach depends on the location and size of the lesion.

STAGE I AND II ANAL CANCERS

Patients with stage I anal cancer should be offered primary radiation therapy plus chemotherapy with 5-FU and mitomycin. Salvage approaches (chemoradiation therapy with 5-FU and cisplatin with radiation therapy or surgical resection) should be reserved for patients with incomplete responses or recurrent disease. Patients who are not candidates for chemoradiation therapy or surgery may be treated with interstitial radiation alone.

STAGE IIIA ANAL CANCER

Stage IIIA anal cancer often appears to be stage II until involvement of perirectal lymph nodes or an adjacent organ is demonstrated by diagnostic imaging. Frequently, these patients can be treated as outlined for stages I and II, with chemoradiation therapy, although the response rates are lower and the need for salvage is more likely.

STAGE IIIB ANAL CANCER

The presence of metastases to inguinal nodes is a poor prognostic sign, although long-term disease-free survival can be achieved in up to 55% of patients. Primary therapy should still involve chemoradiation therapy as outlined for patients with earlier-stage disease. Surgical resection of residual disease at the primary site and both superficial and deep inguinal node dissection for residual or recurrent tumor should be performed. Because of the relatively poor prognosis, patients with stage IIIB disease should be referred to clinical trials whenever possible.

STAGE IV ANAL CANCER

There is no standard chemotherapy for patients with metastatic disease. These tumors are sensitive to a variety of chemotherapeutic agents, including 5-FU, cisplatin, doxorubicin, and vincristine. Cisplatin plus 5-FU has demonstrated responses in up to 50% of patients in a very small series. Palliation of symptoms from the primary lesion with surgery, radiation therapy, or chemoradiation therapy is appropriate.

RECURRENT ANAL CANCER

As previously mentioned, local recurrences or residual disease after chemoradiation therapy can be effectively controlled in a substantial number of patients with either (a) salvage chemoradiation therapy with 5-FU plus cisplatin and low-dose radiation or (b) surgical resection.

BIBLIOGRAPHY

Cummings BJ. Anal cancer. Int J Radiat Oncol Biol Phys 1990;19:1309–1315.

Flam M, John M, Pajak TF, et al. Role of mitomycin in combination with fluo-rouracil and radiotherapy, and of salvage chemoradiation in the definitive non-surgical treatment of epidermoid carcinoma of the anal canal: results of a phase III randomized intergroup study. J Clin Oncol 1996;14:2527–2539.

Longo WE, Vernava AM, Wade TP, et al. Recurrent squamous cell carcinoma of the anal canal: predictors of initial treatment failure and results of salvage ther-apy. Ann Surg 1994;220:40–49.

Martenson JA, Lipsitz SR, Lefkopoulou M, et al. Results of combined modality therapy for patients with anal cancer (E7283): an Eastern Cooperative Oncology Group study. Cancer 1995;76:1731–1736.

UKCCCR Anal Cancer Trial Working Party. Epidermoid anal cancer: results from the UKCCCR randomised trial of radiotherapy alone versus radiotherapy, 5-fluorouracil, and mitomycin. Lancet 1996;348:1049–1054.

Zucali R, Doci R, Bombelli L. Combined chemotherapy-radiotherapy of anal cancer. Int J Radiat Oncol Biol Phys 1990;19:1221–1223.

Adrenal Gland Cancer

Victoria J. Dorr

INCIDENTAL ADRENAL TUMORS

Incidental adrenal tumors are a frequent finding in this era of improved CT resolution. They are noted in up to 2% of abdominal scans. As these tumors can account for both benign and malignant conditions, additional evaluation is necessary. The differential diagnosis of an incidental adrenal tumor includes the following:

1. Functional and nonfunctional adrenal cortical adenomas
2. Functional and nonfunctional adrenal cortical carcinomas
3. Pheochromocytomas
4. Adrenal cysts
5. Myelolipomas
6. Congenital adrenal hyperplasia
7. Adrenal hemorrhage
8. Metastases from other tumors

A careful history and physical examination may provide clues to the diagnosis. Evidence of weakness, weight change, and Cushing's syndrome suggest a functional adrenal cortical tumor. The diagnosis of a primary adrenal malignancy in such cases depends on surgical removal. Virilization, feminization, or menstrual changes indicate a sex hormone–secreting tumor. Hypertension and the triad of headache, sweating, and palpitation make pheochromocytoma likely.

Additional clues to the cause of the adrenal mass can be found on CT. The size of the tumor is a key factor; it is rare to see a primary adrenal cortical carcinoma smaller than 5 cm. Bilateral adrenal abnormalities are more commonly seen in patients with metastatic disease, nodular adrenal hyperplasia, congenital adrenal hyperplasia, or adrenal hemorrhage. Fat within a tumor suggests a myelolipoma. MRI of the adrenal gland can help to distinguish adrenal carcinomas from adenoma, pheochromocytoma, and metastasis. This is based on specific characteristics of T1- and T2-weighted images that can occur with each of these conditions.

Assessment for adrenal hormone secretion should be undertaken to determine whether the tumor is functional. This includes 24-hour urine for free cortisol, vanilmandelic acid (VMA), metanephrines, and catecholamines. A low-dose dexamethasone suppression test should also be performed. (Dexamethasone 1 mg is given orally at 11 P.M., and the plasma cortisol is measured at 8 AM the following morning. Normally the plasma cortisol suppresses to less than 5 μg/dL.) Serum potassium should be checked; if this is low and the patient is hypertensive, both aldosterone and renin levels should be obtained. If on physical examination there is evidence of virilization or feminization, 24-hour urinary 17-ketosteroids and 17-hydroxy steroids should be checked. Additionally, serum testosterone or estrogen should be determined according to physical findings.

Adrenal biopsies offer no proven benefit in differentiating benign from malignant primary tumors of the adrenal gland. Biopsies of an adrenal gland, either by CT or ultrasound guidance, may be useful only in patients with a known primary malignancy. In these patients a tumor larger than 3 cm indicates metastases in only 75 to 85% of cases. Adrenal biopsy is contraindicated in pheochromocytoma. Recommendations:

1. Assess functional status of tumors.
2. If metastasis from a separate primary site is suspected, a CT- or ultrasound-guided biopsy is indicated, as even tumors as large as 3 cm may be benign.
3. Tumors that are less than 5 cm and nonfunctional should be evaluated with MRI. If the MRI is not diagnostic, repeat imaging in 6 months is indicated. At that time if no change has occurred, adenoma is likely and no further evaluation is required unless clinically indicated.
4. Tumors that are smaller than 5 cm and functional should be resected.
5. Tumors that are larger than 5 cm should be resected en bloc. They are associated with a 33% chance of carcinoma and a 33% chance of pheochromocytoma.

ADRENAL CORTICAL CARCINOMAS

INCIDENCE

The annual incidence of adrenal cortical carcinomas is 2 per 100,000 persons worldwide. Women are more likely to develop functional tumors, and men are more likely to develop nonfunctional adrenal tumors. There is a bimodal distribution. Peaks are seen at less than 5 years and again at the fourth and fifth decades of life.

ETIOLOGY AND RISK FACTORS

Adrenal cortical carcinomas are associated with several familial syndromes. These include multiple endocrine neoplasia (MEN) type 1, Li-Fraumeni syndrome, familial adenomatous polyposis, and familial adrenal cortical carcinomas.

SIGNS AND SYMPTOMS

At presentation, 50 to 80% of patients have functional tumors manifesting as adrenocortical excess. Most commonly this is in the form of excessive cortisol production. Signs and symptoms of excessive cortisol production include progressive weight gain, particularly in a truncal distribution, the buffalo hump (fat deposition in the interscapular region), moon facies, mild blood pressure elevation, muscle wasting and weakness, easy bruisability, emotional lability, depression, psychosis, diabetes mellitus (in up to 10% of patients), hirsutism (fine hair on the face, upper arms, and back), virilization, menstrual irregularities or amenorrhea, decreased libido, striae, ruddy complexion, hypokalemia, and impaired immune function with opportunistic infections occurring.

Sex hormone–producing adrenal cortical carcinomas are rare. Signs and symptoms of excess sex hormone production include virilization in women, feminization in men, precocious puberty, and gynecomastia. Aldosterone-producing adrenal cortical carcinomas are rare but may be associated with hypertension and hypokalemia.

DIAGNOSIS

Please see Incidental Adrenal Tumors in this subchapter.

Laboratory testing should be performed to assess function of the tumor. The gold standard for evaluation of hypercortisolism is a 24-hour urinary free cortisol. This can be supplemented by a dexamethasone suppression test. (Dexamethasone 1 mg is given orally at 11 P.M. and the plasma cortisol is measured at 8 AM the following morning. Normally, the plasma cortisol suppresses to less than 5 $\mu g/dL$.) There is a 3% false-positive and a 3% false-negative rate with the dexamethasone suppression test. If a sex hormone–producing tumor is suspected, 24 hour urinary 17-ketosteroids and 17-hydroxy steroids should be obtained. Additionally, serum testosterone or estrogen should be obtained according to physical findings. If hyperaldosteronism is suspected, serum aldosterone and renin levels should be obtained.

Radiologic evaluation should include CT. This can be useful in some cases to distinguish benign from malignant conditions. Adrenal cortical carcinomas are usually larger than 6 cm. The CT is also important to assess for nodal or distant metastases. In cases of doubt, MRI can be useful to help distinguish adrenal cortical carcinoma from pheochromocytoma, metastatic disease, or benign adenoma based on signal characteristics.

Fine-needle aspiration cannot reliably distinguish benign from malignant primary tumors and should be avoided except in cases of known primary distant tumors when the question is metastasis. Biopsy of an adrenal nodule is particularly dangerous in cases of pheochromocytoma.

The pathologic determination of malignancy is difficult with adrenal tumors. The diagnosis is based on several criteria. A weight of the tumor of 100 to 5000 g suggests a malignancy or a tumor larger than 6 cm in diameter. A high mitotic activity similarly suggests malignancy. The definitive diagnosis of malignancy requires vascular or capsular invasion or distant metastases. Adrenal cortical carcinomas may also be difficult to differentiate from renal cell carcinomas; however, the vimentin stain is usually positive in adrenal cortical carcinomas and negative with renal cell carcinoma.

STAGING

CT of the chest and abdomen is indicated to assess for distant or nodal metastasis. This is also helpful in evaluating resectability. An intravenous pyelogram (IVP) of the kidney may be required if complete resection of the tumor requires a nephrectomy. The usual pattern of metastases include lymph nodes, lung, and liver. The staging criteria are shown in Table 1B.28.

PROGNOSIS

The median survival for patients with adrenal cortical carcinoma is 14 months. The 5-year overall survival is 22%. Most patients with stage II disease have disease recurrence or metastases, 50% within 2 years. The overall survival for stage II disease is 30 to 40% at 5 years. All patients with stage III disease have disease recurrence or metastases within 5 years. The overall survival at 5 years is less than 30% for stage III disease and less than 15% for stage IV disease. Age over 40 is associated with a poorer prognosis; younger patients with stage I and II disease have a better resection after complete surgical resection.

Table 1B.28. Staging System for Adrenal Gland Cancer

Stage
I   Tumor less than 5 cm without local invasion, nodal metastases, or distant metastases.
II Tumor greater than 5 cm without local invasion, nodal metastases, or distant metastases.
III Tumor with local invasion or positive lymph nodes.
IV Tumor with both local invasion and positive lymph nodes or distant metastases.

TREATMENT

Complete surgical resection is the only curative therapy. Every effort should be made to resect all disease at the time of initial surgery. A transabdominal approach is preferred because of large size of these tumors in general. In cases of hepatic, cerebral, or pulmonary metastases, initially or at the time of recurrence, aggressive surgical resection may yield a long-term remission. If complete surgical resection is not feasible, surgical debulking is indicated to decrease the amount of functionally secreting tumor and complications due to the tumor mass.

Postoperatively, follow-up measurement of steroid hormones is indicated to assess for recurrence. It is recommended that dexamethasone rather than hydrocortisone be used for replacement to prevent interference with testing. CT should be done routinely to assess for surgically removable recurrences.

Radiation therapy has little role in adrenal cortical carcinoma, but abdominal radiation has been used with palliative intent. It is successful in improving the symptoms of hormone excess and/or tumor mass symptoms in approximately 65% of patients. Radiation for bone metastases is similarly beneficial. Unfortunately, no improvement in survival has been seen.

Several chemotherapeutic agents have some success in the treatment of adrenal cortical carcinomas. In lieu of appropriate clinical trials, the usual first-line chemotherapy agent is mitotane (o,p-DDD). Mitotane is adrenolytic. An initial dose of 1 g twice daily is recommended, taken with fatty foods to aid absorption. The dose is escalated until adverse effects occur or until symptomatic improvement is seen. Monitoring serum o,p-DDD levels may have some benefit, as no responses have been seen with levels below 10 μg/mL. Generally levels of more than 14 μg/mL are considered therapeutic. The dose-limiting toxicity of mitotane is gastrointestinal (anorexia, nausea, vomiting, and diarrhea). Neuromuscular side effects (depression, dizziness, tremors, headache, confusion, and weakness) and skin rashes may also occur. Mitotane may also prolong the bleeding time and is associated with abnormal platelet aggregation.

Responses to mitotane are generally seen in the first 6 weeks. Overall, a steroid response of 80% and a measurable tumor response of 35% have been seen. No effect on survival has been seen, although a few long-term survivors are reported. There is no proven benefit of mitotane in an adjuvant setting.

Second-line chemotherapy commonly consists of cisplatin-based combination chemotherapy. The most common combination includes etoposide (VP-16). Response rates of 50 to 100% are seen in very small series of patients. The responses are short.

Doxorubicin (Adriamycin) has also been evaluated. When used as first-line chemotherapy, a 19% measurable tumor response has been seen. However, doxorubicin is not effective as second-line therapy when mitotane has failed. Finally, suramin, which is adrenolytic, is under investigation. Partial or minor remissions have been seen in 50% of patients thus treated.

PHEOCHROMOCYTOMA

INCIDENCE

Pheochromocytomas occur in 0.1% of hypertensive patients. They are associated with sudden death. Malignancy associated with pheochromocytoma is variable and is reported in 5 to 46% of cases. Extra-adrenal pheochromocytomas are more likely to be malignant.

ETIOLOGY AND RISK FACTORS

Pheochromocytomas may be associated with several familial syndromes. These include multiple endocrine neoplasia (MEN) types 2a and 2b, von Recklinghausen's neurofibromatosis, and von Hippel-Lindau's retinal cerebellar hemangioblastomatosis. Bilateral pheochromocytoma is almost always familial. Pheochromocytoma can be associated with the rule of tens: 10% occur in children, 10% are associated with familial syndromes, 10% of sporadic cases are bilateral, 10% are extra-adrenal, and 10% are malignant.

SIGNS AND SYMPTOMS

The most common symptom of pheochromocytoma is hypertension. More than 90% of patients have hypertension. Postural hypotension is also common. Hypertensive crises may be precipitated by physical stress, increased intra-abdominal pressure, or drugs (phenothiazine, metoclopramide, naloxone, and droperidol). The triad of headache, sweating, and palpitations occur so frequently that the lack of these symptoms makes the diagnosis of pheochromocytoma unlikely. Other symptoms include anxiety attacks, pallor, nausea, weakness, dyspepsia, visual disturbance, abdominal pain, tremor, and weight loss.

DIAGNOSIS

Laboratory evaluation for pheochromocytoma includes a 24-hour urine for vanilmandelic acid (VMA), metanephrines, and catecholamines. If the metanephrines are more than 3 mg/24 hours or plasma catecholamines are more than 2000 pg/mL, pheochromocytoma is likely and patients should proceed with radiologic evaluation. In patients with borderline results (metanephrines 1.4 to 3 mg/24 hours or plasma catecholamines 400 to 2000 pg/mL) further biochemical testing should be performed. If the plasma catecholamines are more than 1000 pg/mL, a clonidine suppression test should be performed. (Plasma catecholamines are sampled before and 3 hours after a 0.3 mg dose of clonidine. Normally the plasma catecholamines fall below 500 pg/mL.) If the plasma catecholamines are 400 to 1000 pg/mL, a glucagon provocative test should be performed. (Plasma catecholamines are sampled 1 to 3 minutes after 1 to 2 mg of glucagon is given. A threefold increase in plasma catecholamines is diagnostic of pheochromocytoma.)

Radiologic evaluation by CT or MRI should be performed if the diagnosis of pheochromocytoma is suspected because of clinical symptoms or biochemical evaluation. Evaluation for resectability, bilateral tumors, and metastatic disease should be performed. [31]I-metaiodobenzylguanidine (MIBG) scanning is helpful when other imaging techniques are negative and symptoms or biochemical evaluation suggest a pheochromocytoma. MIBG scanning may also be of use if an extra-adrenal occurrence is suspected. MIBG has 90% sensitivity and 100% specificity for pheochromocytoma. It is less sensitive, however, in malignant pheochromocytoma. Fine-needle aspiration of a pheochromocytoma should not be done because of a high risk of hypertensive complications.

Pathologic determination of malignancy is difficult. In general, malignant tumors are larger. A higher DNA ploidy and a higher mitotic rate are also seen with malignant pheochromocytoma. Benign tumors may actually have a higher nuclear pleomorphism than malignant cells. The only absolute criteria for malignancy, however, are the presence of chromaffin cells where they are not expected or distant metastases.

STAGING STUDIES

CT should be performed to evaluate for bilateral, nodal, or distant metastases. MIBG scanning should be done to assess for extra-adrenal disease and metastases. A bone scan should also be done because MIBG has low sensitivity in bone.

PROGNOSIS

The median overall survival is 4 years in malignant pheochromocytoma. Tumor recurrence occurs in 10 to 46% of patients within 5 years. The 5-year overall survival is 52% in malignant pheochromocytoma.

THERAPY

Complete surgical resection is the primary treatment goal. To prevent complications of surgery in patients with pheochromocytoma, careful preparation for surgery must be done. Preoperative therapy is recommended to be started at least 2 weeks prior to surgery. α-Adrenergic blockade with phenoxybenzamine at a starting dose of 10 mg orally twice a day is recommended to control hypertension. Volume replacement is indicated to prevent postural hypotension. β-Blockers should be added as needed to control tachycardia and arrhythmia. If patients fail to achieve blood pressure control or are unresectable, metyrosine has been effective. Metyrosine depletes tumor catecholamines. The usual starting dose is 250 mg by mouth four times a day.

In patients with local recurrences or limited metastasis, surgical resection has been shown to be beneficial. For patients with MEN-2, strong consideration should be given to bilateral adrenalectomy due to the high frequency of bilateral disease.

Radiation therapy has a limited role in malignant pheochromocytoma. It is generally reserved for palliative management. MIBG-targeted radiation therapy was a potentially exciting, unique way to target therapy to affected sites. Unfortunately, malignant cells did not take up enough MIBG for this to be therapeutically efficacious.

Chemotherapy also has a limited role. For metastatic disease cyclophosphamide plus vincristine and dacarbazine was reported to have a 61% response rate with a median duration of response of 22 months. Streptozocin has been reported to have less than a 10% response rate in malignant pheochromocytoma.

BIBILOGRAPHY

Adrenocortical carcinoma. PDQ Treatment for Health Professionals. National Cancer Institute. http://cancernet.nci.nih.gov/clinpdq/soa/Adrenocortical_carcinoma_Physician.html; 1/18/98.

Flack MR, Chrousos GP. Neoplasms of the adrenal cortex. In: Cancer medicine. 4th ed. Holland JF, Frei E, Bast RC, et al., eds. Baltimore: Williams & Wilkins, 1997;1551–1562.

Landis SH, Murray T, Bolden S, Wingo PA. Cancer statistics 1998. CA Cancer J Clin 1998;48:6–29.

McKittrick RJ, Stephens RL. Chemotherapy of endocrine tumors. In: Perry MC, ed. The chemotherapy source book. 2nd ed. Baltimore: Williams & Wilkins, 1997;1201–1214.

Norton JA. Adrenal tumors. In: DeVita VT, Hellman S, Rosenberg SA, eds. Cancer: principles & practice of oncology. 5th ed. Philadelphia: Lippincott-Raven, 1997;1617–1729.

Bladder Cancer

Victoria J. Dorr

INCIDENCE

Bladder cancer accounts for 2% of cancers. In 1998, approximately 54,400 cases occurred in the United States, with 12,500 deaths secondary to bladder cancer. At the time of diagnosis 75% of bladder cancers are superficial. Bladder cancer mortality is decreasing slightly each year.

EPIDEMIOLOGY

The peak incidence of bladder cancer occurs in the seventh decade of life. A number of chemical compounds have been identified as carcinogenic to bladder epithelium. Aniline dyes and aromatic amines have been identified as carcinogenic. Contact with these compounds occurs in the dye, textile, printing, rubber, electrical cable, hair dressing, dry cleaning, and leather industries. Other risk factors include a prior exposure to cyclophosphamide or pelvic irradiation. Heavy phenacetin abuse has been associated with bladder cancer as well. Cigarette smoking is a risk factor. Bladder schistosomiasis is associated with an increased risk of squamous cell bladder cancer. Artificial sweeteners have been investigated as possible causative factors, but four studies have failed to demonstrate any link.

SIGNS AND SYMPTOMS

Most patients present with painless hematuria.

DIAGNOSIS AND STAGING

Most bladder cancers (95%) are transitional cell carcinomas. Squamous cell carcinoma accounts for 3% of bladder tumors. Small cell and adenocarcinoma histologies can also rarely be seen.

Cystoscopy is the standard diagnostic test for bladder cancer. Cytology on urinary sediment may yield a diagnosis in up to 50% of cases. The clinical staging of bladder cancer is determined by depth of invasion of bladder cancer through the bladder wall (Table 1B.29). This determination requires examination under anesthesia to assess the size and mobility of palpable masses, the degree of induration of the bladder wall, and the presence of extravesical extension or invasion of adjacent organs as well as a cystoscopic examination that includes a biopsy. Intravenous pyelogram (IVP) imaging is commonly performed if resection is planned. Clinical staging in patients presenting with advanced bladder cancer should include computed tomography (CT) of the abdomen and pelvis, chest radiography, and bone scan.

CARCINOMA IN SITU

Carcinoma in situ (CIS) most commonly presents as a small focus surrounding a papillary or sessile tumor. When CIS is

Table 1B.29A. TNM Staging System for Bladder Cancer

Primary tumor[a]

TX	Primary tumor cannot be assessed.
T0	No evidence of primary tumor.
Ta	Noninvasive papillary carcinoma.
Tis	Carcinoma in situ (flat tumor).
T1	Tumor invades subepithelial connective tissue.
T2	Tumor invades muscle.
T2a	Tumor invades superficial muscle (inner half).
T2b	Tumor invades deep muscle (outer half).
T3	Tumor invades perivesical fat.
T3a	Tumor invades perivesical fat microscopically.
T3b	Tumor invades perivesical fat macroscopically (extravesical mass).
T4	Tumor invades prostate, uterus, vagina, pelvic wall, or abdominal wall.
T4a	Tumor invades the prostate, uterus, or vagina.
T4b	Tumor invades the pelvic wall or abdominal wall.

Nodal involvement[b]

NX	Regional lymph nodes cannot be assessed.
N0	No regional lymph node metastasis.
N1	Metastasis in a single lymph node 2 cm or less in greatest dimension.
N2	Metastasis in a single lymph node, more than 2 cm but not more than 5 cm in greatest dimension; or multiple lymph nodes, none more than 5 cm in greatest dimension.
N3	Metastasis in a lymph node more than 5 cm in greatest dimension.

Distant metastasis

MX	Presence of distant metastasis cannot be assessed.
M0	No distant metastasis.
M1	Distant metastasis.

[a]The suffix "m" should be added to the appropriate T category to indicate multiple lesions. The suffix "is" may be added to any T to indicate associated carcinoma in situ.

[b]Regional lymph nodes are those within the true pelvis; all others are distant nodes.

Table 1B.29B. AJCC Stage Groupings for Bladder Cancer

Stage	Tumor	Nodes	Metastasis
0a	Ta	N0	M0
0is	Tis	N0	M0
I	T1	N0	M0
II	T2a	N0	M0
	T2b	N0	M0
III	T3a	N0	M0
	T3b	N0	M0
	T4a	N0	M0
IV	T4b	N0	M0
	Any T	N1	M0
	Any T	N2	M0
	Any T	N3	M0
	Any T	any N	M1

identified next to a superficial bladder tumor, there is an increased likelihood of muscle invasion. Approximately 26 to 40% of CIS occurs next to a papilloma. When this occurs, 83% of those patients will develop carcinoma within 5 years. In 140 patients followed for 14 to 21 years with CIS, 40% developed muscle invasive bladder cancer in 5 years and 60% at 10 years.

THERAPY

SUPERFICIAL BLADDER CANCER (TIS, TA, OR T1)

The most important feature predicting progression of disease is tumor grade. Patients with high-grade lesions have a worse prognosis. Other predictors of recurrence include multiple sites or multiple prior occurrences, a positive urine cytology, T1 disease, hematuria, and p53 abnormalities. The standard treatment is transurethral resection of the tumor (TURB). Recurrent disease is treated with TURB, intravesicular therapy with either chemotherapy or immune agents, or intravesicular photodynamic therapy. Intravesicular therapy is indicated to prevent recurrence of superficial disease. The definitive therapy for multiple inaccessible papillary neoplasms, it has been shown to prolong disease-free survival. Overall relapse is decreased 50% by the use of intravesicular therapy. Intravesical Bacillus Calmette-Guérin (BCG) appears to be the most effective agent in use.

MUSCLE-INVASIVE BLADDER CANCER

Stage II bladder cancer may be controlled in some cases by TURB, but often more aggressive forms of treatment are dictated by recurrent tumor or by the large size, multiple foci, or undifferentiated grade of the neoplasm. Radical cystectomy is the standard of care for muscle-invasive disease; however, due to the significant percentage of patients who are upstaged at the time of surgery (30 to 40% of patients with clinical stage T2 or T3a are found to have T3b or node positive disease), discussion about the addition of chemotherapy and radiation therapy is warranted. The most troublesome side effect of cystectomy is the loss of urinary continence; options include the traditional ileostomy with external collection, the surgical creation of continent pouches that allow the patient to catheterize on a regular schedule, and the creation of a neobladder sutured to the urethra. Another side effect is total impotence for both men and women. Nerve-sparing surgeries have been devised to prevent this complication. Table 1B.30 shows the historic 5-year survival with radical cystectomy.

Radiation therapy alone has resulted in a 10 to 23% 5-year survival rate. In randomized studies of radiation compared with surgery, radical cystectomy offers a survival advantage. Definitive radiation therapy with salvage cystectomy allows some patients to preserve bladder and sexual function. Chemotherapy alone has been evaluated in a select group of patients who were not candidates for surgery or who were more than 70 years of age. Chemotherapy was given with 5-FU, epirubicin, and cisplatin. A 54% response rate was seen, and average survival was 11.6 months.

Neoadjuvant chemotherapy has also been investigated. It has the potential advantages of earlier treatment of micrometastatic disease, down-staging of tumors to allow easier surgical removal, and assessment of efficacy of chemotherapy in individual tumors. Overall, 10 to 43% of patients treated with neoadjuvant therapy have a pathologic complete response (CR) at the time of cystectomy. Bladder preservation with neoadjuvant chemotherapy occurred in 13 to 45%. A meta-analysis of 479 patents treated in this fashion demonstrated a 2% increase in relative risk of death with chemotherapy. This effect may be due in

Table 1B.30. Historic 5-Year Survival Rate with Radical Cystectomy

TNM Stage	5-Year Overall Survival (%)
T2	40–70
T3a	40–50
T3b	20–25
T4 or node +	5

part to the choice of agents (usually MVAC [methotrexate plus vincristine, doxorubicin, and cisplatin]). The chemotherapy resulted in significant toxicity, and in fact 25 to 33% of patients were unable to tolerate chemotherapy in these studies. Patients who did have a response to chemotherapy had significantly improved survival. The use of adjuvant postoperative chemotherapy has also been evaluated. In patients who were at high risk for recurrence (node positive disease, extravesicular tumor extension or vascular or lymphatic incision), a significant benefit was seen in 5-year disease-free survival with CAP (cyclophosphamide plus doxorubicin and cisplatin) (70% with chemotherapy versus 35% with observation). Patients outside the study who were treated at the same time and at the same institution and who were considered at low risk for recurrence had a 76% 5-year disease-free survival.

METASTATIC BLADDER CANCER

For metastatic bladder cancer, combination chemotherapy is superior to single-agent therapy. The standard combination chemotherapy in advanced bladder cancer is MVAC. The overall response to MVAC is 48.8%, with an average survival of 9.8 months. MVAC, however, has substantial toxicity, and the

Table 1B.31. Options for Treatment of Metastatic or Recurrent Bladder Cancer

Treatment	Response Rate (CR + PR) (%)	Duration of Response
MVAC (methotrexate, vincristine, doxorubicin, cisplatin)	48.8	9 mo
Carboplatin and 5-FU in patients with poor performance status	24	8 mo
CAP (cyclophosphamide, doxorubicin, cisplatin)	13 α	
CAP-M (Cyclophosphamide, Doxorubicin, Cisplatin, and Methotrexate)	38	
5-FU and α-interferon	30	
Vinblastine, ifosfamide, and gallium nitrate	67 (41 CR)	20 wk; 19% long-term survivors
CMV (Cisplatin, Methotrexate, and Vinblastine)	35–48	
Carboplatin and paclitaxel	66 (33 CR)	5 mo
Piritrexim	23	
Gemcitabine	24	8 mo
Paclitaxel	42	

Radiation therapy is effective for palliation of symptomatic disease.

search for better-tolerated effective agents continues. Table 1B.31 lists several options for treatment of metastatic or recurrent bladder cancer.

RECURRENT BLADDER CANCER

The prognosis for any patient with progressive or recurrent invasive bladder cancer is generally poor. Salvage therapy with one of the regimens in Table 1B.29 may be an option.

BIBLIOGRAPHY

Bladder cancer. PDQ treatment for health professionals. National Cancer Institute. http://cancernet.nci.nih.gov/clinpdq/soa/Bladder_cancer_Physician. html; 1/18/98.

Brockstein BE and Vogelzang NJ. Chemotherapy of genitourinary cancer. In: Perry MC, ed. The chemotherapy source book. 2nd ed. Baltimore: Williams & Wilkins, 1997;1234–1241.

Landis SH, Murray T, Bolden S, Wingo PA. Cancer statistics 1998. CA Cancer J Clin 1998;48:6–29.

Kantoff PW, Zietman AL, Wishnow K. Bladder cancer. In: Holland JF, Frei E, Bast RC, et al., eds. Cancer medicine. 4th ed. Baltimore: Williams & Wilkins, 1997;2105–2124.

Scher HI, Shipley WU, Herr HW. Cancer of the bladder. In: DeVita VT, Hellman S, Rosenberg SA, eds. Cancer: principles & practice of oncology. 5th ed. Philadelphia: Lippincott-Raven, 1997;1253–1395.

Renal Cancer

Victoria J. Dorr

INCIDENCE

Approximately 29,000 cases of renal cell cancer (RCC) are diagnosed each year in the United States, with 12,000 deaths annually due to metastatic disease. Renal cell cancer has slowly been increasing in incidence over the past 30 years. The median age of diagnosis is the sixth decade. Up to 20% of patients have metastatic disease at presentation. RCC is one of the few cancers in which spontaneous remission may occur.

ETIOLOGY

Both sporadic and hereditary forms of RCC involve alteration of chromosome 3p. Familial RCC is transmitted in an autosomal dominant fashion. Von Hippel-Lindau (VHL) disease is an autosomal dominant disorder, with up to a third of patients developing RCC. VHL disease is a familial cancer syndrome in which affected persons have a predisposition to develop tumors in a number of organs, including the kidneys, brain, spine, eyes, adrenal glands, pancreas, inner ear, and epididymis. Hereditary papillary renal cell carcinoma (HPRC) is an inherited disorder with an autosomal dominant inheritance pattern in which affected persons develop bilateral, multifocal papillary renal carcinoma. In all forms of hereditary RCC, the malignancy tends to be multifocal and bilateral, and it occurs at a relatively young age.

Smoking is clearly associated with RCC, with up to 30% of cases believed to be attributable to smoking. Obesity, particularly in women, and analgesic abuse (primarily phenacetin) are also associated with an increased risk of RCC. Patients exposed to Thorotrast have an increased incidence of RCC. There is an increased incidence of renal carcinoma in patients with end-stage renal disease who develop acquired cystic disease of the kidney. The risk of developing kidney cancer has been estimated to be 30 times as high in dialysis patients with cystic changes in their kidney as in the general population.

SIGNS AND SYMPTOMS

The most frequent complaint at the time of presentation is of pain, occurring in up to 40% of patients. Up to a third of patients present with hematuria. Weight loss, fatigue, and fever occur in fewer than 15% of patients. Abnormal liver function, increased alkaline phosphatase levels, hypercalcemia, polycythemia, neuromyopathy, and amyloidosis have all been reported in association with renal cell carcinoma. A flank mass is palpable in up to 30% of patients.

DIAGNOSIS

Approximately 85% of RCCs are adenocarcinoma. Adenocarcinoma is divided into several subtypes. The most common histologic subtype of adenocarcinoma RCC is clear cell. Granular cell carcinoma has a higher nuclear grade. The sarcomatoid variant has a worse prognosis than either the clear cell or granular cell subtype. A unique subtype of RCC is the oncocytoma, which has a survival rate of more than 99%. Papillary cell subtype tumors tend to progress more slowly than the other types of RCC. Most of the remaining 15% of tumors are transitional cell cancer.

The diagnostic modalities used to evaluate and stage renal mass lesions include excretory urography (IVP), CT, arteriography, venography, ultrasound, and MRI (Table 1B.32). Another commonly used staging system is as follows:

Table 1B.32A. TNM Staging System for Renal Cancer

Primary tumor

TX   Primary tumor cannot be assessed.

T0   No evidence of primary tumor.

T1   Tumor 7 cm or less in greatest dimension limited to the kidney.

T2   Tumor more than 7 cm in greatest dimension limited to the kidney.

T3   Tumor extends into major veins or invades adrenal gland or perinephric tissues but not beyond Gerota's fascia.

T3a   Tumor invades adrenal gland or perinephric tissues but not beyond Gerota's fascia.

T3b   Tumor grossly extends into renal vein(s) or vena cava.

T3c   Tumor grossly extends into the vena cava above the diaphragm.

T4   Tumor invades beyond Gerota's fascia.

Regional lymph nodes[a]

NX   Regional lymph nodes cannot be assessed.

N0   No regional lymph node metastasis.

N1   Metastasis in a single lymph node 2 cm or less in greatest dimension.

N2   Metastasis in a single lymph node more than 2 cm but not more than 5 cm in greatest dimension or multiple lymph nodes, none more than 5 cm in greatest dimension.

N3   Metastasis in a lymph node more than 5 cm in greatest dimension.

Distant metastasis

MX   Presence of distant metastasis cannot be assessed.

M0   No distant metastasis.

M1   Distant metastasis.

[a]Laterality does not affect the N classification.

Table 1B.32B. AJCC Stage Groupings for Renal Cancer

Stage	Tumor	Nodes	Metastasis
I	T1	N0	M0
II	T2	N0	M0
III	T1–3	N1	M0
	T3	N0	M0
IV	T4	Any N	M0
	Any T	N2	M0
	Any T	N3	M0
	Any T	Any N	M1

Stage I. Tumor confined to the kidney. This stage corresponds to AJCC stages I and II (T1 or T2, N0). It is associated with a 66% 5-year survival.

Stage II. Perirenal and/or adrenal tissues are involved with tumor but are still within Gerota's fascia. This stage corresponds to AJCC TNM stage T3a, N0. It is associated with a 64% 5-year survival.

Stage III. Regional invasion; tumor involves renal vein or inferior vena cava, regional lymph nodes, or both. This stage corresponds to AJCC TNM stages T3b, N0, M0; any T, N1–N3, M0. It is associated with a 42% 5-year survival if it involves renal vein or inferior vena cava and 18% if disease involves the hilar lymph nodes.

Stage IV. Advanced disease with direct extension to adjacent organs other than adrenal tissue or with distant metastases. This stage corresponds with AJCC TNM stages T4, any N, M0; or any T, any N, M1.

TREATMENT OPTIONS

LOCAL DISEASE

Surgical resection is the only accepted curative therapy for stage I renal cell cancer. Resection may be simple or radical. Radical resection includes removal of the kidney, adrenal gland, perirenal fat, and Gerota's fascia, with or without a regional lymph node dissection. Some, but not all, surgeons believe the radical operation yields superior results. In patients who are not candidates for surgery, external radiation therapy or arterial embolization can provide palliation.

ADVANCED DISEASE

For patients with stage II and T3b, N0, M0 renal cell cancer, radical resection is the only accepted curative therapy. Lymphadenectomy is commonly performed, but its effectiveness has not been definitively proved. Preoperative and postoperative radiation therapy has been investigated in the management of stage II disease. Its benefit has not been proved, although some benefit may be derived in patients with extensive disease.

In patients with any T, N1 to N3, M0 RCC, surgery is curable in a small minority of cases. A radical nephrectomy and lymph node dissection are necessary. The value of preoperative and postoperative external irradiation has not been demonstrated, but external beam radiation therapy may be used for palliation in patients who are not candidates for surgery.

Almost all patients with stage IV disease are incurable. Tumor embolization, external beam irradiation, and nephrectomy can aid in the palliation of symptoms due to the primary tumor or related ectopic hormone production. There is minimal evidence that nephrectomy induces regression of distant metastases. Spontaneous regressions occur in up to 7% of patients whether or not nephrectomy is performed. Selected patients with solitary or a limited number of distant metastases can achieve prolonged survival with nephrectomy and surgical resection of the metastases.

Chemotherapy has been tested in clinical trials in more than 3500 patients in 72 regimens. Overall, a disheartening response rate of 5.6% was seen. FUDR appeared to have the highest response rate, with responses occurring in 27%. Other agents that have been investigated include continuous infusion 5-FU, vinblastine, and gemcitabine, all with about a 5% response rate. Tamoxifen has a reported response rate of 1.7% to 12% in metastatic RCC. Megestrol acetate (Megace) has had a response rate of 1 to 2%. Cimetadine (Tagamet) has a response rate similar to that of many chemotherapeutic agents (5%), and in one study produced a response rate of 13% when combined with coumarin.

Spontaneous remissions of renal cell cancer suggest an immune phenomenon. Thus, immune therapy with interleukin-2 (IL-2) and interferon have been investigated. α-Interferon has approximately a 15 to 20% objective response rate in appropriately selected individuals. In general, these patients have non-bulky pulmonary and/or soft tissue metastases with excellent performance status (ECOG 0 or 1) and no weight loss. The interferon doses used in studies reporting good response rates have been in an intermediate range of 6 to 20 million units three times weekly. These responses are rarely complete or durable.

Administration of IL-2 appears to have an overall response rate similar to that of interferon but with approximately 5% of the responding patients having durable complete remissions. The optimal dosing of IL-2 is unknown. High-dose therapy appears to be associated with higher response rates but more toxicity. Outpatient subcutaneous administration has also demonstrated responses with acceptable toxicity.

The most promising regimen for metastatic RCC appears to be an outpatient regimen of interferon, IL-2, and 5-FU. Overall response rates of 22 to 39% have been reported, with up to 33% CR seen. Patients who achieved a complete response had a significantly improved chance of long-term survival. Patients who achieved a partial response had a median duration of response of 22 months.

BIBLIOGRAPHY

Brockstein BE, Vogelzang NJ. Chemotherapy of genitourinary cancer. In: Perry MC, ed. The chemotherapy source book. 2nd ed. Baltimore: Williams & Wilkins, 1997;1229–1234.

Landis SH, Murray T, Bolden S, Wingo PA. Cancer statistics 1998. CA Cancer J Clin 1998;48:6–29.

Linehan WM, Shipley WU, Parkinson DR. Cancer of the kidney and ureter. In: DeVita VT, Hellman S, Rosenberg SA, eds. Cancer: principles & practice of oncology. 5th ed. Philadelphia: Lippincott-Raven, 1997;1253–1395.

Renal cell cancer. PDQ Treatment for Health Professionals. National Cancer Institute. http://cancernet.nci.nih.gov/clinpdq/soa/Renal_cell_cancer_Physician.html; 1/18/98.

Richie JP, Kantoff PW, Shapiro CL. Renal cell carcinoma. In: Cancer medicine. 4th ed. Holland JF, Frei E, Bast RC, et al., eds. Baltimore: Williams & Wilkins, 1997;2085–2096.

Prostate Cancer

Victoria J. Dorr

INCIDENCE

Prostate cancer is the most common cancer in men and the second most common cause of cancer death in men. In 1998, about 184,500 men were diagnosed with prostate cancer, and it caused about 39,200 deaths. The incidence of prostate cancer continues to increase. Occult prostate cancer is a common finding at autopsy, with approximately two-thirds of men having occult prostate cancer by age 80. The lifetime risk of developing occult prostate cancer is 1 in 3, the lifetime risk of developing clinical prostate cancer is 1 in 6, and the lifetime risk of dying of prostate cancer is 1 in 28.

ETIOLOGY

The causation of prostate cancer is unknown, although racial and genetic risk factors have been identified. At autopsy the occult incidence of prostate cancer is noted in all ethnic groups; however, African-Americans are more likely than whites to develop clinical prostate cancer, and clinical prostate cancer is rare in Asian populations. One factor identified as a promoter of prostate cancer development is diet. A statistically significant association of prostate cancer risk exists with total fat intake for all ethnic groups.

In men with a first-degree relative with prostate cancer, there is a twofold increased risk of developing prostate cancer; in men with more than two first-degree relatives with prostate cancer, the risk is increased fourfold. The autosomal dominant genes associated with breast and ovarian cancer (BRCA1 and BRCA2) have both been associated with an increased risk of prostate cancer. Vasectomy is not considered a risk factor for prostate cancer.

SCREENING

The American Cancer Society recommends that an annual digital rectal examination and prostate specific antigen (PSA) be performed in all men over age 50. These two tests are complementary; in 25% of patients a rectal examination detects a lesion that is not detected by PSA; conversely, PSA detects 14% of prostate cancers that would have been missed on rectal examination. An elevation in PSA is due to malignancy in 33%. The chance of an elevation in PSA being secondary to prostate cancer increases with the PSA value. Unfortunately, the likelihood that the cancer is advanced also increases with the PSA value.

CHEMOPREVENTION

Studies evaluating the efficacy of several agents for their ability to prevent prostate cancer are under way. These include finasteride and retinoid agents.

DIAGNOSIS AND STAGING

An abnormality on rectal examination or PSA is usually further evaluated by the use of a transrectal ultrasound and biopsy of suspicious lesions. Transrectal ultrasound can be used to assess location, size, and local extent of prostate cancer (Table 1B.33). Ultrasound cannot accurately assess lymph nodes. Lymph node status also is an important prognostic factor. Computed tomography (CT) can detect grossly enlarged nodes but poorly defines intraprostatic features; therefore, it is less reliable for staging of disease than surgical staging. Radical pelvic lymph node dissection is routinely carried out in patients undergoing a radical prostatectomy. Some evidence suggests that in patients undergoing a perineal prostatectomy for nonpalpable, ultrasound-detected lesions with a PSA less than 20 and a low Gleason score, lymph node dissection may be omitted. Alternatively, laparoscopic lymph node dissection may be performed. Preoperative seminal vesicle biopsy may be useful in patients with palpable nodules who are being considered for radical prostatectomy, since seminal vesicle involvement may affect the choice of primary therapy and predicts for pelvic lymph node metastasis. MRI using an endorectal coil to assess for extent of local disease may be considered; MRI cannot accurately assess lymph node status. Bone scans to evaluate for asymptomatic bone lesions have been commonly performed. However, the PSA test may have a role in choosing which patients require bone scans. In one series of patients, a bone scan was positive in only 0.23% of patients who were asymptomatic and who had PSA values less than 20 ng/mL. Chest radiography is necessary in initial staging, since 6% of patients have pulmonary metastases at the time of presentation. Bone scans are reserved for patients who have PSA above 20 or T3 or Gleason grade 8 to 10 lesions. CT to assess for extent of local disease is performed in patients with a PSA above 20, or T3 or Gleason grade 8 to 10 lesions as well.

THERAPY

LOCALIZED DISEASE

There is substantial controversy about the appropriate therapy for localized prostate cancer. Options include surgery, radiation therapy, and observation with or without hormone ther-

Table 1B.33A. TNM and Jewett Staging Systems for Prostate Cancer

TNM System

Primary tumor[a]

TX	Primary tumor cannot be assessed.
T0	No evidence of primary tumor.
T1	Clinically inapparent tumor not palpable or visible by imaging.
T1a	Tumor incidental histologic finding in 5% or less of tissue resected.
T1b	Tumor incidental histologic finding in more than 5% of tissue resected.
T1c	Tumor identified by needle biopsy (e.g., performed because of elevated PSA).
T2	Palpable tumor confined within the prostate.[b]
T2a	Tumor involves one lobe.
T2b	Tumor involves both lobes.
T3	Tumor extends through the prostatic capsule.[c]
T3a	Extracapsular extension.
T3b	Tumor invades seminal vesicle(s).
T4	Tumor is fixed or invades adjacent structures other than seminal vesicles (bladder neck, external sphincter, rectum, levator muscles) and/or is fixed to pelvic wall.

Regional lymph nodes[d]

NX	Regional lymph nodes cannot be assessed.
N0	No regional lymph node metastasis.
N1	Metastasis in regional lymph node or nodes.

Distant metastasis[e]

MX	Presence of distant metastasis cannot be assessed.
M0	No distant metastasis.
M1	Distant metastasis.
M1a	Nonregional lymph node(s).
M1b	Bone(s).
M1c	Other site(s).

Histopathologic grade

GX	Grade cannot be assessed.
G1	Well differentiated (slight anaplasia).
G2	Moderately differentiated (moderate anaplasia).
G3–4	Poorly differentiated or undifferentiated (marked anaplasia).

continued

Table 1B.33A. TNM and Jewett Staging Systems for Prostate Cancer *continued*

Jewett Staging System

A	Clinically undetectable tumor confined to the prostate gland; an incidental finding at prostatic surgery.
A1	Well-differentiated with focal involvement, usually left untreated.
A2	Moderately or poorly differentiated or involves multiple foci in the gland.
B	Tumor confined to the prostate gland.
B0	Non-palpable, PSA-detected.
B1	Single nodule in one lobe of the prostate.
B2	More extensive involvement of one lobe or involvement of both lobes.
C	Tumor clinically localized to the periprostatic area but extending through the prostatic capsule; seminal vesicles may be involved.
C1	Clinical extracapsular extension.
C2	Extracapsular tumor producing bladder outlet or ureteral obstruction.
D	Metastatic disease.
D0	Clinically localized disease (prostate only) but persistently elevated enzymatic serum acid phosphatase titers.
D1	Regional lymph nodes only.
D2	Distant lymph nodes, metastases to bone or visceral organs.
D3	D2 prostate cancer patients who relapsed after adequate endocrine therapy.

*a*There is no pathologic T1 classification; T1 staging is clinical only.
*b*Tumor found in one or both lobes by needle biopsy but not palpable or reliably seen on imaging is classified as T1c.
*c*Tumor invasion into the prostatic apex or into but not beyond the prostatic capsule is classified as T2.
*d*Regional lymph nodes are the nodes of the true pelvis, those below the bifurcation of the common iliac arteries. They include the following groups (laterality does not affect the N classification): pelvic (NOS), hypogastric, obturator, iliac (internal, external, NOS), periprostatic, and sacral (lateral, presacral, promontory [Gerota's], or NOS). Distant lymph nodes are outside the confines of the true pelvis, and their involvement constitutes distant metastasis. They can be imaged using ultrasound, computed tomography, magnetic resonance imaging, or lymphangiography. They include aortic (para-aortic, periaortic, lumbar), common iliac, inguinal, superficial inguinal (femoral), supraclavicular, cervical, scalene, and retroperitoneal (NOS) nodes.
*e*When more than one site of metastasis is present, the most advanced category (pM1c) is used.

apy. The American Urological Association Prostate Cancer Clinical Guidelines Panel considers these "interventions to be options because the data from the literature do not provide clear-cut evidence for the superiority of any one treatment." (American Urological Association Prostate Cancer Clinical Guidelines Panel.

Table 1B.33B. AJCC Stage Groupings for Prostate Cancer

Stage	Tumor	Nodes	Metastasis	Histopathologic Grade
I	T1a	N0	M0	G1
II	T1a	N0	M0	G2, 3–4
	T1b	N0	M0	Any G
	T1c	N0	M0	Any G
	T1	N0	M0	Any G
	T2	N0	M0	Any G
III	T3	N0	M0	Any G
IV	T4	N0	M0	Any G
	Any T	N1	M0	Any G
	Any T	Any N	M1	Any G

Report on the management of clinically localized prostate cancer. Baltimore: American Urological Association, 1995) This panel reviewed 12,501 papers, of which only 165 (1.3%) provided acceptable information. The lack of clear evidence of superiority for one modality versus another is because there are no randomized trials of comparably staged patients on which to base recommendations; there are inherent biases in series of selected patients; and there are different definitions of failure and differences in the follow-up intervals and follow-up routines used to monitor outcomes. Table 1B.34 presents the historical survival rate for each modality. An important point regarding these data is that patients undergoing surgery have pathologic staging, whereas patients receiving radiation or deferred therapy have clinical staging. The significance of this is that at the time of surgery as many as 40% of patients may be found to have locally advanced (stage III or C disease), which is rarely cured, and thus the populations of clinical and pathologically staged patients are not comparable.

SURGERY

Surgery is usually reserved for patients in good health who are under age 70 and who elect surgery after discussion of the potential complications. These patients should have a negative bone scan and tumors confined to the prostate gland (stages I and II). Prostatectomy can be performed by the perineal or retropubic approach. Pelvic node dissection is not considered therapeutic, but it spares patients with positive nodes the morbidity of prostatectomy. Radical prostatectomy is usually not performed if frozen section reveals metastases in the pelvic lymph nodes, and such patients should be considered for entry into existing clinical trials or receive radiation therapy to control

Table 1B.34. Survival in Prostate Cancer

Survival (years) %									
	Disease Free			Disease Specific			Overall		
Stage	5	10	15	5	10	15	5	10	15
Deferred Therapy									
A		74						65	
C	76	63		88	70		64	37	
A		84							
A–C	72	64		94	89		67	44	
A				82	78		75	65	
Radical Prostatectomy									
A–C		57						72	54
B1								63	51
B	87	67	48					74	55
B–C	91	71	58					78	67
A–D$_1$	88	73		85	70		90	75	
B$_2$		38	25						
B–C				33					
Radiation Therapy									
A–C	71	50					69	47	
A–D$_1$	63						77		
A$_2$–B	90								
A$_2$–B	78	60							
C	60	40							
A	97	97					83	62	
B	86	74					73	46	
C	74	69					58	38	
A	84						96		
B	68						77		
C	53						61		

Adapted with permission from Dorr VJ, Williamson SK, Stephens RL. An evaluation of prostate-specific antigen as a screening test for prostate cancer. Arch Intern Med 1993;153:2529–2537.

local symptoms. Patients with pathologic organ-confined disease have a less than 10% chance of recurrence. Patients with either lymph node involvement or extension beyond the prostate may be candidates for additional adjuvant therapy. Postoperative radiation therapy, androgen deprivation, and adjuvant chemotherapy are being investigated.

Early complications of radical prostatectomy include rectal injury, myocardial infarction, thromboembolic disease, lymphocele formation, anastomotic urinary leakage, and sepsis. The mortality associated with radical prostatectomy is less than 2%. Late complications of radical prostatectomy can include bladder neck contractures, postoperative hernia, and hydrocele formation. The most important long-term complications are stress incontinence and impotence. It has been reported that 10% of patients are incontinent at 6 months and 5% at 1 year following radical prostatectomy. The risk of impotence is reported at 30 to 40% at 6 months and 15 to 25% at 1 year. A recent study of a survey sent to 757 patients identified as having had a radical prostatectomy from Medicare claims (92% response rate) had men self-report complications. In this series, 31% reported wearing pads or clamps for incontinence and 47% reported daily incontinence with cough or full bladder. Additionally, 61% reported no partial or full erection since surgery, and only 11% had erections sufficient for intercourse. Some 20% had also had surgery for urethral stricture. Finally, 18% at 2 years, 22% at 3 years, and 29% at 4 years reported receiving additional radiation or hormone therapy for progressive disease.

Cryosurgery entails destruction of prostate cancer cells by intermittent freezing of the prostate tissue with cryoprobes followed by thawing. It is less well established than standard prostatectomy, and long-term outcomes are not known. Serious toxic effects include bladder outlet injury, urinary incontinence, sexual impotence, and rectal injury.

RADIATION THERAPY

Candidates for definitive radiation therapy must have a confirmed pathological diagnosis of cancer that is clinically confined to the prostate and/or surrounding tissues (stages I, II, and III). In addition, patients considered poor medical candidates for radical prostatectomy can be treated with acceptably low complications if care is given to delivery technique. An initial serum PSA level above 15 ng/mL predicts probable failure with conventional radiation therapy. Interstitial brachytherapy has been used in several trials for treatment of stage I and II carcinoma of the prostate. Potential major side effects of radiation therapy include small bowel obstruction, vesicle fistula, hemorrhagic cystitis, urethral stricture (8.5%), and pubic bone necrosis. Minor sequelae include proctitis, rectal ulceration, rectal and anal stricture, and chronic cystitis. Additionally, 3% report incontinence and 39% report impotence after radiation.

FOLLOW-UP AFTER LOCAL THERAPY

After local therapy patients should be monitored with PSA values. An elevated or rising PSA after definitive local treatment requires a repeat value in 1 to 2 months. If the value is still elevated or increasing, repeat staging procedures, including a bone scan and pelvic CT, should be performed. If these studies are normal, repeat biopsy should be performed if the patient received radiation, and if the patient underwent surgery, the prostatic fossa and urethra should be biopsied. If disease is detected, androgen deprivation therapy is usually recommended.

OBSERVATION

The rationale for observation is that cancer-specific survival for stage I and II patients who are observed is 90% at 5 years and 80% at 10 years. Prostate cancer is also most likely to occur in an elderly man who may suffer from other comorbid diseases. Care should be taken in choosing deferred therapy, as progression eventually occurs in about half of cases by 7 years; and with follow-up past 10 years the risk of metastatic disease increases. For patients over age 70, the risk of dying of prostate cancer is 10% because of other competing causes of death. Patients who are candidates for observation alone should have low-volume, low Gleason grade disease with life expectancy in general of 10 to 15 years.

Few data on the efficacy of hormone therapy for the primary treatment of prostate cancer are available. Neoadjuvant hormone therapy with androgen blockade prior to prostatectomy or radiation therapy is under investigation.

TREATMENT OF ADVANCED PROSTATE CANCER

Treatment choices in patients with disease confined to regional lymph nodes (stage D1) are vexing. The use of prostatic and pelvic irradiation results in only rare long-term survivors. Hormone therapy may be considered in conjunction with radiation. Several studies have investigated its utility, and a debate remains about whether early hormone treatment provides a survival advantage or just a delay to progression.

The primary treatment of metastatic or locally advanced prostate cancer has been hormone ablation. Initial results from a randomized study of immediate hormonal treatment (orchiectomy or luteinizing hormone-releasing hormone [LHRH] analogue) versus deferred treatment (watchful waiting with hormone therapy at progression) in men with locally advanced or asymptomatic metastatic prostate cancer showed a better overall survival and an improved prostate cancer-specific survival with the immediate treatment. The incidence of pathologic fractures, spinal cord compression, and ureteric obstruction were also lower in the immediate treatment arm.

Androgen ablation can be achieved by surgical removal of the testes or chemically with gonadotropin-releasing hormone

(GnRH) analogues, exogenous estrogens, progestational agents, antiandrogens, or adrenal enzyme synthesis inhibitors such as ketoconazole and aminoglutethimide. Overall, all agents that block androgen production are comparable in terms of their antitumor effect. The difference comes in their side effect profiles. A duration of response of 12 to 18 months is expected, although a 5-year disease free survival of 20% has been reported. Orchiectomy, the gold standard, should result in a rapid improvement in patients with symptomatic disease. Approaches using LHRH agonists and/or antiandrogens in patients with stage IV prostate cancer have produced response rates similar to those of standard hormone treatments. The concept of total androgen blockade (TAB) relates to the fact that 90% to 95% of androgens originate in the testicles and the remainder are synthesized in the adrenal gland. The latter may contribute up to 40% of the active androgens in the prostate. On balance, the literature does not show a survival advantage associated with TAB over and above standard castration, but TAB may improve the more subjective end point of response rate.

Appropriate primary treatment options for patients with stage IV prostate cancer include the following:

1. Orchiectomy alone or with an androgen blocker. Orchiectomy plus nilutamide produces better objective response rates, bone pain relief, and freedom from progression rates than orchiectomy alone. However, the addition of an antiandrogen to surgical castration has not been shown to improve survival in a meta-analysis.
2. LHRH agonists such as leuprolide in daily or depot preparations. These agents may be associated with tumor flare when used alone, and therefore the concomitant use of antiandrogens should be considered in the presence of bone pain, ureteral obstruction, or impending spinal cord compression.
3. Leuprolide plus flutamide. However, the addition of an antiandrogen to leuprolide has not been shown to improve survival in a meta-analysis.
4. Estrogens: (diethylstilbestrol, chlorotrianisene, ethinyl estradiol, conjugated estrogens USP, DES-diphosphate).
5. External beam irradiation for attempted cure of highly selected stage M0 patients. Definitive radiation therapy should be delayed 4 to 6 weeks after transurethral resection to reduce incidence of stricture. Hormone therapy may be considered in addition to external beam irradiation.
6. Palliative radiation therapy.
7. Careful observation without further immediate treatment in selected patients.

RECURRENT OR PROGRESSIVE DISEASE

Second-line hormone therapy produces few responses. A beneficial response to flutamide withdrawal has recently been seen in 20 to 40% of men after the drug was discontinued. This response not only is important as a treatment option but also is a confounding factor in many studies, as time must be allowed to ensure that the response is to the agent tested and not to the flutamide withdrawal. Responses to second-line hormone therapy are rare.

The role of chemotherapy in prostate cancer remains controversial. Most studies fail to demonstrate an improvement in survival when chemotherapy is compared with controls. One study of cyclophosphamide 1 g intravenously every 3 weeks did demonstrate a 3-month improvement in survival over observation. Other active chemotherapeutics in patients with hormone-refractory disease (response rates of 5 to 30%) include doxorubicin, cisplatin, mitoxantrone, vinblastine, and trimetrexate. Estramustine as a single agent has a poor response rate, but in combination with vinblastine it has produced response rates of 25%. Caution must be used in interpreting these results, however, because PSA response is frequently used to judge overall response to an agent. Suramin remains under investigation as an active agent in prostate cancer.

The primary goal of chemotherapy in these patients is palliation; therefore, studies that evaluate quality of life with chemotherapy are important. A study comparing prednisone against mitoxantrone plus prednisone showed significantly improved pain control in the chemotherapy-treated arm. However, there were no statistically significant differences in overall survival, well-being, or measured global quality of life between the two treatments.

Both strontium and samarium may have a role in the palliation of bone pain. Given as intravenous radionuclide, subjective responses are seen in bone pain with both agents. Dose-limiting toxicity is myelosuppression.

BIBLIOGRAPHY

Bladder cancer. PDQ Treatment for Health Professionals. National Cancer Institute.   http://cancernet.nci.nih.gov/clinpdq/soa/Prostate_cancer_Physician.html; 1/18/98.

Brockstein BE and Vogelzang NJ. Chemotherapy of genitourinary cancer. In: Perry MC, ed. The chemotherapy source book. 2nd ed. Baltimore: Williams & Wilkins, 1997;1215–1222.

Fowler FJ, Barry MJ, Lu-Yao G, et al. Patient-reported complications and follow-up treatment after radical prostatectomy: the National Medicare experience: 1988–1990 (updated June 1993). Urology 1993;42:622–629.

Landis SH, Murray T, Bolden S, Wingo PA. Cancer statistics 1998. CA Cancer J Clin 1998;48:6–29.

Oesterling J, Fuks Z, Lee CT, Scher HI. Cancer of the prostate. In: DeVita VT, Hellman S, Rosenberg SA, eds. Cancer: principles & practice of oncology. 5th ed. Philadelphia: Lippincott-Raven, 1997;1253–1395.

Trump DL, Shipley WU, Dillioglugil O, Scardino PT. Neoplasms of the prostate. In: Cancer medicine. 4th ed. Holland JF, Frei E, Bast RC, et al., eds. Baltimore: Williams & Wilkins, 1997;2125–2164.

Penile Cancer

Victoria J. Dorr

INCIDENCE AND ETIOLOGY

Penile cancer effects only 1 in 100,000 men in the United States. There were approximately 1500 cases and 200 deaths attributable to penile cancer in 1998. Most penile cancers occur in uncircumcised men, suggesting the effect of a local irritant. Carcinoma is rare among men who were circumcised at birth, but circumcision performed at puberty or in adulthood does not have the same protective potential. The lifetime risk of penile cancer may be as high as 1 in 600 in uncircumcised men. There are no data to confirm a relation between penile cancer and sexually transmitted disease.

SIGNS AND SYMPTOMS

Generally, penile cancer presents with a painless mass or nonhealing ulcer on the penis. Some patients have inguinal lymphadenopathy.

DIAGNOSIS AND STAGING

Diagnosis is made by incisional or excisional biopsy. Most penile cancers are squamous cell carcinoma. Staging for penile cancers is shown in Table 1B.35.

THERAPY

STAGE I

Stage I penile cancer is curable. For lesions limited to the foreskin, wide excision and circumcision may be sufficient. For carcinoma in situ of the glans, microscopic directed surgery (MOHS) or local applications of fluorouracil can be recommended.

For infiltrating tumors, options include penile amputation, radiation therapy, and microscopic-directed limited surgery. The choice may depend on size and location of the lesion. Microscopic node metastases are common, so consideration may be given to elective adjuvant inguinal node dissection in poorly differentiated tumors. The influence of prophylactic lymphadenectomy on survival is not known.

STAGE II

Stage II penile cancer is most frequently managed by penile amputation for local control. Whether the amputation is partial,

Table 1B.35A. TNM Staging System for Penile Cancer

Primary tumor

TX	Primary tumor cannot be assessed.
T0	No evidence of primary tumor.
Tis	Carcinoma in situ.
Ta	Noninvasive verrucous carcinoma.
T1	Tumor invades subepithelial connective tissue.
T2	Tumor invades corpus spongiosum or cavernosum.
T3	Tumor invades urethra or prostate.
T4	Tumor invades other adjacent structures.

Regional lymph nodes

NX	Regional lymph nodes cannot be assessed.
N0	No regional lymph node metastasis.
N1	Metastasis in a single superficial inguinal lymph node.
N2	Metastasis in multiple or bilateral superficial inguinal lymph nodes.
N3	Metastasis in deep inguinal or pelvic lymph node(s), unilateral or bilateral.

Distant metastasis

MX	Presence of distant metastasis cannot be assessed.
M0	No distant metastasis.
M1	Distant metastasis.

Table 1B.35B. AJCC Stage Groupings for Penile Cancer

Stage	Tumor	Nodes	Metastasis
0	Tis	N0	M0
	Ta	N0	M0
I	T1	N0	M0
II	T1	N1	M0
	T2	N0	M0
	T2	N1	M0
III	T1	N2	M0
	T2	N2	M0
	T3	N0	M0
	T3	N1	M0
	T3	N2	M0
IV	T4	Any N	M0
	Any T	N3	M0
	Any T	Any N	M1

total, or radical depends on the extent and location of the neoplasm. Primary radiation therapy with surgical salvage may be an alternative approach. Microscopic node metastases are common, so consideration may be given to elective adjuvant inguinal node dissection in poorly differentiated tumors. The influence of prophylactic lymphadenectomy on survival is not known.

STAGE III

Stage III penile cancer is by definition lymph node positive; however, clinically positive inguinal lymph nodes may be due to infection. Thus, a course of antibiotics and observation for 2 to 3 weeks can be used before lymphadenectomy. In patients with proven lymph node–positive disease, bilateral ilioinguinal dissection is the treatment of choice. Postoperative irradiation may decrease the incidence of inguinal recurrence. Radiation to involved lymph nodes may be an alternative in patients who are not candidates for surgery.

Chemotherapy with vincristine, bleomycin, and methotrexate has been effective in both an adjuvant and neoadjuvant role. Another regimen with cisplatin plus continuous-infusion 5-FU has also been found to be effective in a neoadjuvant setting.

STAGE IV

There is no curative treatment for patients with stage IV penile cancer, so treatment should be aimed at palliation. Palliative surgery may be used for control of symptomatic local disease. Radiation may be used for palliative measures as well. Chemotherapy for penile carcinoma varies with the histology of the lesion. For patients with pure transitional tumors, cisplatin-combination regimens have shown efficacy. For patients with squamous cell histology, antitumor activity has been demonstrated with the single agents bleomycin, methotrexate, and cisplatin. Overall response is about 30%, with few CRs observed. Combination therapy with cyclophosphamide plus bleomycin and cisplatin produced similar results. Two reports have produced complete remissions lasting 36 months in patients treated with bleomycin and methotrexate, followed by radiation therapy. Cisplatin with 5-FU has produced responses of 25 to 100%, but in very small series of patients.

BIBLIOGRAPHY

Herr HW, Fuks Z, Scher HI. Cancer of the urethra and penis. In: DeVita VT, Hellman S, Rosenberg SA, eds. Cancer: principles & practice of oncology. 5th ed. Philadelphia: Lippincott-Raven, 1997;1253–1395.

Landis SH, Murray T, Bolden S, Wingo PA. Cancer statistics 1998. CA Cancer J Clin 1998;48:6–29.

Marcial VA, Puras A, Marcial-Vega VA. Neoplasms of the penis. In: Holland JF, Frei E, Bast RC, et al., eds. Cancer medicine. 4th ed. Baltimore: Williams & Wilkins, 1997;2165–2176.

Penile cancer. PDQ treatment for health professionals. National Cancer Institute. http://cancernet.nci.nih.gov/clinpdq/soa/Penile_cancer_Physician.html; 1/18/98.

Testicular Cancer

Victoria J. Dorr

INCIDENCE

While germ cell tumors are relatively uncommon, occurring in 3 in 100,000 men annually, they are the most common solid tumor in men aged 15 to 35. Testicular masses in men over age 50 are more commonly lymphoma than germ cell tumors. In 1998 there were about 7,600 cases and 400 deaths from testicular cancer. Testicular cancer is a diagnostic and treatment success story. In 1970 survival of testicular cancer was only 10%, but now more than 90% of men are cured.

ETIOLOGY

Familial cases of testicular cancer have been reported; in these families, testicular cancer is bilateral in 2 to 3% of patients. Genetic abnormalities associated with testicular cancer include an isochrome 12p and a rare p53 abnormality. Mediastinal germ cell tumors have been associated with Klinefelter's syndrome. Cryptorchidism is reported in 10% of men with testicular cancer. Cryptorchidism increases the risk of testicular cancer by a factor of 5 to 40. In these patients, 25% of tumors occur in the contralateral testicle. Orchipexy before puberty appears to prevent testicular cancer. The incidence of testicular cancer is four times as high in the white population as in to the African-American population. Testicular cancer is rare in Asian men.

SIGNS AND SYMPTOMS

The usual presentation of testicular cancer is painless enlargement of one testicle. Patients may also describe a heavy feeling or dull ache in the scrotum, inguinal area, or pelvis. The early detection of testicular cancer is key, and screening is recommended, with monthly self-examination of the testicles. Extragonadal presentation of germ cell tumors occurs in fewer than 10% of cases.

DIAGNOSIS AND STAGING

Physical examination correctly predicts malignancy 60% of the time. Ultrasound is useful to differentiate the mass further. Radical orchiectomy is the primary diagnostic procedure. Testicular ultrasound to evaluate both testicles should be performed prior to surgery. A chest radiograph to evaluate for evidence of thoracic disease should be done. Abdominal CT should be done to assess for the presence of retroperitoneal lymphadenopathy. Staging for testicular cancer is shown in Table 1B.36.

Table 1B.36A. TNM and Surgical Staging Systems for Testicular Cancer

TNM System

Primary tumor[a]

pTX Primary tumor cannot be assessed; if no radical orchiectomy has been performed, TX is used.

pT0 No evidence of primary tumor (e.g., histologic scar in testis).

pTis Intratubular tumor: preinvasive cancer.

pT1 Tumor is limited to testis and epididymis without vascular or lymphatic invasion. Tumor may invade the tunica albuginea but not the tunica vaginalis.

pT2 Tumor is limited to testis and epididymis with vascular or lymphatic invasion or the tumor has involved the tunica vaginalis.

pT3 Tumor invades the spermatic cord.

pT4 Tumor invades the scrotum.

Regional lymph nodes

NX Regional lymph nodes cannot be assessed.

N0 No regional lymph node metastasis.

N1 Metastasis in a lymph node mass or multiple lymph nodes all 2 cm or less in greatest dimension.

N2 Metastasis in a lymph node mass more than 2 cm but not more than 5 cm in greatest dimension; or multiple lymph nodes, none more than 5 cm in greatest dimension.

N3 Metastasis in a lymph node more than 5 cm in greatest dimension.

Distant metastasis

MX Presence of distant metastasis cannot be assessed.

M0 No distant metastasis.

M1 Distant metastasis.

M1a Nonregional nodal or pulmonary metastasis.

M1b Distant metastasis other than M1a.

Serum tumor markers

SX Not available or not performed.

S0 All markers normal.

S1 LDH less than 1.5 times normal, hCG less than 5000, and AFP less than 1000

S2 LDH 1.5–10 times normal or hCG 5000–50,000 or AFP 1000–10,000.

S3 LDH more than 10 times normal or hCG more than >50,000 or AFP more than 10,000.

continued

Table 1B.36A. TNM and Surgical Staging Systems for Testicular Cancer *continued*

Surgical Staging[b]

Stage

I   Testicular cancer is limited to the testis. Invasion of the scrotal wall by tumor or interruption of the scrotal wall by previous surgery does not change the stage but does increase the risk of spread to the inguinal lymph nodes, and this must be considered in treatment and follow-up. Invasion of the epididymis tunica albuginea and/or the spermatic cord also does not change the stage but does increase the risk of retroperitoneal nodal involvement and the risk of recurrence. Stage I corresponds to AJCC stages I and II.

II Testicular cancer involves the testis and the retroperitoneal or para-aortic lymph nodes, usually in the region of the kidney. Retroperitoneal involvement should be further characterized by the number of nodes involved and the size of involved nodes. The risk of recurrence is increased if more than five nodes are involved, if one or more involved nodes is larger than 2 cm, or if there is extranodal fat involvement. Bulky stage II disease describes patients with extensive retroperitoneal nodes (>5 cm) who require primary chemotherapy and who have a less favorable prognosis. Stage II corresponds to AJCC stages III and IV (no distant metastasis).

III Spread beyond the retroperitoneal nodes revealed by physical examination, radiographs, and/or blood tests. In nonbulky stage III metastases are limited to lymph nodes and lung with no mass larger than 2 cm in diameter. Bulky stage III includes extensive retroperitoneal nodal involvement plus lung nodules or spread to other organs such as liver or brain. Stage III corresponds to AJCC stage IV (distant metastasis).

[a]*The extent of primary tumor is classified after radical orchiectomy.*
[b]*In addition to the clinical stage definitions, surgical stage may be designated according to the results of surgical removal and microscopic examination of tissue.*

Germ cell tumors in general produce tumor markers. These can be used to aid diagnosis, for staging, for prognosis, and for follow-up of the patient. α-Fetoprotein (AFP) has a half-life of 5 to 7 days. It is produced by pure embryonal carcinoma, terato-carcinoma, yolk sac tumor, or combined tumors but not by seminoma. It is elevated in 80% of nonseminomas. In seminomas an elevation, seen in 10% of patients, is believed to indicate an unidentified area of nonseminoma. It is recommended that those patients be treated similarly to patients with the same stage of nonseminoma. Human chorionic gonadotropin (HCG) is elevated in both seminoma and nonseminomas. The serum half-life is 18 to 36 hours. Lactic dehydrogenase (LDH) has independent prognostic significance and correlates with tumor burden, growth rate, proliferation, and death.

Table 1B.36B. AJCC Stage Groupings for Testicular Cancer

Stage	Tumor	Nodes	Metastasis	Serum Markers
0	Tis	N0	M0	S0
IA	pT1	N0	M0	S0
IB	pT2–4	N0	M0	S0
IS	Any pT	N0	M0	S1–3
II	Any pT	N1–3	M0	SX
IIA	Any pT	N1	M0	S0–1
IIB	Any pT	N2	M0	S0–1
IIC	Any pT	N3	M0	S0–1
III	Any pT	Any N	M1	SX
IIIA	Any pT	Any N	M1a	S0–1
IIIB	Any pT	N1–3	M0	S2
	Any pT	Any N	M1a	S2
IIIC	Any pT	N1–3	M0	S3
	Any pT	Any N	M1a	S3
	Any pT	Any N	M1b	Any S

HISTOLOGY

Overall, non-seminoma is the most common histologic type, although it is rarely seen in patients under 10 or over 60 years of age. Nonseminomas consist of pure embryonal carcinoma, teratocarcinoma, yolk sac tumor, choriocarcinoma, or combined tumors. Nonseminomas may have areas of seminoma, although the reverse does not hold true.

TREATMENT

For all patients with gonadal disease, the initial diagnostic and therapeutic treatment should be a radical inguinal orchiectomy. The initial route of metastasis is to the retroperitoneal lymph nodes, so imaging and treating this area is important.

SEMINOMA
STAGE I SEMINOMA

Seminomas are highly sensitive to radiation therapy, which is the primary treatment for early-stage disease. Infradiaphragmatic radiation therapy to the retroperitoneal lymph nodes to a dose of 2500 to 3000 Gy results in 98% 5-year survival. The ipsilateral hemiscrotum does not require radiation therapy unless gross tumor spillage occurs.

Observation has also been investigated as an alternative to radiation in part because of the increased risk of gastrointestinal malignancies after radiation therapy. The relapse rate, which is about 15%, occurs usually later than in nonseminomatous germ cell tumors. It can even occur past 5 years from the time of original diagnosis. Observation is not usually recommended.

STAGE II SEMINOMA

For patients with nonbulky (less than 5 cm) lymphadenopathy, radiation therapy should be given as it would be for stage 1 disease, with a boost of 500 to 750 Gy to the involved lymph nodes. Relapse rates range from 5 to 15%, and death is rare. Exceptions to radiation therapy for seminoma include horseshoe kidney, which is associated with an increased risk of radiation-induced renal failure. Observation for stage 1 and chemotherapy for stage 2 disease are indicated for patients with horseshoe kidney. Inflammatory bowel disease also may be a contraindication to radiation. Patients with bulky or extensive lymphadenopathy should be treated with chemotherapy. Cisplatin-based chemotherapy will cure 70 to 90% of these patients.

NONSEMINOMA

STAGE I NONSEMINOMA

Retroperitoneal lymph node dissection (RPLND) is the most common treatment. The number of lymph nodes removed has important therapeutic implications. If fewer than 6 nodes are removed, the risk of recurrence is up to 35%. Current imaging studies used to stage patients clinically underestimate lymph node involvement in 15 to 40% of cases; hence the importance of RPLND from a diagnostic and therapeutic standpoint. Teratoma is also missed by CT in up to 20% of patients. RPLND is curative in 98% and is associated with less than 1% mortality. In-field recurrences can occur in up to 10%; chemotherapy cures 98% of these patients. Infertility secondary to retrograde ejaculation may occur but has been reduced by the use of a modified procedure. Patients with N1 disease are cured by RPLND in 65% of cases with no adjuvant chemotherapy. The addition of two cycles of adjuvant chemotherapy with BEP (bleomycin, etoposide, cisplatin) reduces recurrence below 2%.

Surveillance is an alternative approach for managing the patient with clinical stage I disease. Most patients with stage I disease have pathologic negative lymph nodes at the time of RPLND. Physical examination, chest radiography, and tumor markers should be obtained monthly for the first year, every 2 months for the second year, and every 3 to 6 months thereafter. CT scans should be performed every 2 to 3 months for 2 years and every 6 months thereafter. Surveillance should be continued for at least 5 years. Treatment for relapsed disease is effective if started early. Patients with advanced disease at relapse fare worse. Therefore, patients with poor compliance should be considered for RPLND. Overall, 28% relapse. Of these, 95% enter remission with chemotherapy. Overall, with close observation and treatment at first relapse, there is a cure rate above 99%, similar to the results obtained with RPLND.

Chemotherapy as initial therapy has been investigated in a very small number of patients. Three reports of two cycles of cisplatin-based chemotherapy results in less than 5% recurrence and a 99% cure rate. Patients with prolonged elevations of HCG and AFP after orchiectomy have metastatic disease and should receive initial chemotherapy.

STAGE II NONSEMINOMA

For patients who initially have suprahilar, retrocrural, bilateral retroperitoneal, or contralateral retroperitoneal disease on CT, the risk of metastatic disease is high enough to warrant initial treatment with chemotherapy. Most patients with stage IIa disease undergo RPLND. Surveillance after RPLND is preferred in patients with fewer than 6 nodes involved and no disease over 2 cm. In patients with more than 6 nodes or tumor larger than 2 cm, adjuvant chemotherapy with two cycles of cisplatin-based chemotherapy is generally recommended. Cure rates above 99% are reported with adjuvant chemotherapy.

FOLLOW-UP

Physical examination, chest radiography, and tumor markers should be obtained monthly for the first year, every 2 months for the second year, and every 3 to 6 months thereafter. CT should be performed every 2 to 3 months for the first 2 years and every 6 months thereafter. Surveillance should be continued for at least 5 years. Half of relapses occur in 6 months, 80% by 12 months, and the vast majority by 24 months. However, follow-up to detect late relapses should continue at least 5 to 10 years.

METASTATIC DISEASE

Chemotherapy is the treatment of choice. Between 1974 and 1981, 201 patients were treated on three trials of PVB (cisplatin, vinblastine, bleomycin) chemotherapy. Of these, 74% are alive and considered cured. The Southeastern Cancer Study Group compared PVB with BEP. Chemotherapy with BEP demonstrated an improved response rate, improved survival in patients with advanced disease, and a significant reduction in the neuromuscular toxicity associated with PVB chemotherapy. BEP is the treatment of choice in most institutions.

Table 1B.37. Metastatic Testicular Cancer

	Nonseminoma			Seminoma
	Good Prognosis	Intermediate Prognosis	Poor Prognosis	
Extrapulmonary metastasis	No	No	Yes	If present, DFS 57% and OS 72%
Primary tumor site	Testis or retroperitoneum	Testis or retroperitoneum	Mediastinal	Any
AFP	<1000	1000–10,000	>10,000	Any
HCG	<5000	5000–50,000	>50,000	Any
LDH	<1.5 × norm	1.5–10 × norm	>10 × norm	Any
Progression-free survival 5 years	89%	75%	41%	82%
Overall survival 5 years	92%	80%	48%	86%
Treatment	EP × 4 or BEP × 3 or VAB-6 × 4	EP × 4 or BEP × 3 or VAB-6 × 4	BEP × 4	Same as nonseminoma with same characteristics

AFP, alpha-feto protein; BEP, Bleomycin, Etoposide, Cisplatin; EP, Etoposide, Cisplatin; HCG, human chorionic gonadotropin; LDN, Lactic dehydrogenase; VAB-6, Vinblastine, Dactinomycin, Bleomycin, Cisplatin, Cyclophosphamide.

Overall there is an 80% cure rate. Failures usually occur in the first 2 years. Late relapse carries a poor prognosis. Treatment planning is based on several prognostic factors and is outlined in Table 1B.37.

For the patient with metastatic disease and good to intermediate risk, etoposide plus cisplatin (EP) administered in four cycles was found to be equivalent to four cycles of VAB-6 (Vinblastine, Dactinomycin, Bleomycin, Cisplatin, Cyclophosphamide). Alternatively, three cycles of BEP was found to be equivalent to four cycles. However, three cycles of EP was inferior to three cycles of BEP. In testicular cancer carboplatin produces inferior response to cisplatin. For patients with poor prognosis, four cycles of BEP appears to be the optimal management.

RESIDUAL MASSES AFTER CHEMOTHERAPY

If residual masses are present after chemotherapy and tumor markers are normal, resection should be performed. About 10% of residual masses are malignant. An additional two cycles of chemotherapy are recommended, or consider salvage chemotherapy. Overall, 70 to 90% are ultimately be cured, 45% have fibrosis, and 45% have teratoma.

RELAPSE OR PRIMARY REFRACTORY DISEASE

VeIP (Vinblastine, Ifosphamide, Cisplatin) or VIP (Etoposide, Ifosphamide, Cisplatin) is the usual standard-dose salvage therapy. Between 25 and 45% of patients obtain a complete response, and 15 to 27% remain in durable remission. Autologous stem cell transplantation and high dose chemotherapy may cure an additional 15 to 25%. Transplantation as initial salvage therapy remains investigational, although preliminary data suggest a higher cure rate. If a solitary resectable lesion is chemotherapy resistant with an elevated AFP, surgical resection is indicated. Cure occurs in 20%.

BIBILOGRAPHY

Bosl GJ, Bajorin DF, Sheinfeld J, Motzer RJ. Cancer of the testis. In: DeVita VT, Hellman S, Rosenberg SA, eds. Cancer: principles & practice of oncology. 5th ed. Philadelphia: Lippincott-Raven, 1997;1253–1395.

Brockstein BE, Vogelzang NJ. Chemotherapy of genitourinary cancer. In: Perry MC, ed. The chemotherapy source book. 2nd ed. Baltimore: Williams & Wilkins, 1997;1222–1229.

Landis SH, Murray T, Bolden S, Wingo PA. Cancer statistics 1998. CA Cancer J Clin 1998;48:6–29.

Nichols CR, Timmerman R, Foster RS, et al. Neoplasms of the testis. In: Cancer medicine. 4th ed. Holland JF, Frei E, Bast RC, et al., eds. Baltimore: Williams & Wilkins, 1997;2177–2214.

Testicular cancer. PDQ treatment for health professionals. National Cancer Institute. http://cancernet.nci.nih.gov/clinpdq/soa/Testicular_cancer_Physician .html#3; 1/18/98.

Cervical Cancer

Victoria J. Dorr

INCIDENCE

There were approximately 13,700 new cases of invasive cancer of the cervix and 4900 deaths from it in the United States in 1998. The prognosis for this disease is affected by the extent of disease at the time of diagnosis. Pap smears should detect more than 90% of these cases. Thus, the current death rate is far higher than it should be, reflecting that even today, Pap smears are not done on approximately one-third of women. Death rates from cervical cancer have declined since the 1930s. In many third world countries cervical cancer is the leading cause of cancer death in women.

ETIOLOGY

Squamous cell carcinoma of the cervix follows a pattern of transmission similar to that of a sexually transmitted disease. The risk of cervical cancer is high in prostitutes and in women with first coitus at a young age, with multiple sex partners, with sexually transmitted diseases, and in women with first pregnancy at a young age. Promiscuous male sexual partners also appear to be a risk factor. Other risk factors include cigarette smoking, human immunodeficiency virus (HIV), vitamin A and C deficiency, and possibly oral contraceptive use. Human papillomavirus (HPV) subtypes 16, 18, 31, 32, and 52 are believed to be responsible for more than 90% of cervical cancers and cervical intraepithelial neoplasia (CIN). HPV-18 has been associated with poorly differentiated carcinomas and adenocarcinoma, an increased incidence of lymph node involvement, and a high rate of disease recurrence; HPV-16 has been associated with large cell keratinizing tumors and a lower recurrence rate. HPV types 6 and 11 carry a low risk of carcinogenesis and are primarily associated with condyloma. Other viruses may also play a role; herpes simplex virus and Epstein-Barr virus are also being investigated as cancer promoters in cervical cancer. Cervical cancer occurs in up to 40% of women affected with the HIV virus.

SCREENING AND DIAGNOSIS

Annual pelvic examination with Pap smear beginning at age 18 years or with the onset of sexual activity is recommended. After three or more consecutive normal annual examinations, the cytologic evaluation can be performed less frequently at the discretion of the physician. The false-negative rate of the Pap smear is 10 to 15%. Several premalignant conditions that are identified are presented in Table 1B.38. Generally, patients with class I or II Pap smears should have a repeat smear after appropriate treatment as clinically indicated. Patients with stage III, IV, or V disease should undergo colposcopy and biopsy.

SIGNS AND SYMPTOMS

Early invasive disease is usually asymptomatic. As cervical cancer progresses, abnormal vaginal bleeding may occur, particularly after coitus. A foul-smelling discharge may also be reported. As the disease progresses, pelvic pain may occur. Advanced cases may involve the bladder, with hematuria and vaginal urinary leakage.

STAGING

More than 90% of cervical cancer is squamous cell type, with the remainder primarily adenocarcinoma; rarely adenosquamous and small cell disease may occur. After a diagnosis of malignancy is made, standard laboratory studies should include complete blood count and renal and liver function tests. All patients should have a chest radiograph to rule out lung metastases and an intravenous pyelogram to determine the kidneys' location and to rule out ureteral obstruction by tumor. Cystoscopy

Table 1B.38. Premalignant Conditions of Cervical Cancer

Bethesda System	Dysplasia/CIN System	Papanicolaou System
Within normal limits	Normal	Class I
Infection	Inflammatory atypia	Class II
Squamous cell abnormalities		
Atypical squamous cells of undetermined significance (ASCUS)	Squamous atypia	Class IIR
Low-grade squamous intraepithelial lesion	HPV atypia	Class II R
Low-grade quamous intraepithelial lesion	Mild dysplasia	Class III CIN 1
High-grade squamous intraepithelial lesion	Moderate dysplasia	Class III CIN 2
High-grade squamous intraepithelial lesion	Severe dysplasia	Class III CIN 3
High-grade squamous intraepithelial lesion	Carcinoma in situ	Class IV
Invasive squamous carcinoma	Invasive squamous carcinoma	Class V

CIN, *cervical intraepithelial neoplasia.*

and proctoscopy or barium enema should be obtained in patients with bulky tumors. CT and MRI have been evaluated as an alternative to lymph node dissection, but they are considered inferior to surgical staging, as small tumors may be missed and lymph nodes may be enlarged because of infection. However, there is little evidence to demonstrate overall improved survival with routine surgical staging, and it usually should be performed only as part of a clinical trial. Pretreatment surgical staging in bulky but locally curable disease may be indicated in select cases when a nonsurgical search for metastatic disease is negative. If abnormal nodes are detected by CT or lymphangiography, fine-needle aspiration should be negative before a surgical staging is performed. Table 1B.39 demonstrates the likelihood of lymph node involvement of each International Federation of Gynecology and Obstetrics (FIGO) stage. The FIGO and TNM classification systems for cervical cancer are listed in Table 1B.40.

TREATMENT

PREINVASIVE DISEASE

Patients with noninvasive squamous lesions can be treated with superficial ablative therapy (cryosurgery or laser therapy) or with loop excision. During pregnancy, no therapy is warranted for preinvasive lesions of the cervix, including carcinoma in situ, although colposcopy is recommended to exclude invasive cancer. All of these procedures preserve fertility in the woman. Recurrence rates are low (10 to 15%), and progression to invasive cervical cancer occurs in fewer than 2%; however, these women should be followed up lifelong.

MICROINVASIVE DISEASE (STAGE IA)

For patients with less than 3 mm invasion there is no risk of lymph node involvement. These patients are usually managed with cervical conization or vaginal hysterectomy. Oophorectomy does not have to be performed in premenopausal women. These patients have a 95 to 100% 5-year survival. Intracavitary radiation alone may also be used in patients who are not candi-

Table 1B.39. Effect of Stage on Likelihood of Lymph Node Involvement and Survival

FIGO Stage	Pelvic LN + (%)	Aortic LN + (%)	5 year Overall Survival (%)
I	1–20	0–2	85
II	25–35	2–20	60–80
III	50	30	35–45
IV			2–15

Table 1B.40. Staging Systems for Cervical Cancer

TNM System

Primary tumor

Tis	Carcinoma in situ; intraepithelial carcinoma.
T1	The carcinoma is strictly confined to the uterus (extension to the corpus should be disregarded).
T1a	Microinvasive carcinoma (early stromal invasion) diagnosed only by microscopy; all macroscopic disease is T1b. Stromal invasion with a maximal depth of 5 mm measured from the base of the epithelium and a horizontal spread of no more than 7 mm. Vascular space involvement, venous or lymphatic, does not alter classification.
T1a1	Measured stromal invasion less than 3 mm and less than 7 mm in horizontal spread.
T1a2	Measured stromal invasion 3 mm or more and less than 5 mm with a horizontal spread not more than 7 mm.
T1b	Clinically visible lesion confined to the cervix or microscopic lesion larger than T1a2.
T1b1	Clinically visible lesion not more than 4 cm.
T1b2	Clinically visible lesion larger than 4 cm.
T2	The carcinoma extends beyond the uterus but has not extended to the pelvic wall or lower third of vagina.
T2a	No obvious parametrial involvement.
T2b	Obvious parametrial involvement.
T3	Carcinoma extends to the pelvic wall. On rectal examination, there is no cancer-free space between the tumor and the pelvic wall. The tumor involves the lower third of the vagina. All cases of hydronephrosis or nonfunctioning kidney are included unless they are known to be due to another cause.
T3a	Tumor involves lower third of vagina; no extension to pelvic wall.
T3b	Extension to pelvic wall or hydronephrosis or nonfunctioning kidney.
T4	Carcinoma extends beyond the true pelvis or clinically involves the mucosa of the bladder or rectum. A bullous edema as such does not permit a case to be allotted to T4.
T4a	Spread of the growth to adjacent organs.

Regional nodes

NX	Not possible to assess the regional nodes.
N0	No involvement of regional nodes.
N1	Evidence of regional node involvement.

Distant metastasis

MX	Presence of distant metastases cannot be assessed.
M0	No known distant metastasis.
M1	Distant metastasis present.

continued

Table 1B.40. Staging Systems for Cervical Cancer *continued*

FIGO and AJCC Staging

Stage	
0	N0, M0; carcinoma in situ, intraepithelial carcinoma. There is no stromal invasion.
I	T1a, N0, M0; carcinoma strictly confined to the cervix; extension to the corpus does not advance the stage.
IA	Preclinical carcinomas of the cervix; that is, those diagnosed only by microscopy.
IA1	Measured invasion of the stroma no deeper than 3 mm and no wider than 7 mm.
IA2	Measured invasion of stroma greater than 3 mm but no deeper than 5 mm and no wider than 7 mm.
IB	Clinical lesions confined to the cervix or preclinical lesions greater than stage IA.
IB1	Clinical lesions no greater than 4 cm.
IB2	Clinical lesions larger than 4 cm.
II	Carcinoma extends beyond the cervix but has not extended to the pelvic wall. The carcinoma involves the vagina but not as far as the lower third.
IIA	T2a, N0, M0; no obvious parametrial involvement, upper two thirds of vagina involved.
IIB	T2b, N0, M0; obvious parametrial involvement but not to pelvic sidewall.
III	Either the carcinoma extends to the pelvic wall or the tumor involves the lower third of the vagina. All cases of hydronephrosis or nonfunctioning kidney are included unless hydronephrosis is known to be due to another cause.
IIIA	T3a, N0, M0; no extension to the pelvic wall; tumor extends to the lower third of the vagina.
IIIB	T1–3, N1, M0; extension to the pelvic wall or hydronephrosis or nonfunctioning kidney. T3b, N0–N1, M0.
IV	Carcinoma extends beyond the true pelvis or clinically involves the mucosa of the bladder or rectum. Bullous edema of the bladder as such does not permit a case to be allotted to stage IV.
IVA	T4a, NX–N1, M0; spread of the growth to adjacent organs (positive biopsies from either bladder or rectum).
IVB	Spread to distant organs; any T, any N, M1.

dates for surgery. For patients with 3 to 5 mm of invasion, the risk of lymph node involvement is 3 to 5%. Radical hysterectomy is usually recommended.

STAGES IB AND IIA

Either radical hysterectomy with bilateral pelvic lymphadenectomy or radiation therapy is the recommended treatment.

With this treatment 5-year survival is 80 to 90% for stage IB and 75 to 80% with stage IIA. External beam pelvic irradiation is usually combined with two or more intracavitary applications based on reports indicating improved outcome with two intracavitary implants rather than one. Radiation to para-aortic nodes may be indicated in primaries 4 cm or larger. For patients with adenocarcinomas larger than 3 cm, radiation therapy is the preferred treatment.

If the patient is found to have nodal involvement at the time of surgery, an attempt at resection of gross disease should be made. Resection of gross disease may improve response rates seen with postoperative radiation. Radiation therapy with extended fields to include the para-aortic lymph nodes is usually recommended postoperatively in patients with nodal involvement, although no survival advantage has been seen to date.

STAGE IIB

The preferred treatment is external beam irradiation with two or more intracavitary applications. These patients are expected to have a 50 to 60% 5-year survival. The resection of macroscopically involved pelvic nodes may improve rates of local control with postoperative radiation therapy. Treatment of unresected periaortic nodes with extended field radiation leads to long-term disease control in patients with low volume (less than 2 cm) nodal disease below L3. One study showed a survival advantage in patients who received radiation to para-aortic nodes without histologic evidence of disease.

Adjuvant chemotherapy with hydroxyurea or cisplatin 5-FU has been investigated. The hydroxyurea is given as 80 mg/kg orally twice weekly concurrently with radiation. Combined therapy resulted in an improved response, improved progression-free survival, and improved overall survival. The results with cisplatin and 5-FU were similar, but with increased toxicity.

STAGES IIIA AND IIIB

Treatment is radiation therapy with a chemotherapy sensitizer (hydroxyurea) similar to that of stage IIB. These patients have a 30 to 40% 5-year survival.

STAGE IVA

The treatment for Stage IVA disease is radiation therapy with adjuvant hydroxyurea. Where disease does not extend deeply into the parametrial areas, anterior or posterior exoneration may be advised under certain circumstances.

STAGE IVB

There is no standard chemotherapy treatment for patients with stage IVB cervical cancer that provides substantial palliation. Radiation therapy or local surgery may be used for palliation of locally symptomatic disease. The efficacy of several chemotherapy regimens are listed below. In general, combination chemotherapy demonstrates better response rates than treatment with single agents, although this has not resulted in a survival advantage. Few patients with metastatic disease have long-term survival. Only one of the agents tested to date, cisplatin, has activity in non–squamous cell carcinoma (20% response rate.) Tested drugs include the following:

- Cisplatin (15 to 25% response rate)
- Ifosfamide (31% response rate)
- Paclitaxel (17% response rate)
- Chlorambucil (25% response rate)
- Doxorubicin (17% response rate)
- CPT-11 (24% response rate)
- Docetaxel (14% response rate)
- Ifosfamide- and cisplatin-based combination therapy (50 to 62% response rate)
- Cisplatin plus 5-FU (15 to 60% response rate)
- Bleomycin plus cisplatin and ifosfamide (65 to 100%)
- Irinotecan (21% response rate in patients previously treated with chemotherapy)

Bibilography

Cervical cancer. PDQ Treatment for Health Professionals. National Cancer Institute. http://cancernet.nci.nih.gov/clinpdq/soa/Cervical_cancer_Physician-.html; 1/18/98.

Eifel PJ, Berek JS, Thigpen JT. Cancer of the cervix, vagina and vulva. In: De-Vita VT, Hellman S, Rosenberg SA, eds. Cancer: principles & practice of oncology. 5th ed. Philadelphia: Lippincott-Raven, 1997;1427–1539.

Landis SH, Murray T, Bolden S, Wingo PA. Cancer statistics 1998. CA Cancer J Clin 1998;48:6–29.

Thigpen JT. Chemotherapy of gynecologic cancer. In: Perry MC, ed. The chemotherapy source book. 2nd ed. Baltimore: Williams & Wilkins, 1997;1260–1268.

Wharton JT. Neoplasms of the cervix. In: Cancer medicine. 4th ed. Holland JF, Frei E, Bast RC, et al., eds. Baltimore: Williams & Wilkins, 1997;2227–2262.

Endometrial Cancer

Victoria J. Dorr

Endometrial cancer is the most prevalent gynecologic malignancy. In 1998 there were approximately 36,100 new cases of endometrial cancer and 6300 deaths resulting from it. It is a highly curable tumor.

ETIOLOGY AND RISK FACTORS

Obesity is associated with an increased risk of endometrial cancer. Endometrial cancer is also increased in patients with hypertension, diabetes, or a history of colon cancer. Long-term unopposed estrogen use is linked to endometrial cancer. Patients who are nulliparous, anovulatory patients, patients on hormone replacement therapy with estrogen, and the use of tamoxifen are all associated with an increased risk of endometrial cancer. The addition of progesterone to estrogen replacement prevents the increased risk of endometrial cancer associated with estrogen use.

SIGNS AND SYMPTOMS

The most common presenting symptom of endometrial cancer is extramenstrual bleeding. Occasionally patients have pelvic pain or urinary or bowel complaints, but these are usually associated with more advanced disease. Patients on estrogen or tamoxifen with extramenstrual vaginal bleeding should be evaluated.

DIAGNOSIS

A technique that directly samples the endometrial tissue is mandatory to detect endometrial cancer. The Pap smear is not reliable as a screening procedure in endometrial cancer.

STAGING

Surgical staging includes total abdominal hysterectomy and bilateral salpingo-oophorectomy, cytology on peritoneal washings, and lymph node sampling from pelvic and para-aortic lymph nodes. Surgical staging is required to assess the depth of myometrial invasion. Spread to the pelvic and para-aortic nodes is common. Distant metastases most commonly involve the lungs, inguinal and supraclavicular nodes, liver, bones, brain, and vagina.

Endometrioid endometrial histology is the most frequent type seen, in up to 75% of cases. Histology types associated with a worse prognosis include serous papillary adenocarcinoma, clear cell type, undifferentiated tumors, and squamous cell tumors. Other prognostic factors include tumor grade; myometrial, vascular, or lymphatic invasion; positive peritoneal cytology washings; more than eight mitoses per high-powered field; and negative progesterone receptors. Staging for endometrial cancer is shown in Table 1B.41.

TREATMENT

Primary treatment of endometrial cancer is surgery with total abdominal hysterectomy and bilateral salpingo-oophorectomy, cytology on peritoneal washings, and lymph node sampling from pelvic and para-aortic lymph nodes. Surgery with or without radiation therapy is curative for most patients with localized disease. Radiation therapy is the second most effective modality. Intracavitary radiation combined with external beam radiation is used in patients who are inoperable.

STAGE I

Primary therapy for stage I should be surgery. Adjuvant radiation is recommended in stage I endometrial cancer with poor

Table 1B.41. Staging System for Endometrial Cancer

Stage I is carcinoma confined to the corpus uteri.

IA	Tumor limited to endometrium.
IB	Invasion to less than one-half of the myometrium.
IC	Invasion to greater than one-half of the myometrium.

Stage II involves the corpus and the cervix but has not extended outside the uterus.

IIA	Endocervical glandular involvement only.
IIB	Cervical stromal invasion.

Stage III extends outside of the uterus but is confined to the true pelvis.

IIIA	Invades serosa and/or adnexa and/or has positive peritoneal cytology.
IIIB	Vaginal metastases.
IIIC	Metastases to pelvic and/or para-aortic lymph nodes.

Stage IV involves the bladder or bowel mucosa or has metastasized to distant sites.

IVA	Tumor invasion of bladder and/or bowel mucosa.
IVB	Distant metastases, including intra-abdominal and/or inguinal lymph nodes.

Grade

G1	5% or less of a nonsquamous or nonmorular solid growth pattern.
G2	6–50% of a nonsquamous or nonmorular solid growth pattern.
G3	More than 50% of a nonsquamous or nonmorular solid growth pattern.

Most patients with endometrial carcinoma present with stage I disease. The 5-year survival rate for stage 1A is 93.8%; for stage 1B, 95.4%; for stage 1C, 75%; for stage II, 60%; for stage III, 40%; and for stage IV, 5%.

prognostic factors (grade 2 or 3 or myometrial invasion more than 50% in depth). Adjuvant radiation reduces pelvic relapses by 60% and improves overall survival by 12%. Progestational agents have been evaluated as adjuvant therapy in a randomized clinical trial of stage I disease and have not shown any benefit.

STAGE II

Patients with stage II disease should be considered for preoperative external beam radiation followed by surgical resection, particularly in patients with extensive cervical involvement. If surgical resection is performed first, adjuvant irradiation should be administered. Since radiation therapy has been used extensively to treat high-risk endometrial carcinomas for many years, few unselected series of patients treated with surgery alone have been reported. For this reason, the true risk of recurrence in unirradiated patients with high-grade or deeply invasive tumors is unknown, but it is thought to be as high as 25%.

STAGE III

In patients with stage III disease and no extension beyond the ovaries, initial surgery should be considered. This is followed with radiation therapy of the whole abdomen and pelvis in most cases. The 5-year disease-free survival rate is 35 to 60%. In patients with parametrial or sidewall disease, the 5-year disease-free survival is 10 to 15%.

ADJUVANT CHEMOTHERAPY

Cytotoxic chemotherapy has been considered as an adjuvant treatment in certain circumstances. These include patients with stage II tumors, clear cell or papillary serous histology, absence of hormone receptors, a preoperative finding of elevated cancer antigen CA125, and stage I disease with deep myometrial invasion. The only randomized trial failed to demonstrate a benefit with adjuvant therapy.

ADJUVANT HORMONE THERAPY

While adjuvant therapy with progestins seems attractive in theory, unfortunately, in practice no benefit has been found when medroxyprogesterone was used in an adjuvant setting.

ADVANCED OR RECURRENT DISEASE

Patients with local recurrences may be candidates for additional surgery or irradiation. For patients with advanced or recurrent disease, chemotherapy may be used. Single agents with efficacy include cisplatin, carboplatin, doxorubicin, or 5-FU.

Response rates of 20 to 30% are usually seen. Combination chemotherapy appears to be more effective than single agents, offering response rates of 40 to 60%. Hormone therapy with progestational agents can also be considered. An overall response of 34% is expected, with a duration of response of 20 months and an average overall survival of 25 months.

BIBLIOGRAPHY

Endometrial cancer. PDQ Treatment for Health Professionals. National Cancer Institute. http://cancernet.nci.nih.gov/clinpdq/soa/Endometrial_cancer_Physician.html; 1/18/98.

Landis SH, Murray T, Bolden S, Wingo PA. Cancer statistics 1998. CA Cancer J Clin 1998;48:6–29.

Thigpen JT. Chemotherapy of gynecologic cancer. In: Perry MC, ed. The chemotherapy source book. 2nd ed. Baltimore: Williams & Wilkins, 1997; 1253–1288.

Gestational Trophoblastic Tumors

Victoria J. Dorr

INCIDENCE

Gestational trophoblastic tumors (GTT) are made up of four distinct subtypes: molar pregnancy, including complete and partial hydatidiform moles; invasive mole (chorioadenoma destruens); placental trophoblastic tumors; and choriocarcinoma. Hydatidiform mole occurs in 1 in 500 pregnancies when an empty egg is fertilized. An invasive mole occurs in 20% of hydatidiform moles, when the molar pregnancy becomes invasive. Choriocarcinoma can occur with any pregnancy; 50% are associated with molar pregnancies. Placental trophoblastic tumors, which are rare, are derived from intermediate trophoblast cells. They present clinically as nodules in the endometrium and myometrium following removal of a mole.

ETIOLOGY AND RISK FACTORS

Gestational trophoblastic disease can occur after any pregnancy, abortion, or molar pregnancy. Women over age 40 have a fivefold increased risk, and women under 20 also have an increased risk of GTT. Patients with a history of molar pregnancies, lower socioeconomic status, and blood group A in whom the partner is blood group O also have an increased risk. Diets deficient in vitamin A are thought to be a risk factor. HCG (human chorionic gonadotropin) above 100,000 mIU/mL or more, a uterus larger than expected for gestational age, and the presence of theca lutein ovarian cysts larger than 6 cm identifies a woman with a 31% risk of nonmetastatic disease and an 8.8% risk of developing metastatic GTT. Women without these risk factors have only a 3.1% risk of developing invasive disease and a 0.6% risk of developing metastatic disease.

SIGNS AND SYMPTOMS

A molar pregnancy presents with first trimester bleeding in up to 97% of cases and a uterus that is larger than expected for gestational age. On examination fetal heart tones are absent. A lack of body parts is seen on ultrasound. HCG levels tend to be much higher than expected, and hyperemesis is common. Iron deficiency anemia, hyperthyroidism, and toxemia may occur. Rupture of the uterus can occur with invasive moles. In malignant gestational trophoblastic disease, 46% of patients have metastatic disease, primarily of lung (80%), vagina (30%), CNS

(10%), gastrointestinal system, liver, and kidney. Pulmonary hypertension may arise from pulmonary artery occlusion.

DIAGNOSIS

Molar pregnancy is readily diagnosed by ultrasound. After a molar pregnancy the diagnosis of gestational trophoblastic disease is made by following HCG. A persistently elevated HCG strongly suggests GTT. Biopsy of metastatic lesions may be dangerous, as they have a high tendency to bleed.

STAGING

A careful history and physical examination, baseline HCG, chest radiography, and CT of head, chest, abdomen, and pelvis should be performed. Staging for gestational trophoblastic tumors is shown in Table 1B.42. A scoring system is shown in Table 1B. 43.

TREATMENT

MOLAR PREGNANCY

Surgical evacuation is the treatment of choice; usually this is performed via suction curettage. Prophylactic chemotherapy in patients with high-risk disease has been evaluated. Prophylactic methotrexate reduced the risk of subsequent GTT from 47% to 14%. Single-agent actinomycin D had similar results.

GESTATIONAL TROPHOBLASTIC TUMOR OF ALL SUBTYPES

All patients should undergo a staging workup for metastatic disease as described earlier. Surgery is used in all stages as clinical symptoms warrant (e.g., hysterectomy if bleeding, thoracotomy for removal of resistant disease). Placental trophoblastic tumors should be treated primarily with surgery, as they usually resist chemotherapy.

Stage I

Primary therapy for stage I GTT should include hysterectomy with adjuvant single-agent chemotherapy with methotrexate or actinomycin D. In patients with stage I disease who wish to preserve fertility, single-agent chemotherapy alone is a viable alternative. Chemotherapy is expected to induce complete response in 93%. Placental trophoblastic tumor should be treated with hysterectomy, however, because of its poor response to chemotherapy.

Patients with disease-resistant to single-agent chemotherapy should be treated with combination chemotherapy (EMA-CO) or salvage surgical resection. All patient should attain a remission with salvage therapy.

Table 1B.42. Staging System for Gestational Trophoblastic Tumors

AJCC Stage

I	Lesion confined to uterus.
II	Lesion outside uterus but confined to vagina, ovary, tube, broad ligament.
III	Lung metastasis with or without genital tract involvement.
IV	Metastasis to other sites.

TNM Stage

TX	Primary tumor cannot be assessed.
T0	No evidence of primary tumor.
T1	Disease limited to uterus.
T2	Disease outside the uterus but limited to genital structures (ovary, tube, vagina, broad ligament).

Distant Metastasis

M0	No clinical metastasis.
M1a	Lung metastasis.
M1b	All other distant metastasis.

Risk factors

hCG > 100,000 IU/24 hour urine.
Detection of disease more than 6 months from termination of the antecedent pregnancy.

IA	T1, M0, no risk factors.
IB	T1, M0, one risk factor.
IC	T1, M0, two risk factors.
IIA	T2, M0, no risk factors.
IIB	T2, M0, one risk factor.
IIC	T2, M0, two risk factors.
IIIA	Any T, M1a, no risk factors.
IIIB	Any T, M1a, one risk factor.
IIIC	Any T, M1a, two risk factors.
IVA	Any T, M1b, no risk factors.
IVB	Any T, M1b, one risk factor.
IVC	Any T, M1b, two risk factors.

Stages II and III

Patients with stage II and III disease should have their risk calculated according to the scoring system shown in Table 1B.43. Patients at low or intermediate risk (fewer than 8 points) may be treated with single-agent chemotherapy with methotrexate or actinomycin D. Single-agent therapy induces

Table 1B.43. Scoring system for GTT

	Score			
	1	2	3	4
Age (years)	≤39	>39		
Prior pregnancy	Hydatidiform mole	Abortion	Term	
Time from pregnancy to start of chemotherapy (mo)	<4	4–6	7–12	>12
HCG level	<1000	1000–10,000	10,000–100,000	>100,000
ABO blood type		O or A	B or AB	
Largest size (cm)	<3	3–5	>5	
Site of metastasis		Spleen, kidney	GI, liver	Brain
# of metastases		1–3	4–8	>8
Prior chemotherapy			1 Drug	>1 Drug

Total scores: low risk, not more than 4; intermediate risk, 5–7; high risk, 8 or more.

complete response in 80 to 85% of patients. Patients who fail to respond to single-agent chemotherapy should receive combination chemotherapy with EMA-CO (etoposide plus methotrexate, leucovorin, actinomycin D, cyclophosphamide, and vincristine). All patients should be salvageable with combination chemotherapy.

Patients with high-risk disease (more than 8 points) should be treated with EMA-CO initially. Patients with disease resistant to EMA-CO should receive combination chemotherapy with PVB (cisplatin, vinblastine, bleomycin) or EMA-CE.

Stage IV

Patients with stage IV disease should be treated primarily with EMA-CO. Patients with brain metastasis should receive methotrexate at a higher dose of $1 \, \text{g/m}^2$. Whole-brain irradiation should be given concurrently with chemotherapy for brain metastasis. Resistant disease should receive salvage chemotherapy with EMA-CE or PVB. Approximately 75% of patients achieve a remission with this program. Early data suggest that paclitaxel or stem cell transplant with high-dose therapy may also have a role in relapsed or refractory disease.

Follow-up

HCG levels are important after GTT. HCG should return to normal within 8 to 10 weeks; it should be measured weekly until three consecutive negative values are obtained. It should be measured monthly thereafter for at least 6 months in molar pregnancy, for 12 to 18 months in GTT, and for 24 months in patients with brain metastasis. Effective birth control should be used to prevent pregnancy, which may confuse the picture.

BIBLIOGRAPHY

Berkowitz RS, Goldstein DP. Gestational trophoblastic neoplasia. In: Cancer medicine. 4th ed. Holland JF, Frei E, Bast RC, et al., eds. Baltimore: Williams & Wilkins, 1997;2327–2336.

Gestational trophoblastic tumor. PDQ treatment for health professionals. National Cancer http://cancernet.nci.nih.gov/clinpdq/soa/Gestational_trophoblastic_tumor_Physician.html; 1/18/98.

Landis SH, Murray T, Bolden S, Wingo PA. Cancer statistics 1998. CA Cancer J Clin 1998;48:6–29.

Muggia FM, Eifel PJ, Burke TW. Gestational trophoblastic disease. In: DeVita VT, Hellman S, Rosenberg SA, eds. Cancer: principles & practice of oncology. 5th ed. Philadelphia: Lippincott-Raven, 1997;1427–1539.

Thigpen JT. Chemotherapy of gynecologic cancer. In: Perry MC, ed. The chemotherapy source book. 2nd ed. Baltimore: Williams & Wilkins, 1997; 1268–1277.

Ovarian Cancer

Victoria J. Dorr

INCIDENCE

Epithelial carcinoma of the ovary is one of the most common gynecological malignancies and the fourth most frequent cause of cancer death in women, with half of cases occurring in women over age 65. In 1998 there were approximately 24,500 cases and 15,400 deaths due to epithelial ovarian cancer. Any of several types of tumors may affect the ovary. The common epithelial tumors account for 60% of all ovarian neoplasms and for 80 to 90% of ovarian malignancies.

CLASSIFICATION

The epithelial carcinomas include the following cellular classifications:

Serous cystomas

- Serous benign cystadenomas
- Serous cystadenomas with proliferating activity of the epithelial cells and nuclear abnormalities but with no infiltrative destructive growth (low potential or borderline malignancy)
- Serous cystadenocarcinomas

Mucinous cystomas

- Mucinous benign cystadenomas
- Mucinous cystadenomas with proliferating activity of the epithelial cells and nuclear abnormalities but with no infiltrative destructive growth (low potential or borderline malignancy)
- Mucinous cystadenocarcinomas

Endometrioid tumors similar to adenocarcinomas in the endometrium

- Endometrioid benign cysts
- Endometrioid tumors with proliferating activity of the epithelial cells and nuclear abnormalities but with no infiltrative destructive growth (low malignant potential or borderline malignancy)
- Endometrioid adenocarcinomas

Clear cell (mesonephroid) tumors

- Benign clear cell tumors
- Clear cell tumors with proliferating activity of the epithelial cells and nuclear abnormalities but with no infiltrative

destructive growth (low malignant potential or borderline malignancy)
- Clear cell cystadenocarcinomas

Malignant tumors other than those of the common epithelial types are not included with the categories listed here.

ETIOLOGY

Approximately 5 to 10% of ovarian tumors are familial. Most are thought to be secondary to BRCA1 and BRCA2. The risk of hereditary ovarian cancer increases when a first-degree relative has ovarian or breast cancer, particularly when young, or when multiple family members have breast or ovarian cancer. (For a more thorough discussion see the subchapter on breast cancer, discussion of etiology, earlier in this chapter) For patients at increased risk for ovarian carcinoma, prophylactic oophorectomy may be considered after age 35 if childbearing is complete. However, the benefit of prophylactic oophorectomy has not yet been established. A small percentage of women may develop a primary peritoneal carcinoma similar in appearance to ovarian cancer despite prophylactic oophorectomy. A history of endometrial or colon cancer also increases the risk of ovarian carcinoma.

The risk of ovarian carcinoma increases with age. The median age of onset is 58, with a peak at age 75 to 79. Pregnancy is protective, with nulliparous women at a higher risk of ovarian cancer. Patients with North American or European ancestry are at greater risk; the risk of ovarian carcinoma is lower in the African-American and Asian population. The use of oral contraceptives is protective in part (relative risk of 0.75). Fertility drugs are associated with an increased risk of ovarian cancer (relative risk of 2 to 3). Hormone replacement therapy has not been associated with an increased risk of ovarian cancer.

SCREENING

At present routine screening for ovarian carcinoma cannot be recommended. A laparotomy is usually required to evaluate an abnormal screening test result, making false-positives less attractive from a morbidity and cost standpoint. Pelvic examination with ovarian palpation at the time of a Pap smear has not proved useful as a screening test. Transvaginal ultrasound and CA-125 are commonly recommended for screening women at high risk for ovarian carcinoma, although there is little evidence to support their use.

SIGNS AND SYMPTOMS

Unfortunately, epithelial ovarian cancer rarely produces any symptoms until it has progressed, and approximately 70% of cancers are stage III or IV at the time of diagnosis. Conversely, patients with germ cell tumors tend to have pain, and 70% of these patients are diagnosed with stage I disease. Bloating and abdominal discomfort are the most frequent complaints of women with epithelial ovarian cancer. Vaginal bleeding, gastrointestinal symptoms, and urinary symptoms may also occur. Complaints of abdominal pain and bloating should prompt a pelvic examination with rectovaginal examination.

DIAGNOSIS

A palpable adnexal or ovarian mass on pelvic examination should be further evaluated with an endovaginal ultrasound. Masses in a premenarchal girl should be evaluated promptly, as functional cysts do not occur. Characteristics of the adnexal mass on ultrasound help to determine whether additional evaluation is warranted. A CA-125 may be helpful as well. Postmenopausal women with complex pelvic masses, simple cysts in association with elevated serum CA-125 levels, or simple cysts in association with abnormal color Doppler flow studies should undergo prompt surgery. Enlarged ovaries are frequent in the premenopausal woman; in these cases a CA-125 with a cutoff of 65 may be helpful in identifying patients who require additional evaluation. A rising CA-125 also suggests that a malignancy may be present. Serum α-fetoprotein (AFP) and human chorionic gonadotropin (HCG) have been helpful in recognizing preoperatively the presence of an endodermal sinus tumor, embryonal carcinoma, choriocarcinoma, or mixed germ cell tumors.

Preoperative CT of the abdomen and pelvis may be helpful in defining the extent of the tumor and in identifying locally metastatic disease. A chest radiograph should be obtained to rule out metastatic disease.

A suspicious lesion is most commonly evaluated laparoscopically. The risk is in rupturing a malignant tumor. Malignant tumors that are ruptured generally receive adjuvant therapy. If disease appears to be limited to the ovaries or pelvis, it is essential at laparotomy to examine and sample for biopsy the diaphragm, both paracolic gutters, the pelvic peritoneum, para-aortic and pelvic nodes, and infracolic omentum and to obtain peritoneal washings. Understaging occurs frequently at the initial surgery for ovarian malignancies, especially when the preoperative diagnosis is benign process. The simplest solution for such patients is to return the patient for a properly performed staging laparotomy. However, if this is not possible, an alternative is to obtain CT and CA-125. If CT and CA-125 are normal and the tumor has low malignant potential, no further therapy is recommended. If the tumor is an invasive epithelial tumor, adjuvant chemotherapy should be considered. If CT demonstrates residual disease, resection should be attempted.

If ascites is present, paracentesis obtaining fluid for cytology can be diagnostic.

STAGING AND TREATMENT

Staging for ovarian cancer is shown in Table 1B.44. The primary treatment of all stages except IV is surgery. The goal should be optimal cytoreduction to remove all tumor or to debulk to less than 1 cm. Overall, optimal surgery is possible in about 35% of cases. A total abdominal hysterectomy and bilateral salpingo-oophorectomy with omentectomy should accompany adequate surgical staging.

STAGE I

A few patients do not require additional treatment after surgical resection. Patients with stage IA and stage IB with well to moderately differentiated tumors have more than a 90% 5-year survival rate without additional therapy. In selected patients who desire further childbearing and who have grade I tumors, unilateral salpingo-oophorectomy may be used.

The chance of relapse and death from ovarian cancer is up to 20% if the tumor is grade III, densely adherent, or stage IC, although the importance of tumor rupture as the only adverse characteristic is not clear. Adjuvant therapy options in this population include (a) intraperitoneal radioisotopic ^{32}P; (b) total pelvic and abdominal radiation; (c) systemic chemotherapy; or (d) careful observation. Cisplatin- or paclitaxel-based chemotherapy is the usual treatment. Studies comparing one modality with another do not demonstrate a benefit of one treatment over another. Patients with intra-abdominal adhesions are not candidates for ^{32}P therapy. One study comparing ^{32}P with cisplatin did demonstrate an increased rate of complications with ^{32}P.

STAGE II

Surgery (total abdominal hysterectomy, bilateral salpingo-oophorectomy, tumor debulking, and appropriate staging) to remove all or most of the tumor is the initial treatment for stage II disease. Adjuvant therapy with a number of options should then be instituted. Most patients should receive systemic chemotherapy. Total abdominal and pelvic radiation therapy is

Table 1B.44. Staging System for Ovarian Cancer

Stage I is growth limited to the ovaries.

IA   Growth limited to one ovary; no ascites. No tumor on the external surface; capsule intact.

IB   Growth limited to both ovaries; no ascites. No tumor on the external surfaces; capsules intact.

IC   Tumor either stage IA or IB, but with tumor on the surface of one or both ovaries; or with capsule ruptured; or with ascites present containing malignant cells or with positive peritoneal washings.

Stage II is growth involving one or both ovaries with pelvic extension.

IIA   Extension and/or metastases to the uterus and/or tubes. No malignant cells in ascites or peritoneal washing.

IIB   Extension to other pelvic tissues.

IIC   Tumor either stage IIA or stage IIB but with tumor on the surface of one or both ovaries; or with capsule(s) ruptured; or with ascites containing malignant cells or with positive peritoneal washings.

Stage III is tumor involving one or both ovaries with peritoneal implants outside the pelvis and/or positive retroperitoneal or inguinal nodes. Superficial liver metastasis constitutes stage III. Tumor is limited to the true pelvis but with histologically verified malignant extension to small bowel or omentum.

IIIA   Tumor grossly limited to the true pelvis with negative nodes but with histologically confirmed microscopic seeding of abdominal peritoneal surfaces.

IIIB   Tumor of one or both ovaries with histologically confirmed implants of abdominal peritoneal surfaces, none exceeding 2 cm in diameter. Nodes negative.

IIIC   Abdominal implants greater than 2 cm in diameter and/or positive retroperitoneal or inguinal nodes.

Stage IV is growth involving one or both ovaries with distant metastasis. If pleural effusion is present, there must be positive cytology findings. Parenchymal liver metastasis constitutes stage IV.

Favorable prognostic factors include clear cell histology, clinically occult disease, good performance status, younger age, lower stage, no ascites.

Overall 5-year survival for epithelial ovarian carcinoma is 73% for stage I, 46% for stage II, 19% for stage III, and 5% for stage IV.

an option only if there is minimal residual pelvic disease of less than 0.5 cm and no macroscopic upper abdominal disease.

STAGE III

Surgical debulking is the initial course of action for stage III disease. The goal of surgery should be removal of all lesions with less than 1 cm residual disease. There is considerable evidence that the volume of disease left after surgery correlates with survival. A recent review of current literature showed that patients with optimal cytoreduction had a median survival of 39 months compared with a survival of only 17 months in patients with suboptimal cytoreduction.

Surgery should be followed by chemotherapy. Combination chemotherapy regimens containing cisplatin have been shown to produce higher response rates and in some studies have produced a statistically significant improvement in survival compared with drug regimens without cisplatin. A recent meta-analysis addressing this comparison in 1400 patients reveals a strong trend in favor of platinum-containing combinations with respect to response but not survival. A meta-analysis shows that carboplatin and cisplatin are equivalent in terms of survival. Two additional studies confirm that cisplatin and carboplatin are equivalent and that both are superior to cyclophosphamide in response rates, disease-free survival and overall survival; however, carboplatin is associated with a more favorable toxicity profile than cisplatin.

The Gynecological Oncology Group (GOG) has conducted a randomized phase III clinical trial comparing paclitaxel plus cisplatin (TP) against cyclophosphamide plus cisplatin (CP) in suboptimally debulked (more than 1 cm residual mass) stages III and IV patients who had no prior chemotherapy. There was a statistically significant improvement in response in the TP arm (73%) versus the CP arm (60%). Median survival was also significantly better in the TP arm (24 months versus 38 months; p = .001). There are no data on whether modifications (substitution of carboplatin for cisplatin or alterations in length of infusion time of paclitaxel) to the TP regimen affect the benefit seen with the original.

A second-look laparotomy can be considered after completion of chemotherapy for stage III patients who have CT without residual disease and whose CA-125 is normal. Its use is generally reserved for clinical trials.

STAGE IV

Optimal surgical debulking may be indicated in a select few stage IV patients. Patients with parenchymal liver disease, enlarged retrocrural lymph nodes, supraclavicular lymph nodes, mediastinal metastases, and parenchymal lung metastases are not candidates for optimal cytoreductive surgery. In addition, women who have disease on CT that involves the porta hepatis, suprarenal lymphadenopathy, or omental metastases that extend into the hilum of the spleen usually have such advanced disease at the time of surgery that optimal cytoreduction is virtually impossible. Women with malignant pleural effusion alone can undergo cytoreductive surgery, but its effect on survival is unknown. Chemotherapy is generally given as for stage III disease.

RECURRENT DISEASE

In patients in whom a significant time (5 to 12 months) has passed since chemotherapy and who have responded to chemotherapy with one of the platinum compounds, treatment with cisplatin or carboplatin should be considered. In patients who are platinum refractory (progression while on therapy or relapse shortly after completion of therapy), therapy with drugs that are non–cross-resistant, such as paclitaxel, docetaxel, ifosfamide, hexamethylmelamine, oral etoposide, gemcitabine, topotecan, liposomal doxorubicin, or tamoxifen, should be considered. Participation in clinical trials should also be considered.

BORDERLINE OVARIAN TUMORS

Borderline ovarian tumors account for 15% of ovarian neoplasms. Of these, 90% present as stage I disease, and a single-side oophorectomy can be performed with a 90% cure rate. For patients who present with stage II or III disease, treatment is complete surgical resection. There is no evidence of benefit with adjuvant chemotherapy in this population.

BIBLIOGRAPHY

Berek JS, Thomas GM, Ozols RF. Ovarian cancer. In: Cancer medicine. 4th ed. Holland JF, Frei E, Bast RC, et al., eds. Baltimore: Williams & Wilkins, 1997; 2289–2326.

Landis SH, Murray T, Bolden S, Wingo PA. Cancer statistics 1998. CA Cancer J Clin 1998:48:6–29.

Ovarian epithelial cancer. PDQ treatment for health professionals. National Cancer Institute. http://cancernet.nci.nih.gov/clinpdq/soa/Ovarian_epithelial _cancer_Physician.html; 1/18/98.

Ozols RF, Schwartz PE, Eifel PJ. Ovarian cancer, fallopian tube carcinoma, and peritoneal carcinoma. In: DeVita VT, Hellman S, Rosenberg SA, eds. Cancer: principles & practice of oncology. 5th ed. Philadelphia: Lippincott-Raven, 1997;1427–1539.

Thigpen JT. Chemotherapy of gynecologic cancer. In: Perry MC, ed. The chemotherapy source book. 2nd ed. Baltimore: Williams & Wilkins, 1997; 1268–1277.

Ovarian Germ Cell Tumors

Victoria J. Dorr

INCIDENCE

Germ cell malignancies are made up of dysgerminoma, ter-atoma, endodermal sinus tumor, embryonal carcinoma, poly-embryoma, choriocarcinoma, and mixed forms. Approximately 25% of ovarian tumors have germ cell origin, but only 3% are malignant. In women under age 20 germ cell tumors constitute 70% of tumors, with a third being malignant.

SIGNS AND SYMPTOMS

Symptoms of germ cell tumor may include pelvic fullness or bloating, dysuria or urinary frequency, rectal pressure, or men-strual abnormalities. Acute pain associated with torsion or rup-ture of the adnexa is more common in germ cell tumors than in epithelial ovarian tumors.

DIAGNOSIS

A careful history and physical examination, including a pelvic examination, should be performed. Adnexal masses larger than 2 cm in postmenopausal patients with or larger than 8 cm in premenopausal women should undergo surgical explo-ration. Elevations in AFP and HCG are common. Transvaginal ultrasound may also be useful. A routine complete blood count and chemistry profile, including liver function testing, should be performed, as well as chest radiography. Karyotyping should be performed on all premenarchal girls because of a predisposition for these tumors to arise in dysgenetic gonads.

STAGING

Staging is the same as for ovarian epithelial carcinomas.

TREATMENT

DYSGERMINOMAS

These are the most common germ cell tumors, accounting for 30 to 40% of germ cell tumors. This tumor is analogous to the tes-ticular seminoma in men. The primary treatment is surgical re-section. Surgery should include palpation of retroperitoneal lymph nodes, with biopsy if enlarged, and peritoneal washings sent for cytology. The minimum surgery if fertility is desired re-quires unilateral oophorectomy. Dysgerminoma has a tendency to be bilateral, so careful evaluation of the opposite ovary must be performed.

Stage IA

For state IA disease surgery alone with careful observation is a treatment option, with additional therapy withheld until progression. Results similar to that of initial adjuvant therapy can be obtained by salvage irradiation or surgical excision. Approximately 5 to 15% of patients develop recurrence over 2 to 3 years.

Stages IB, II, III, and IV

Patients with stage IB disease may be candidates for bilateral oophorectomy with uterus preservation to preserve the chance that a woman may be able to carry a pregnancy later. For all other patients the treatment is primary surgery followed by radiation therapy. Patients with advanced disease may be treated with chemotherapy regimens similar to those used in testicular germ cell tumors (BEP, PVB, or doxorubicin plus cyclophosphamide). Ovarian germ cell tumors appear to be more chemotherapy sensitive than the testicular germ cell tumors.

IMMATURE TERATOMAS AND ENDODERMAL SINUS TUMORS

Primary surgery is performed as it would be for a dysgerminoma. Bilateral disease is rare. Cisplatin-based chemotherapy should be used for any patient with stage IA grade 2 or 3 disease and for stage II, III, or IV disease. The most commonly used regimens are VAC and BEP. While no comparative studies are complete, BEP chemotherapy appears to have a superior response.

BIBLIOGRAPHY

Berek JS, Thomas GM, Ozols RF. Ovarian cancer. In: Cancer medicine. 4th ed. Holland JF, Frei E, Bast RC, et al., eds. Baltimore: Williams & Wilkins, 1997; 2289–2326.

Landis SH, Murray T, Bolden S, Wingo PA. Cancer statistics 1998. CA Cancer J Clin 1998;48:6–29.

Ovarian germ cell tumor. PDQ Treatment for Health Professionals. National Cancer Institute. http://cancernet.nci.nih.gov/clinpdq/soa/Ovarian_germ_cell_tumor_Physician.html; 1/18/98.

Ozols RF, Schwartz PE, Eifel PJ. Ovarian cancer, fallopian tube carcinoma, and peritoneal carcinoma. In: DeVita VT, Hellman S, Rosenberg SA, eds. Cancer: principles & practice of oncology. 5th ed. Philadelphia: Lippincott-Raven, 1997; 1427–1539.

Thigpen JT. Chemotherapy of gynecologic cancer. In: Perry MC, ed. The chemotherapy source book. 2nd ed. Baltimore: Williams & Wilkins, 1997;1268–1277.

Adult Soft Tissue Sarcomas

John D. Wilkes

BACKGROUND

Adult soft tissue sarcomas are uncommon and histologically diverse malignant tumors that may arise at any anatomic location. If approached correctly, many of these tumors are curable, although the identification of optimal treatments has been hampered by the rarity and diversity of these tumors. This chapter reviews the general management of adult soft tissue sarcomas with emphasis on the role of chemotherapy. Pediatric sarcomas (osteogenic, primitive neuroectodermal tumor, Ewing's, and rhabdomyosarcomas) and Kaposi's sarcoma are reviewed elsewhere in this textbook.

EPIDEMIOLOGY

It is estimated that 7600 new diagnoses of soft tissue sarcoma occurred in 1998 in the United States, with approximately 4300 deaths. Soft tissue sarcomas account for only about 1% of all cancer diagnoses in this country. While soft tissue sarcomas may occur at any age, slightly more than 50% are diagnosed in adults over 50 years of age. There is also a slight male predominance.

ETIOLOGY

The precise causation of adult soft tissue sarcomas is unknown. A variety of occupational and therapeutic exposures (polyvinyl chloride, Thorotrast, arsenic, herbicides, chlorophenols, radiation, alkylating agents) have been implicated in the minority of sarcomas. Chronic immunosuppression (AIDS, allogeneic organ transplantation) and inflammatory conditions (Paget's disease, postmastectomy lymphedema, trauma) may also give rise to soft tissue and bone sarcomas. Finally, inherited conditions such as the Li-Fraumeni syndrome, neurofibromatosis, and hereditary retinoblastoma are associated with a significant increase in the incidence of soft tissue sarcomas.

CLINICAL MANIFESTATIONS

The clinical manifestations of adult sarcomas depend largely on the anatomic location of the tumor. Most sarcomas present as a palpable mass on an extremity or the trunk. Retroperitoneal sarcomas, which account for approximately 15% of diagnoses, usually present with abdominal or back pain and a palpable mass.

In general, low-grade tumors tend to recur locally, with

approximately 50% transforming to higher-grade lesions. High-grade lesions often fail at distant sites, with the lungs being the most frequent location of metastatic disease. Bone or soft tissue metastases occur less frequently. Lymph node and brain metastases are uncommon.

STAGING EVALUATION

The diagnosis and staging of sarcomas is often challenging and must be individualized to the patient. After taking a careful history and performing a physical examination with attention to the location of the tumor mass and its relation to vascular and neurologic structures, diagnostic imaging should be obtained. Depending on the clinical presentation, plain radiographs, CT, MRI (exceptionally useful for extremity sarcomas), and nuclear medicine imaging studies all may provide useful information. A carefully planned biopsy is important. Since treatment is determined, to some extent, by the histology of the tumor, it is essential to have a careful pathologic review by an experienced histopathologist. Routine microscopy, immunohistochemistry, electron microscopy, and/or cytogenetic evaluations may be required to establish the diagnosis. Unfortunately, the histologic diagnosis of soft tissue sarcomas is highly subjective, and concordance between experienced pathologists is only about 66%.

The stage of a soft tissue sarcoma is determined by the histologic grade, size of the tumor, lymph node involvement, and distant metastases (GTNM system). Staging for adult soft tissue sarcomas is shown in Table 1B.45.

PROGNOSIS

The prognosis for adult soft tissue sarcomas depends on several factors, including the patient's age and the size, histologic grade, and stage of the tumor. In general, the factors that predict local recurrence (age above 50 years, microscopic positive margin, fibrosarcoma or peripheral nerve tumor histologies) are different from those associated with distant recurrence (size larger than 5 cm, high-grade histology, deep location, leiomyosarcoma, nonliposarcomas).

TREATMENTS

PRIMARY THERAPY

Many adult soft tissue sarcomas are curable at the time of diagnosis. The choice of treatment depends significantly on the location of the primary tumor and its relation to other structures. Complete staging and treatment planning by a multidisciplinary team of cancer specialists is required to determine optimal treatment for patients with soft tissue sarcoma. For stage I soft tissue

Table 1B.45A. Staging System for Adult Soft Tissue Sarcomas

Tumor grade

GX	Grade cannot be assessed.
G1	Well differentiated.
G2	Moderately well differentiated.
G3	Poorly differentiated.
G4	Undifferentiated.

Primary tumor

TX	Primary tumor cannot be assessed.
T0	No evidence of primary tumor.
T1	Tumor 5 cm or less in greatest dimension.
T1a	Superficial tumor.
T1b	Deep tumor.
T2	Tumor more than 5 cm in greatest dimension.
T2a	Superficial tumor.
T2b	Deep tumor.

Nodes

NX	Regional lymph nodes cannot be assessed.
N0	No regional lymph node metastasis.
N1	Regional lymph node metastasis.

Distant metastasis

MX	Presence of distant metastasis cannot be assessed.
M0	No distant metastasis.
M1	Distant metastasis.

Table 1B.45B. Stage Grouping for Adult Soft Tissue Sarcomas

Stage	Grade	Tumor	Nodes	Metastasis
IA	G1,G2	T1a/b	N0	M0
IB	G1,G2	T2a	N0	M0
IIA	G1,G2	T2b	N0	M0
IIB	G3,G4	T1a/b	N0	M0
IIC	G3,G4	T2a	N0	M0
III	G3,G4	T2b	N0	M0
IV	Any G	Any T	N1	M0
	Any G	Any T	N0	M1

Adapted with permission from American Joint Committee on Cancer. Cancer staging manual. 5th ed. Philadelphia: Lippincott-Raven, 1997.

sarcomas at most anatomic sites, complete surgical resection with 2-cm negative tissue margins is the treatment of choice. For patients who cannot be completely operated with adequate margins, radiation therapy may decrease the local recurrence rate.

EXTREMITY SARCOMAS

For select patients with sarcomas of the extremities, either pre-operative or postoperative radiation and limb-sparing surgery have become standard. The 5-year survival rates are comparable with those achieved with more radical surgical procedures. Low-grade sarcomas are often cured with aggressive surgery alone. Higher-grade sarcomas are associated with increased local and distant treatment failure. These patients may be considered for more aggressive approaches incorporating surgery and adjuvant radiation. Regional intra-arterial chemotherapy in conjunction with radiation therapy and limb-sparing surgery has been evaluated for patients with extremity soft tissue sarcoma but remains investigational.

TRUNK, HEAD, AND NECK

Surgery alone can achieve local control of soft tissue sarcomas of the trunk or the head and neck in some adults. Most patient are candidates for adjuvant or neoadjuvant radiation therapy because of close margins, high-grade histology, or possibly significant disfigurement.

RETROPERITONEUM

The prognosis for retroperitoneal sarcomas is less favorable than for other sites because of the advanced stage at presentation and incomplete resectability. Nonetheless, surgical resection, often including adjacent structures or organs, should be attempted and followed by adjuvant radiation therapy.

ADJUVANT CHEMOTHERAPY

The role of adjuvant chemotherapy in adult soft tissue sarcomas remains extremely controversial. Several prospective trials examine the role of adjuvant doxorubicin as a single agent or in combination. Analysis of these prospective trials is complicated by their small sizes, diverse chemotherapy regimens, and variable inclusion criteria. As yet there is no convincing evidence to support the use of adjuvant chemotherapy for soft tissue sarcomas.

METASTATIC DISEASE

Soft tissue sarcomas that have spread to distant sites require special attention. Patients with stage IV disease because of regional lymph node metastases are often best managed with resection of the primary lesion, regional lymphadenectomy, and postoperative radiation therapy. Some 20 to 30% of patients with stage IV soft tissue sarcomas with isolated pulmonary metastases may be curable with aggressive treatment of the primary tumor and resection of the pulmonary metastases.

For patients with stage IV disease who are not candidates for surgical intervention, systemic chemotherapy or radiation may provide palliation. Active chemotherapeutic agents for advanced adult soft tissue sarcomas include doxorubicin, ifosfamide, dacarbazine, methotrexate, and actinomycin D. There appears to be a dose–response relation with doxorubicin, with improved responses seen at doses of 60 to 70 mg/m^2.

Combination regimens such as MAID (doxorubicin, ifosfamide, DTIC, mesna), AI (doxorubicin, ifosfamide), and CYVADIC (cyclophosphamide, vincristine, doxorubicin, dacarbazine) achieve response rates of 30 to 50% but are associated with increased toxicity and have not proved a survival advantage over single-agent doxorubicin. Responses can be achieved in approximately 30% of patients treated with high-dose ifosfamide (10 to 15 gm/m2) after failure of first-line treatments. Newer agents with some promise include docetaxel, edatrexate, and epirubicin. As always, referral to clinical trials evaluating new agents is recommended.

BIBLIOGRAPHY

Geer RJ, Woodruff J, Casper ES, et al. Management of small soft-tissue sarcoma of the extremity in adults. Arch Surg 1992;127:1285–1289.

Karakousis CP, Perez RP. Soft tissue sarcomas in adults. CA Cancer J Clin 1994;44:200–210.

Karakousis CP, Proimakis C, Walsh DL Primary soft tissue sarcoma of the extremities in adults. Br J Surg 1995;82:1208–1212.

Le Doussal V, Coindre JM, Leroux A, et al. Prognostic factors for patients with localized primary malignant fibrous histiocytoma. Cancer 1996;77:1823–1830.

Lewis JJ, Leung D, Heslin M, et al. Association of local recurrence with subsequent survival in extremity soft tissue sarcoma. J Clin Oncol 1997;15:646–652.

Marcove RC, Sheth DS, Healey J, et al. Limb-sparing surgery for extremity sarcoma. Cancer Invest 1994;12:497–504.

Marcus SG, Merino MJ, Glastein E, et al. Long-term outcome in 87 patients with low-grade soft-tissue sarcoma. Arch Surg 1993;128:1336–1343.

Pisters PT, Leung DY, Woodruff J, et al. Analysis of prognostic factors in 1,041 patients with localized soft tissue sarcomas of the extremities. J Clin Oncol 1996;14:1679–1689

Santoro A, Tursz T, Mouridsen H, et al. Doxorubicin versus CYVADIC versus doxorubicin plus ifosfamide in first-line treatment of advanced soft tissue sarcomas: a randomized study of the European Organization for Research and Treatment of Cancer Soft Tissue and Bone Sarcoma Group. J Clin Oncol 1995;13: 1537–1545.

Tierney JF, Mosseri V, Stewart LA, et al. Adjuvant chemotherapy for soft-tissue sarcoma: review and meta-analysis of the published results of randomised clinical trials. Br J Cancer 1995;72:469–475.

van Geel AN, Pastorino U, Jauch KW, et al. Surgical treatment of lung metastases: the European Organization for Research and Treatment of Cancer: Soft Tissue and Bone Sarcoma Group study of 255 patients. Cancer 1996;77:675–682.

Ewing's Sarcoma and Primitive Neuroepithelial Tumors

Victoria J. Dorr

Ewing's sarcoma accounts for 10 to 14% of primarily bone tumors. It is rare in African-Americans. The peak incidence of Ewing's sarcoma occurs between ages 10 and 25. Primitive neuroepithelial tumors (PNETs) have been called by various terms, depending on their location and extent of neural differentiation: peripheral neuroepithelioma, Askin's tumor, adult neuroblastoma, peripheral neuroblastoma, and primitive neuroectodermal tumors. PNETs and Ewing's sarcoma are a biologic spectrum of the same disease. An 11:22 translocation is commonly seen in PNETs and may also be seen in Ewing's sarcoma.

SIGNS AND SYMPTOMS

Patients usually present with fever, weight loss, malaise, poorly localized bone pain, and a rapidly enlarging mass. An elevated sedimentation rate and leukocytosis may occur. The most common sites are the femur (27%), pelvis (18%), and tibia and fibula (17%).

DIAGNOSIS

Plain films show a fusiform enlargement of the long bones with onion skin layering of the periosteum and central mottling cracked ice appearance. CT or MRI may be used to evaluate the local tumor further. CT of the chest should be obtained to look for pulmonary metastases. A bone marrow aspirate and biopsy and a bone scan should also be performed.

STAGING

LOCALIZED DISEASE

Localized Ewing's sarcoma and PNET are defined as not demonstrable by clinical imaging techniques beyond the primary site. The tumor may invade directly into adjacent tissues and still be considered in this category. Actually, most of these patients have microscopic metastatic disease at diagnosis. Among patients with localized tumors, location of the primary site is related to outcome, with the least favorable sites being the pelvis and ribs and the most favorable sites being distal bones.

METASTATIC DISEASE

Metastatic Ewing's sarcoma is defined as a tumor that has distant spread. The sites of metastatic disease are most commonly lung, bone, and bone marrow. Lymph node and in particular central nervous system metastases are less common.

PROGNOSIS

Age is a significant prognostic factor. Survival and recurrence are higher in patients over 10 years of age. An elevated lactose dehydrogenase (LDH) also carries a poor prognosis. Chemotherapy-induced necrosis in the primary tumor has been shown to be a statistically significant prognostic factor for disease-free and overall survival.

TREATMENT

Current therapy results in a 70% cure in children under age 10 with localized disease and 33% in those with metastatic disease at the time of diagnosis. The initial treatment is multiagent chemotherapy. The use of doxorubicin in clinical trials has significantly improved survival. Ifosfamide plus etoposide has shown activity in Ewing's sarcoma and PNET, and a large randomized clinical trial demonstrated that outcome was improved when the ifosfamide plus etoposide combination was given in alternating courses with vincristine, doxorubicin or dactinomycin, and cyclophosphamide.

Radiation therapy to the primary disease in the fifth or sixth cycle of chemotherapy controls local disease in 70% of patients under age 10 years and 46% of patients older than 16 years. Radiation of more than 6000 rad is associated with a higher risk of secondary sarcomas. Recurrence rates remain high locally, so resection may be deemed appropriate where feasible. Although there have been no randomized trials of surgery versus radiation therapy versus surgery plus radiation therapy, survival and disease-free survival have been the same for these treatment modalities. Surgical resection of pulmonary metastases has not proved beneficial in Ewing's sarcoma.

BIBLIOGRAPHY

Ewing's sarcoma/primitive neuroepithelial tumors. PDQ treatment for health professionals. National Cancer Institute. http://cancernet.nci.nih.gov/clinpdq/soa/Ewing's_sarcoma-primitive_neuroepithelial_tumor_Physician.html; 1/18/98.

Raftopoulos H, Antman KH. Chemotherapy of sarcomas of bone and soft tissue. In: Perry MC, ed. The chemotherapy source book. 2nd ed. Baltimore: Williams & Wilkins, 1997;1289–1315.

Neuroblastoma

Victoria J. Dorr

INCIDENCE

Neuroblastoma is the most common extracranial solid tumor in children less than 5 years of age. Two-thirds of these tumors occur before age 5. Neuroblastoma can arise from any site along the sympathetic nervous system. Primarily these tumors occur in the abdomen, although chest and neck are common sites in infants.

SIGNS AND SYMPTOMS

Symptoms attributable to tumor mass are the most common complaints at the time of presentation. Patients may have proptosis, periorbital ecchymoses, spinal cord compression, bone pain, anemia, fever, hypertension, cerebellar ataxia, or severe watery diarrhea. An opsoclonus-myoclonus syndrome usually associated with low-grade disease and a superior survival rate has been reported.

DIAGNOSIS

The diagnosis of neuroblastoma can be difficult. The differential diagnosis includes lymphoma, rhabdomyosarcoma, and PNET. The minimum requirement to diagnose neuroblastoma is one of the following:

1. An unequivocal pathologic diagnosis made from tumor tissue by light microscopy with or without immunohistology, electron microscopy, or increased levels of urine or serum catecholamines or metabolites. Catecholamines and metabolites include dopamine, homovanillic acid (HVA), and/or vanillylmandelic acid (VMA). To be considered increased, at least two of these must have levels greater than three standard deviations above the mean per milligram creatinine for age.
2. Bone marrow aspirate or biopsy must contain unequivocal tumor cells and increased levels of urine or serum catecholamines or metabolites as described earlier.

STAGING

Recommended evaluations for neuroblastoma include a careful history and physical examination; CT of the chest, abdomen, pelvis, and any other site that is clinically involved; bilateral bone marrow aspiration; and biopsy. Bone metastases should be assessed by metaiodobenzylguanidine (MIBG) scan; if the results of the MIBG scan are negative or unavailable, by ^{99}Tc scan (plain radiographs of positive lesions are recommended); and by urinary catecholamine levels. The three distinct staging systems currently in practice are shown in Table 1B.46.

PROGNOSTIC FACTORS

The most important prognostic factors are the extent of tumor and the patient's age, with children under age 1 who have localized disease having the best prognosis. A variety of other prognostic factors have been evaluated.

Low-risk neuroblastoma includes all patients with stage I disease; infants less than 1 year of age with stage 2, 3, or 4S disease; and those whose tumors are hyperdiploid. A 90% disease-free survival is expected in this group of patients. Intermediate-risk neuroblastoma includes all patients who do *not* have N-*myc* amplification and who are older than 1 year and have stage 2 or 3 disease; who are less than 1 year with diploid stage 2, 3, or 4S disease; and who are less than 1 year with hyperdiploid stage 4 disease. This group of patients has an 85% disease-free survival rate. High risk is assigned to any patients who have stage 2A disease and N-*myc* amplification or who are infants less than 1 year with diploid stage 4 disease. This group of patients has a 70% cure rate. Finally, the very high risk neuroblastoma group includes children more than 1 year with stage 4 disease; children with N-*myc* amplification and stage 2B, 3, or 4 disease; and infants less than 1 year with N-*myc* amplifications and stage 4 disease. Only about a third of these patients are cured.

TREATMENT

Patients with stage I disease and low-risk characteristics should be treated with curative resection alone. Adjuvant chemotherapy is not recommended. Infants with low-risk disease (less than 1 year of age and stage 2, 3, or 4S disease with hyperdiploidy and no N-*myc* amplification) should be candidates for surgical removal of all gross disease. Studies of adjuvant therapy are under way. Studies to date have demonstrated a reduction in local recurrence but no difference in survival with the use of adjuvant therapy. This is because recurrent disease is usually local and is curable with additional surgery. Microscopic disease remaining in the tumor bed is not an indication for adjuvant therapy. Trials conducted in patients with no or only microscopic residual disease have not demonstrated that chemotherapy improves survival. Patients who are N-myc positive or who have large bulky symptomatic disease that is not resectable should be considered for chemotherapy or radiation therapy. A retrospective analysis suggested that patients with

Table 1B.46. Staging Systems for Neuroblastoma

Children's Cancer Group

Stage

I	Tumor confined to the organ or structure of origin.
II	Tumor extending in continuity beyond the organ or structure of origin but not crossing the midline. Regional lymph nodes on the ipsilateral side may be involved.
III	Tumor invasively extending in continuity beyond the midline. Regional lymph nodes may be involved bilaterally.
IV	Remote disease involving skeleton, parenchymatous organs, soft tissues, distant lymph node groups, etc. (See stage IVS.)
IVS	Patients who would otherwise be stage I or II but have remote disease confined to one or more of the following sites only: liver, skin, or bone marrow (without radiographic evidence of bone metastases on complete skeletal survey).

Pediatric Oncology Group

Stage

A	Complete gross resection of the primary tumor with or without microscopic residual disease. Intracavitary lymph nodes, not adherent to but removed with the primary, must be histologically free of tumor. Nodes adherent to the surface of or within the primary tumor may be positive. If the primary tumor is in the abdomen or pelvis, the liver must be histologically free of tumor.
B	Incomplete gross resection of the primary tumor. Nodes and liver must be histologically free of tumor.
C	Complete or incomplete gross resection of the primary tumor. Intracavitary nodes not adherent to the primary must be histologically positive for tumor. Liver must be histologically free of tumor.
D	Any dissemination of disease beyond intracavitary nodes (e.g., extracavitary nodes, liver, skin, bone marrow, bone).
DS	Infants less than 1 year of age with stage IVS disease in Children's Cancer Group staging system.

International Neuroblastoma

Stage

1	Localized tumor with complete gross excision with or without microscopic residual disease; representative ipsilateral lymph nodes negative for tumor microscopically; nodes attached to and removed with the primary tumor may be positive.
2A	Localized tumor with incomplete gross excision; representative ipsilateral nonadherent lymph nodes negative for tumor microscopically.

continued

Table 1B.46. Staging Systems for Neuroblastoma *continued*

International Neuroblastoma

2B	Localized tumor with or without complete gross excision with ipsilateral nonadherent lymph nodes positive for tumor. Enlarged contralateral lymph nodes must be negative microscopically.
3	Unresectable unilateral tumor infiltrating across the midline with or without regional lymph node involvement; or localized unilateral tumor with contralateral regional lymph node involvement; or midline tumor with bilateral extension by infiltration (unresectable) or by lymph node involvement. The midline is defined as the vertebral column. Tumors originating on one side and crossing the midline must infiltrate to or beyond the opposite side of the vertebral column.
Stage 4	Any primary tumor with dissemination to distant lymph nodes, bone, bone marrow, liver, skin, and/or other organs except as defined for stage 4S.
Stage 4S	Localized primary tumor as defined for stage 1, 2A, or 2B with dissemination limited to skin, liver, and/or bone marrow (limited to infants less than 1 year of age). Marrow involvement should be minimal (i.e., <10% of total nucleated cells identified as malignant by bone biopsy or by bone marrow aspirate). More extensive bone marrow involvement constitutes stage IV disease. The results of any metaiodobenzylguanidine (MIBG) scan should be negative for disease in the bone marrow.

locally unresected disease whose treatment included teniposide and cisplatin had better survival (93%) than those whose treatment did not include these two drugs (42%; p = .02).

Patients at intermediate risk should be treated with surgery alone if complete resection is feasible or with biopsy followed by chemotherapy and a second-look surgery to remove any residual disease. In patients with unresectable gross disease a biopsy should be obtained; then neoadjuvant chemotherapy should be followed by second-look surgery with resection of residual disease. Disease remaining after surgery may require irradiation. The 3-year event-free survival percentage was 32% for patients with stage III (Evans) disease randomized to treatment with combination chemotherapy; this compares with 59% for those randomized to the same chemotherapy plus local radiation therapy (p = .009). Patients at high risk or very high risk (all children with N-myc amplification regardless of stage and all children younger than 1 year of age with stage IV neuroblastoma) have a substantial risk of disease progression. Clinical trials or consideration of high-dose chemotherapy with autologous stem cell rescue may be warranted.

BIBLIOGRAPHY

Green DM, Tarbell NJ, Shamburger RC. Cancers of childhood. In: DeVita VT, Hellman S, Rosenberg SA, eds. Cancer: principles & practice of oncology. 5th ed. Philadelphia: Lippincott-Raven, 1997;2083–2130.

Landis SH, Murray T, Bolden S, Wingo PA. Cancer statistics 1998. CA Cancer J Clin 1998:48:6–29.

Neuroblastoma. PDQ treatment for health professionals. National Cancer Institute. http://cancernet.nci.nih.gov/clinpdq/soa/Neuroblastoma_Physician. html; 1/18/98.

Strickland DK, Hakami N. Chemotherapy of pediatric solid tumors. In: Perry MC, ed. The chemotherapy source book. 2nd ed. Baltimore: Williams & Wilkins, 1997;1333–1344.

Osteosarcoma

Victoria J. Dorr

INCIDENCE

Osteosarcoma is a tumor of the bone that occurs predominantly in adolescents and young adults. It accounts for approximately 5% of the tumors in childhood. This is the second most common tumor of bone; multiple myeloma is the most common. Approximately 900 cases occur in adults annually, with a peak in adults at age 20 to 30 and again in the sixth decade.

ETIOLOGY

Osteosarcoma classically arises in growth plates around the epiphyses of long bones during adolescent growth spurts; 80% of these tumors arise from the bones around the knee. In adults, osteosarcoma may be seen in previously irradiated sites or in areas of benign bone lesions, such as pagetoid bone or osteochondromas. Paget's disease is associated with a 0.2% risk of sarcoma.

SIGNS AND SYMPTOMS

Patients typically present with severe rapid-onset pain. A firm-to-hard mass with overlying stretched and shiny skin and prominent vascular markings is the hallmark presentation.

DIAGNOSIS

Expert evaluation should be sought prior to biopsy. Plain radiographs and CT or MRI of primary lesions should be performed. Periosteal elevation produces the classic Codman's triangle on radiograph. Sclerotic ossification transversing or radiating from an area may result in a characteristic sunburst appearance. CT of the chest should be considered to evaluate for pulmonary metastases. Bone scans should be performed to evaluate for skip metastases or distant bony lesions. An elevated alkaline phosphatase has prognostic value. Levels that are persistently elevated or increasing after surgical resection increase the likelihood of residual disease. The biopsy should be done by the surgeon who will perform the definitive surgery. An improper biopsy may make limb-sparing surgery impossible.

STAGING

The site of the primary tumor is a significant prognostic factor in localized disease. Distal tumors have been associated with a more favorable prognosis, whereas axial skeleton primary tumors have a poor prognosis. Resectability of the tumor is the most important prognostic feature because this tumor is very resistant to radiation therapy.

The recognition of intraosseous well-differentiated osteosarcoma and parosteal osteosarcoma is important because these are associated with the most favorable prognosis and can be treated successfully with radical excision of the primary tumor. Periosteal osteosarcoma has an intermediate prognosis. All other histology types are associated with a similarly worse prognosis.

LOCALIZED DISEASE

Localized tumors are limited to the bone of origin, although local skip metastases may be apparent within the bone, possibly indicating a worse prognosis. Approximately half of tumors arise in the femur, with 80% of these arising around the knee joint in young patients. Other primary sites in descending order of frequency are tibia, humerus, pelvis, jaw, fibula, and ribs.

METASTATIC DISEASE

Metastatic tumors (tumors with detectable disease that has spread distantly) are found in 10 to 20% of patients at diagnosis; 85% of metastatic disease is in the lungs. The second most common site of metastasis is another bone.

TREATMENT

Randomized studies demonstrate a significant disease-free survival with the addition of chemotherapy to surgical resection. The optimal combination of agents is not yet established. Preoperative chemotherapy has been evaluated in an attempt to improve the rate of limb-sparing surgery. In general, 70 to 90% of extremity osteosarcomas can be treated with a limb-sparing operation after preoperative chemotherapy; they do not require amputation. Theoretically, preoperative chemotherapy also addresses the risk of microscopic metastases earlier. Furthermore, preoperative chemotherapy allows for evaluation of the patient's individual tumor with an eye to modification of therapy if a suboptimal response is seen. Patients who have more than 90% necrosis at the time of surgery have a significantly better survival rate than others. In patients with less than 90% necrosis, the addition of other effective agents postoperatively improves disease-free survival to 40%. Intra-arterial therapy may provide higher local concentrations of chemotherapeutic drugs but has not improved response rates.

Osteosarcoma is radioresistant, and postoperative therapy with radiation therapy alone has failed to demonstrate a benefit in local recurrence rates or to improve the rate of limb-sparing surgery when given preoperatively.

The progression-free survival rate for patients with metastatic or unresectable osteosarcoma is 20 to 40%. The prognosis for these patients depends on the site of metastatic disease and potential resectability. Patients with bony metastases have a poor prognosis. Aggressive management, including surgical removal of primary and/or metastatic disease at the time of diagnosis or after intensive multiagent regimens, is necessary. All patients should receive intensive multiagent chemotherapy whether or not the primary and metastatic lesions are surgically resectable.

BIBLIOGRAPHY

Osteosarcoma. PDQ treatment for health professionals. National Cancer Institute. http://cancernet.nci.nih.gov/clinpdq/soa/Osteosarcoma_Physician.html; 1/18/98.

Raftopoulos H, Antman KH. Chemotherapy of sarcomas of bone and soft tissue. In: Perry MC, ed. The chemotherapy source book. 2nd ed. Baltimore: Williams & Wilkins, 1997;1289–1315.

Retinoblastoma

Victoria J. Dorr

INCIDENCE

Retinoblastoma affects 1 in 18,000 children. Although it may occur at any age, it most often occurs in young children, with 80% of cases diagnosed before age 5 years.

ETIOLOGY

Patients with sporadic retinoblastoma have unilateral disease with no family history. An autosomal dominant form of familial retinoblastoma has been recognized. This is associated with bilateral disease and a risk of second malignancies. Bone tumors are the most frequent second malignancy. Deletions or mutations of the retinoblastoma gene within the q 14 band of chromosome 13 are strongly associated with a predisposition to retinoblastoma. Genetic counseling should be recommended for all patients with retinoblastoma.

STAGING

There are several staging systems in use. The simplest involves classification into intraocular and extraocular disease. Two additional systems are shown in Table 1B.47.

INTRAOCULAR DISEASE

Intraocular retinoblastoma is localized to the eye and may be confined to the retina or may extend to involve the globe; however, it does not extend beyond the eye into the tissues around the eye or to other parts of the body. The 5-year disease-free survival is more than 90%.

EXTRAOCULAR DISEASE

Extraocular retinoblastoma extends beyond the eye. It may be confined to the tissues around the eye or it may spread, typically to the central nervous system (CNS) or to other parts of the body. The 5-year disease-free survival is less than 10%.

TREATMENT

INTRAOCULAR TUMORS

The primary treatment is local, with enucleation, photocoagulation, cryotherapy, or radiation therapy.

EXTRAOCULAR TUMORS

There is no clearly proven effective therapy for the treatment of extraocular retinoblastoma, although orbital irradiation and

Table 1B.47. Staging Systems for Retinoblastoma

Reese-Ellsworth Classification for Intraocular Tumors

This generally adopted classification for intraocular retinoblastoma has prognostic significance for maintenance of sight and control of local disease. The system is relevant to decisions about the use of local treatment modalities.

Group I	Very favorable for maintenance of sight.
Ia	Solitary tumor, smaller than 4 disc diameters in size, at or behind the equator.
Ib	Multiple tumors, none larger than 4 disc diameters in size, all at or behind the equator.
Group II	Favorable for maintenance of sight.
IIa	Solitary tumor, 4–10 disc diameters in size, at or behind the equator.
IIb	Multiple tumors, 4–10 disc diameters in size, behind the equator.
Group III	Possible for maintenance of sight.
IIIa	Any lesion anterior to the equator.
IIIb	Solitary tumor, larger than 10 disc diameters, behind the equator.
Group IV	Unfavorable for maintenance of sight.
IVa	Multiple tumors, some larger than 10 disc diameters.
IVb	Any lesion extending anteriorly to the ora serrata.
Group V	Very unfavorable for maintenance of sight.
Va	Massive tumors involving more than one half the retina.
Vb	Vitreous seeding. Approximately 90% of patients present with one or both eyes categorized as group V.

St. Jude Children's Research Hospital Clinical Staging System

This system attempts to relate the extent of the disease within and outside the eye to prognosis for sight and for freedom from systemic disease. This system is based on histology; it may be used with ophthalmologic examination, computed tomography, and/or magnetic resonance imaging.

Stage

I	Tumor confined to the retina.
IA	Occupying one quadrant or less.
IB	Occupying two quadrants or less.
IC	Occupying more than 50% of the retinal surface.
II	Tumor confined to globe.
IIA	With vitreous seeding.
IIB	Extension to optic nerve head.
IIC	Extension to choroid.
IID	Extension to choroid and optic nerve head.

continued

Table 1B.47. Staging Systems for Retinoblastoma *continued*

St. Jude Children's Research Hospital Clinical Staging System

IIE	Extension to emissaries.
III	Regional extraocular extension of tumor.
IIIA	Extension beyond cut ends of optic nerve.
IIIB	Extension through sclera into orbital contents.
IIIC	Extension to choroid beyond cut end of optic nerve (including subarachnoid extension).
IIID	Extension through sclera into orbital contents and beyond cut end of optic nerve (including subarachnoid extension).
IV	Distant metastases.
IVA	Extension via optic nerve to brain (i.e., gross tumor in the CNS or tumor cells in the cerebrospinal fluid).
IVB	Blood-borne metastases to soft tissue, bone, or viscera.
IVC	Bone marrow metastases.

Approximately 80% of patients present with one or both eyes classified as stage I or II.

chemotherapy have been used. In general, palliative therapy with radiation and/or intrathecal chemotherapy with methotrexate, cytarabine, and hydrocortisone have been used. Systemic chemotherapy with vincristine, cyclophosphamide, and doxorubicin is usually initially tried. Carboplatin, ifosfamide, and etoposide have also been used. Systematic adjuvant chemotherapy is unproven.

BIBLIOGRAPHY

Green DM, Tarbell NJ, Shamburger RC. Cancers of childhood. In: DeVita VT, Hellman S, Rosenberg SA, eds. Cancer: principles & practice of oncology. 5th ed. Philadelphia: Lippincott-Raven, 1997;2083–2130.

Landis SH, Murray T, Bolden S, Wingo PA. Cancer statistics 1998. CA Cancer J Clin 1998;48:6–29.

Retinoblastoma. PDQ treatment for health professionals. National Cancer Institute. http://cancernet.nci.nih.gov/clinpdq/soa/Retinoblastoma_Physician.html; 1/18/98.

Strickland DK, Hakami N. Chemotherapy of pediatric solid tumors. In: Perry MC, ed. The chemotherapy source book. 2nd ed. Baltimore: Williams & Wilkins, 1997;1333–1344.

Rhabdomyosarcoma

Victoria J. Dorr

INCIDENCE AND PROGNOSTIC FACTORS

Childhood rhabdomyosarcoma, a soft tissue malignant tumor of skeletal muscle origin, accounts for 5 to 8% of cases of childhood cancer. Primary sites of tumor with a more favorable prognosis include nonparameningeal head and neck disease, especially the orbit, and nonbladder, nonprostate genitourinary disease, especially of the paratesticular and vaginal region. Patients with tumors less than 5 cm have best survival. In the Intergroup Rhabdomyosarcoma Study (IRS) III, patients with gross residual disease after initial surgery (clinical group III) had a 5-year survival rate of approximately 70%. Patients with no residual tumor after surgery (clinical group I) had more than a 90% 5-year survival rate. Those with microscopic residual tumor following surgery (clinical group II) had approximately 80% 5-year survival. Patients with lymph node involvement had a worse prognosis. The alveolar subtype of histology is inconclusively associated with a worse prognosis. Hyperdiploidy confers the best and diploidy the worst prognosis.

STAGING

A new classification system proposed by pathologists categorizes the histopathologic groups as superior prognosis (I), intermediate prognosis (II), poor prognosis (III), and not evaluable (IV). Botryoid and spindle cell sarcomas are in category I, having survival rates above 80%. Embryonal sarcoma, in category II, has a survival rate of 64%. Alveolar and undifferentiated sarcomas are in category III, with a survival rate of 53% for alveolar sarcoma, and rhabdomyosarcoma with rhabdoid features is in category IV. The first three IRS studies used the clinical staging system shown in Table 1B.48.

TREATMENT

SURGERY

Surgery remains the primary treatment for most tumors. The goal of surgery is removal of abnormal tissue with a rim of surrounding normal tissue where anatomy and tumor stage allow.

RADIATION THERAPY

Radiation therapy is an effective method for achieving local control of tumor for patients with microscopic or gross residual disease following initial surgical resection or chemotherapy.

Table 1B.48. Staging System for Rhabdomyosarcoma

Clinical Group

I	Localized disease that is completely resected with no regional nodal involvement. Approximately 13% of patients are in this group.
IIA	Grossly resected tumor with microscopic residual disease but no regional nodal involvement.
IIB	Regional disease with involved nodes; complete resection and no residual disease.
IIC	Regional disease with involved nodes, grossly resected but with evidence of microscopic residual and/or histologic involvement of the regional node most distal from the primary site. Approximately 20% of patients are in this group.
III	Incomplete resection or biopsy only of the primary site and therefore gross residual disease. Approximately 48% of patients are in this group.
IV	Distant metastatic disease at the time of diagnosis. Approximately 18% of patients are in this group.

The IRS-IV protocols use a newly developed TNM-based pretreatment staging system for randomization to chemotherapy regimens.

Stage

I	Localized disease involving the orbit or head and neck but not parameningeal sites or nonbladder, nonprostate genitourinary region.
II	Localized disease of any primary site not included in stage I. Primary tumors must be less than 5 cm in diameter, and there must be no regional nodal involvement.
III	Localized disease of any primary site not included in stage I. These patients differ from stage II patients by having primary tumors greater than 5 cm and/or regional nodal involvement.
IV	Metastatic disease at diagnosis.

The IRS-IV protocols use a newly developed TNM-based pretreatment staging system for randomization to chemotherapy regimens.

CHEMOTHERAPY

Chemotherapy is required in all groups and histologic variants of rhabdomyosarcoma (Table 1B.49). Multiagent regimens generally use vincristine, dactinomycin, cyclophosphamide, doxorubicin, cisplatin, ifosfamide, etoposide, and dacarbazine (Table 1B.50). Patients with favorable histology and group I disease have 5-year survival rates above 90% with the usual adjuvant therapy of vincristine and dactinomycin postoperatively. No benefit has been seen with the addition of radiation. Patients with group II disease and favorable histology should be approached initially with surgery. This is followed with adjuvant

Table 1B.49. Chemotherapy Regimens for Rhabdomyosarcoma

Group	Anatomic Location	Histology	IRS Regimen
I	All	Favorable	31
I	All	Unfavorable	38
II	All except special group A	Favorable	32 or 33
II	Special group A	Favorable	32
II	All	Unfavorable	38
III	All except special groups A and B		34
III	Special group A		32
III	Special group B		37A, 37B
IV	All		34

Regimens are described in Table 1B.50.
Special group A comprises the orbit, scalp, parotid, oral cavity, larynx, oropharynx, and cheek primary. Special group B comprises the bladder, vagina, uterus, and prostate.

chemotherapy and radiation therapy. The 5-year survival for this group is 80%.

Patients with group I and II disease with unfavorable histology should receive postoperative adjuvant therapy with combination chemotherapy. Combination therapy consists of vincristine plus dacarbazine and cyclophosphamide (VAC) with cisplatin and doxorubicin. An 80% 5-year survival rate can be achieved. Group III patients are treated with repeat cycles of VAC for 5-year survival of 80%. Patients specifically with pelvic disease should receive VAC plus doxorubicin and cisplatin or dactinomycin and etoposide. Patients with head and orbital tumors that are group II and III have 91% survival with radiation plus vincristine and dactinomycin. Patients with parameningeal disease should receive CNS irradiation combined with intrathecal methotrexate, hydrocortisone, and cytarabine. Patients with overt parameningeal disease have a 69% 5-year survival rate.

RECURRENT DISEASE

Patients with recurrent or progressive disease have a poor long-term prognosis. Ifosfamide plus etoposide has considerable activity in the treatment of recurrent rhabdomyosarcoma for children not previously treated with these agents. Dose-intensive therapy with autologous stem cell transplant is also under investigation for patients with recurrent rhabdomyosarcoma.

Table 1B.50. Chemotherapy Regimens for Rhabdomyosarcoma

Regimen 31

DAC 0.015 mg/kg/day, day 1–5 of week 0, 9, 18, 27, 36, 45 (max 0.5 mg/day)

VCR 1.5 mg/m^2 IV day 1 of weeks 3–8, 12–17, 21–26, 30–35, 39–45, 48–53 (max 2 mg)

Regimen 32

Same as regimen 31 with radiation therapy starting day 14

Regimen 33

Same as regimen 32 with DOX

DOX 30 mg/m^2 IV days 1, 2 on weeks 3, 6, 12, 15, 21, 24

Regimen 34

DAC 0.015 mg/kg/day, days 1–5 of weeks 0–12, 16 (max 0.5 mg)

VCR 1.5 mg/m^2 IV day 1 of weeks 0–12, 16 (max 2 mg)

CTX 10 mg/kg/day, days 1–3 of weeks 0, 12, 16; 20 mg/kg day 1 of weeks 3, 6[a], 9[a]

Radiation starts week 6

—Repeat DAC, VCR, CTX every 4 weeks after radiation if clinical or pathologic CR through week 104

Regimen 38

VCR 1.5 mg/m^2 IV weeks 0–11 (max 2 mg)

CDDP 90 mg/m^2 IV over 8 hr weeks 0, 3, 6, 9

DOX 30 mg/m^2 IV days 1, 2 after CDDP wk 0, 3

CTX 20 mg/kg day 1 of week 0, 6[a], 9[a]

Radiation starts week 6

—VCR, CDPP, Dox alternate with DAC as in regimen 31 every 4 weeks for weeks 12–52

IRS-IV Pilot

IFOS 1 0.8 g/m^2/day IV days 1–5 every 3 weeks × 3 with mesna; repeat weeks 9, 12, 16

ETOP 100 mg/m^2/day IV days 1–5 every 3 weeks × 3

VCR 1.5 mg/m^2/week IV day 1 weekly × 9; then weeks 9, 10, 11, 12, 16 (max 2 mg)

XRT weeks 9–16

Weeks 20–29, IFOS, ETOP, VCR repeated every 3 weeks × 2 (VCR is given every week).

Weeks 29+ Repeat ETOP and VCR (3-week cycle) every 9 weeks × 4 cycles.

Regimens 31, 32, 33, 34, 38 reprinted with permission from Strickland DK, Hakami N. Chemotherapy of pediatric solid tumors. In: Perry MC, ed. The chemotherapy source book. 2nd ed. Baltimore: Williams & Wilkins, 1997; 1333–1344. IRS-IV pilot reprinted with permission from Arndt C, Tefft M, Gehan E, et al. A feasibility, toxicity, and early response study of etoposide, ifosfamide, and vincristine for the treatment of children with rhabdomyosarcoma: a report from the Intergroup Rhabdomyosarcoma Study (IRS) IV pilot study. J Pediatr Hematol Oncol 1997; 19: 124–129.

DAC, dactinomycin; VCR, vincristine; DOX, doxorubicin; CTX, cyclophosphamide; IFOS, ifosfamide; ETOP, etoposide; XRT,

[a]*Hold cyclophosphamide if bladder or extensive bone radiation.*

BIBLIOGRAPHY

Childhood rhabdomyosarcoma. PDQ treatment for health professionals. National Cancer Institute. http://cancernet.nci.nih.gov/clinpdq/soa/Childhood_rhabdomyosarcoma_Physician.html; 1/18/98.

Green DM, Tarbell NJ, Shamburger RC. Cancers of childhood. In: DeVita VT, Hellman S, Rosenberg SA, eds. Cancer: principles & practice of oncology. 5th ed. Philadelphia: Lippincott-Raven, 1997;2083–2130

Landis SH, Murray T, Bolden S, Wingo PA. Cancer statistics 1998. CA Cancer J Clin 1998:48:6–29.

Strickland DK, Hakami N. Chemotherapy of pediatric solid tumors. In: Perry MC, ed. The chemotherapy source book. 2nd ed. Baltimore: Williams & Wilkins, 1997;1333–1344.

Wilm's Tumor

Victoria J. Dorr

Wilm's tumor is the second most common malignancy in children under age 15. Approximately a third of Wilm's tumors have loss of genetic material in the tumor cells from the short arm of chromosome 11, encompassing one or both of the Wilm's tumor gene regions on this chromosome. Genes on other chromosomes may also have a causative role in Wilm's tumor, and loss of genetic material from chromosome 16 and/or trisomy of chromosome 1q occurs in some tumors. Hereditary Wilm's tumor (either bilateral tumors or a family history of the neoplasm) is uncommon, with 4 to 5% of patients having bilateral tumors and 1 to 2% of patients having a family history of Wilm's tumor. Staging for Wilm's tumor is shown in Table 1B.51.

PROGNOSIS

Histology types that are associated with a poor prognosis include anaplasia (focal anaplasia may not confer nearly as poor a diagnosis as diffuse anaplasia) and sarcoma (includes clear cell sarcoma of the kidney and malignant rhabdoid tumor of the kidney).

TREATMENT

For the vast majority of patients, therapy consists of surgery followed by chemotherapy and in some patients, radiation therapy. Stage I disease with favorable histology has a disease-free survival rate of more than 90%. Patients should be approached with surgery as the primary treatment. This is followed by 6 months of adjuvant chemotherapy with vincristine plus dactinomycin. Favorable-histology tumors in patients less than 24 months old and with a tumor weight less than 550 g may be candidates for nephrectomy only, with close follow-up, chest radiograph, and abdominal ultrasound every 3 months during the first 2 years after diagnosis. Patients with stage I clear cell sarcoma of the kidney should be considered for nephrectomy, abdominal irradiation, and 24 weeks of chemotherapy with vincristine, doxorubicin, etoposide, cyclophosphamide, and mesna. Patients with rhabdoid tumor of the kidney are candidates for nephrectomy, radiation therapy, and 24 weeks of chemotherapy with cyclophosphamide, mesna, etoposide, and carboplatin.

Stage II patients with favorable histology have a survival similar to those with stage I disease. Initial therapy remains surgical. Adjuvant chemotherapy is usually recommended. Infants have particularly harsh side effects with chemotherapy; it is recommended that doses be reduced for infants. Efficacy was not

Table 1B.51. Staging System for Wilm's Tumor

Stage I (43% of patients) is tumor limited to the kidney and completely excised. The surface of the renal capsule is intact. The tumor is not ruptured before or during removal. The vessels of the renal sinus are not involved. There is no residual tumor apparent beyond the margins of excision.

Stage II (23% of patients) is tumor that extends beyond the kidney but is completely excised. No residual tumor is apparent at or beyond the margins of excision. Any of the following conditions may exist:

1. Regional extension of the tumor, i.e., penetration through the outer surface of the renal capsule into the perirenal soft tissue or more than 1–2 mm of tumor invasion into the renal sinus.
2. Vessels outside the kidney are infiltrated or contain tumor thrombus.
3. The tumor was biopsied or there was local spillage of tumor confined to the flank.

Stage III (23% of patients) is residual tumor confined to the abdomen. One or more of the following conditions may exist:

1. Lymph nodes in the renal hilus, the periaortic chains, or beyond are found to contain tumor on biopsy. Lymph node involvement in the thorax or other extra-abdominal sites is a criterion for stage IV.
2. There is diffuse peritoneal contamination by the tumor, such as by spillage of tumor beyond the flank before or during surgery or by tumor growth that has penetrated through the peritoneal surface.
3. Implants are found on the peritoneal surfaces.
4. Tumor extends beyond the surgical margins either microscopically or grossly.
5. Tumor is not completely resectable because of local infiltration into vital structures.

Stage IV (10% of patients) is defined by hematogenous metastases. There are metastatic deposits beyond stage III, e.g., to the lung, liver, bone, and/or brain.

Stage V (5% of patients) entails bilateral renal involvement at the time of initial diagnosis. An attempt should be made to stage each side according to these criteria on the basis of extent of disease prior to biopsy.

---

compromised by decreasing the dose. Favorable-histology tumors should be treated with nephrectomy and 18 weeks of chemotherapy with vincristine and pulse-intensive dactinomycin. Patients with focal anaplasia should undergo nephrectomy, abdominal irradiation, and 24 weeks of chemotherapy with vincristine, doxorubicin, and pulse-intensive dactinomycin. Patients with diffuse anaplasia should receive nephrectomy, abdominal irradiation, and 24 weeks of chemotherapy with vincristine, doxorubicin, etoposide, cyclophosphamide,

Table 1B.52. Chemotherapy Regimens for Wilm's Tumor

Stage	Histology	Regimen
I	Any	Vincristine
		Dactinomycin 0.015 mg/kg/day IV days 1–5 Weeks 0, 5, 13, 24
II	Favorable	Vincristine 1.5 mg/m^2 IV day 1 weekly weeks 1–10, 15–20, 24–29, 33–38, 42–47, 51–56, 60–65
		Dactinomycin 0.015 mg/kg/day IV days 1–5 Weeks 0, 5, 13, 22, 31, 40, 49, 58
III–IV	Favorable	Vincristine 1.5 mg/m^2 IV day 1 q week of weeks 1–10 and on day 5 q week of weeks 0, 13, 26, 39, 52, 65
		Dactinomycin 0.015 mg/kg/day IV day 1–5 weeks 0, 13, 26, 39, 52, 65
		Doxorubicin 20 mg/m^2 IV days 1–3 of weeks 6, 19, 32, 45, 58
II-IV	Unfavorable	Vincristine 1.5 mg/m^2 IV day 1 q week of weeks 1–10 and on day 5 q week of weeks 0, 13, 26, 39, 52, 65
		Dactinomycin 0.015 mg/kg/day IV day 1–5 of weeks 0, 13, 26, 39, 52, 65
		Doxorubicin 20 mg/m^2 IV day 1–3 of weeks 6, 19, 32, 45, 58
		If diffuse anaplasia: Cyclophosphamide 10 mg/kg/day IV day 1–3

Reprinted with permission of Strickland DK, Hakami N. Chemotherapy of pediatric solid tumors. In: Perry MC. The chemotherapy source book. Baltimore: Williams & Wilkins, 1997;1333–1344.

and mesna. Patients with clear cell sarcoma and rhabdoid tumors of the kidney are treated as they would be for stage I.

All patients with stage III and IV disease should be approached with nephrectomy if feasible and abdominal irradiation followed by 24 weeks of adjuvant therapy. Patients with favorable histology and focal anaplasia may be considered for therapy with vincristine, doxorubicin, and pulse-intensive dactinomycin. Patients with diffuse anaplasia and clear cell sarcoma of the kidney should receive chemotherapy with vincristine, doxorubicin, etoposide, cyclophosphamide, and mesna. Patients with rhabdoid tumors of the kidney should receive adjuvant chemotherapy with cyclophosphamide, mesna, etoposide, and carboplatin. Patients with bulky tumors that are inoperable are treated after biopsy with initial chemotherapy consisting of vincristine and dactinomycin followed by radiation therapy if the tumor has not shrunk within 2 weeks. Surgery is performed as soon as the tumor has shrunk enough, generally within 6 weeks of diagnosis. Patients are subsequently treated as for stage III tumors, which includes postoperative radiation therapy. In stage V disease the initial procedure is usually bilateral biopsy with lymph node sampling. Following chemotherapy with vincristine, dactinomycin, and doxorubicin, a second-look operation may allow complete resection of tumor with maximal preservation of renal mass. Chemotherapy and/or radiation therapy following the second-look operation depends on the response to initial therapy, with more aggressive therapy required for patients with inadequate response to initial therapy observed at the second procedure. Chemotherapy regimens for Wilm's tumor are shown in Table 1B.52.

BIBLIOGRAPHY

Green DM, Tarbell NJ, Shamburger RC. Cancers of childhood. In: DeVita VT, Hellman S, Rosenberg SA, eds. Cancer: principles & practice of oncology. 5th ed. Philadelphia: Lippincott-Raven, 1997;2083–2130.

Landis SH, Murray T, Bolden S, Wingo PA. Cancer statistics 1998. CA Cancer J Clin 1998:48:6–29.

Strickland DK, Hakami N. Chemotherapy of pediatric solid tumors. In: Perry MC, ed. The chemotherapy source book. 2nd ed. Baltimore: Williams & Wilkins, 1997;1333–1344.

Wilm's tumor. PDQ treatment for health professionals. National Cancer Institute. http://cancernet.nci.nih.gov/clinpdq/soa/Wilms_Physician.html; 1/18/98.

Cancer of Unknown Primary Origin

Nasir Shahab and John D. Wilkes

BACKGROUND

Carcinoma of unknown primary origin (CUP) is defined as metastatic cancer in the absence of an identifiable primary site. This entity can be diagnosed only when a malignant tissue diagnosis is inconsistent with a tumor from the organ biopsied and a formal search for a primary (discussed later) is unrevealing. The absence of a known primary produces a diagnostic and therapeutic challenge for the physician and often generates significant anxiety for the patient and family.

EPIDEMIOLOGY

CUP comprises 3 to 5% of all newly diagnosed cancers. The median age at diagnosis is 59 years (range 20 to 89), and there is a slight male predominance. With a few notable exceptions, CUP has a dismal prognosis, with a median survival of only 5 to 6 months and fewer than 10% of patients surviving beyond 5 years. Most unknown primary tumors are adenocarcinomas or poorly differentiated cancers. Less commonly, squamous cell carcinoma, melanoma, sarcoma, and neuroendocrine tumors can present with an occult primary site of origin.

CLINICAL PRESENTATION

Carcinomas of unknown primary site are extremely heterogeneous malignancies with an equally varied clinical presentation depending on the location and extent of metastatic disease. At diagnosis approximately 60% of patients have two or more involved sites, which may include lymph nodes (37%), liver (30%), bone (28%), lung (27%), pleura (11%), brain (8%), peritoneum (6%), adrenals (5%), and/or skin (2%). The pattern of organ involvement may give some clue to the primary site. Lung metastases are twice as likely to arise from an occult primary above the diaphragm, while liver disease is more common with subdiaphragmatic primaries. Often, the metastatic patterns of CUPs vary significantly from the more usual patterns of metastases (i.e., bone metastases from occult pancreatic cancer).

PROGNOSIS

A small minority of patients with CUP have a relatively favorable prognosis. Lymph node involvement and neuroendocrine histology have been associated with longer survival. Male gender, large number of involved organ sites, hepatic involvement, and adenocarcinoma histology are unfavorable prognostic signs.

DIAGNOSTIC STRATEGY

Despite the anxiety of patient and clinician, an extensive anatomic search for a primary site produces little or no clinical benefit and is not cost effective. Even autopsy fails to reveal the primary site in 15 to 25% of cases. Since the survival advantage is limited to a small subset of patients with treatable cancers, the treating oncologist should adopt a limited and rational diagnostic strategy. As mentioned previously, the anatomic search for a primary should be limited to a history and physical examination (including a digital rectal examination with hemoccult testing, prostate examination and testicular examination in men, breast and pelvic examinations in women). Laboratory studies should be limited to a hematology and complete chemistry profile. In addition, all patients should have chest radiographs and all women, mammograms. CT of the abdomen may identify an occult primary tumor, although with the exception of advanced ovarian cancer, the clinical benefit to this additional study is limited. Any further anatomic search should be limited to sites suggested by clues from the history and physical examination or formal pathologic evaluation as discussed later. The pathologist has a key role in the evaluation of CUP. The pathologic specimen should be reviewed with attention to routine histology, immunohistochemical stains, and electron microscopy. Chromosomal analysis and molecular biologic techniques are playing an increasing role in the identification of occult primaries. Any further laboratory testing or diagnostic imaging should be based on clinical presentations and specific histologic subtypes as follows:

Well and moderately differentiated adenocarcinoma: PSA level, transrectal ultrasound of the prostate (men); mammogram, transvaginal pelvic ultrasound (women); for suspicion of prostate, breast, ovarian cancer

Poorly differentiated adenocarcinoma or poorly differentiated carcinoma: CT of chest, abdomen and pelvis, ultrasound of testis or ovaries, β-HCG, AFP for suspicion of germ cell tumor

Squamous cell carcinoma: high cervical lymphadenopathy: CT of head and neck, panendoscopy of the upper aerodigestive tract for suspicion of head and neck cancer; low cervical lymphadenopathy: CT of chest for suspicion of lung cancer

Inguinal lymphadenopathy: anal endoscopy, colposcopy in women for suspicion of cancer of the anus, cervix; neuroendocrine tumor: CT of abdomen, urinary 5-HIAA for suspicion of carcinoid disease

TREATMENT

As mentioned, the overall prognosis for patients with CUP is dismal with some exceptions. It is crucially important that the clinician aggressively pursue distinct clinical and pathologic details of each case in an attempt to identify a treatable and in some cases curable subtype of this disease. If a rational diagnostic evaluation and thorough pathologic review do not yield a primary, management should be based on site-specific histologic diagnosis as follows.

Well-to-moderately differentiated adenocarcinoma with an axillary presentation: While most patients with adenocarcinoma of unknown primary origin with supradiaphragmatic presentations prove to have lung cancer, approximately half of women with isolated axillary lymph nodes have breast cancer. One should consider the possibility of an occult breast primary and treat as stage II breast cancer with axillary lymph node dissection with or without mastectomy or radiation therapy to the breast for curative intent. Adjuvant chemotherapy should then be offered.

Well-to-moderately differentiated adenocarcinoma in a woman: Suspect peritoneal carcinomatosis. This may be an occult ovarian tumor, and treatment with surgical cytoreduction in select patients followed by carboplatin plus paclitaxel chemotherapy may yield favorable results.

Well-to-moderately differentiated adenocarcinoma with blastic bone disease in men: An occult prostate primary is the most effectively treated entity that presents in this fashion. Hormonal manipulations, including bilateral orchiectomy or LHRH analogues with antiandrogens, may provide benefit with limited toxicity.

Well-to-moderately differentiated adenocarcinoma in other sites: These patients should be considered for investigational protocols, as there is no clear chemotherapy regimen of choice. Recently the combination of carboplatin, paclitaxel, and oral etoposide was reported to produce a response rate of 45%.

Poorly differentiated adenocarcinoma or poorly differentiated carcinoma: A minority of these patients have occult germ cell tumors and may respond extremely well to regimens such as etoposide plus cisplatin or bleomycin plus etoposide and cisplatin. In one of the largest series, investigators at Vanderbilt University reported responses of 63% with complete responses of 26% and long-term disease-free survival of 16%. Patients most likely to respond to this approach are often younger than 50 years of age, nonsmokers, have midline tumor distributions, clinical evidence of rapid tumor growth, and/or elevated levels of β-HCG or AFP.

Squamous cell carcinoma in the cervical lymph nodes: After meticulous evaluation of the upper aerodigestive tract, cervical lymph node dissection and/or radiation therapy may yield 5-year survival in the range of about 35 to 59%. If the lower cervical lymph nodes are involved without a lung primary, aggressive local treatment results in 10 to 15% long-term survival.

Squamous cell carcinoma of inguinal lymph nodes: This is almost always from an anogenital primary site. Therapeutic options include local excision alone, superficial groin dissection, or dissection followed by radiation therapy, depending on the clinical presentation.

Poorly differentiated neuroendocrine tumor: In small series of patients treated with intensive platinum-based regimens, a 20% complete response rate was seen, with 14% of patients of patients alive between 19 and 100 months. Standard regimens such as etoposide plus cisplatin are frequently used.

Well-differentiated neuroendocrine tumor: These tumors often have indolent clinical characteristics. Intensive cisplatin-based chemotherapy regimens should be avoided, as historically the responses have been poor. In some cases expectant management is appropriate, but other patients' clinical course justifies the use of systemic chemotherapy. Combination regimens of doxorubicin plus streptozotocin and streptozotocin plus 5-FU have been employed. For patients with isolated symptomatic metastases, surgical debulking or hepatic embolization may afford palliation of symptoms.

Melanoma metastatic to an isolated lymph node: Approximately 5% of patients diagnosed with melanoma have no identifiable primary lesion. Lymph node dissections should be performed, but the role of adjuvant interferon is unknown. The natural history of these patients is similar to that of patients with node-positive melanoma.

BIBLIOGRAPHY

Abbruzzese JL, Abbruzzese MC, Lenzi R, et al. Analysis of a diagnostic strategy for patients with suspected tumor of unknown origin. J Clin Oncol 1995;13:2094–2103.

Davidson BJ, Spiro RH, Patel S, et al. Cervical metastases of occult origin: the impact of combined modality therapy. Am J Surg 1994;168:395–399.

Hainsworth JD, Erland JB, Marshall LA, et al. Carcinoma of unknown primary site: treatment with 1-hour paclitaxel, carboplatin and extended schedule etoposide. J Clin Oncol 1997;15:2385–2393.

Hainsworth JD, Greco FA. Treatment of patients with cancer of an unknown primary site. N Engl J Med 1993;329:257–263.

Hainsworth JD, Johnson DH, Greco FA. Cisplatin-based combination chemotherapy in the treatment of poorly differentiated carcinoma and poorly differentiated adenocarcinoma of unknown primary site: results of a 12-year experience. J Clin Oncol 1992;10:912–922.

Merson M, Andreola S, Galimberti V, et al. Breast carcinoma presenting as axillary nodal metastases without evidence of a primary tumor. Cancer 1992;64: 504–508.

Shapira DV, Jarrett AR. The need to consider survival, outcome, and expense when evaluating and treating patients with unknown primary carcinoma. Arch Int Med 1995;155:2050–2054.

AIDS-Related Malignancies

John D. Wilkes

The median survival for patients with acquired immunodeficiency syndrome (AIDS) continues to increase as a result of improved management of opportunistic infections and more effective antiretroviral strategies. As a consequence, it is estimated that up to 40% of patients with AIDS will develop cancer during their disease course. HIV produces a profound dysfunction of the cell-mediated immune system that predisposes the host to a variety of opportunistic infections and unusual neoplasms. The most common malignancies associated with AIDS are Kaposi's sarcoma, non-Hodgkin's lymphoma, cervical cancer, and anal cancer.

KAPOSI'S SARCOMA

BACKGROUND

Classic Kaposi's sarcoma (KS) is a rare indolent nodular tumor that occurs on the lower extremities of elderly men of Mediterranean or Eastern European Jewish ancestry. In contradistinction, Kaposi's sarcoma associated with AIDS (epidemic KS) is often characterized by an aggressive and fatal clinical course with extensive lymphatic and visceral organ involvement.

EPIDEMIOLOGY

KS occurs in up to 37% of persons with AIDS. Approximately 95% of cases of KS diagnosed in the United States are diagnosed in homosexual or bisexual men. The incidence of KS is highest in homosexual men between 30 and 40 years old. Other factors that appear to be associated with epidemic KS include high number of sexual partners, more sexually transmitted diseases, and the use of recreational drugs. Fewer than 3% of HIV-positive intravenous drug users will develop KS. Recent statistics from the Centers for Disease Control and Prevention (CDC) suggest a decreasing incidence of KS. This decline may reflect changing sexual practices or more effective antiretroviral therapy, or it may be an artifact of the reporting of AIDS-defining illnesses.

ETIOLOGY

Several infectious agents have been implicated in the pathogenesis of epidemic KS, including cytomegalovirus (CMV), hepatitis B, human papillomavirus (HPV), and Epstein-Barr virus (EBV). More recent strong evidence supports a new γ-herpesvirus, KS-associated herpesvirus (KSHV) or human herpesvirus 8 (HHV-8), as playing a role in the development of this cancer. HPV-16 has recently been identified in up to 25% of HIV-negative homosexuals with KS. The mechanisms by which these viruses induce oncogenesis remains to be elucidated.

CLINICAL MANIFESTATIONS

Although the histopathology of the various forms of KS are indistinguishable, the clinical manifestations and disease course vary dramatically. Epidemic KS may arise in the endothelium or lymphatics of any organ but most frequently affects the skin, mucosal surfaces, liver, lung, spleen, and gastrointestinal tract. Multiple organ involvement at the onset is common and may precede the development of skin lesions. The skin lesions of KS include papules, pigmented irregular plaques, and nodules. In contrast to classic KS, these multifocal lesions tend to occur on the face, trunk, and upper extremities. Adenopathy and lymphedema are seen with advanced disease. Submucosal involvement of the gastrointestinal tract occurs in nearly 50% of cases and may manifest as bleeding or obstruction. Pulmonary KS often presents late in the disease course as progressive dyspnea and hemoptysis. Radiographic distinction between KS and infectious processes may be difficult, so bronchoscopy with biopsy is required.

STAGING EVALUATION

A TNM staging system has not been adopted for epidemic KS. In 1989 the AIDS Clinical Trials Group (ACTG) devised a now widely used system based on tumor characteristics, immune function, and systemic illness (Table 1B.53). Thus the appropriate staging of a patient with KS centers on a careful history and physical examination with attention to the oral cavity, skin, and rectum. A CD4 count and chest radiograph are also recommended. Further investigations, including CT or endoscopies, should be performed as indicated by symptoms or physical findings.

PROGNOSIS

In contrast to most malignant processes, the tumor burden in epidemic KS does not appear to be a major prognostic factor. Attempts to validate the ACTG staging system have consistently demonstrated that the CD4 count depletion, history of opportunistic infections, and other AIDS-related diseases have the greatest effect on survival. The median survival for patients with a history of opportunistic infection was 7 months, compared with 20 months in those with no prior opportunistic infection.

Table 1B.53. Staging System for Kaposi's Sarcoma

Characteristic	Good Risk (0) (All of the Following)	Poor Risk (I) (Any of the Following)
Tumor	Confined to skin with or without lymph nodes; with or without minimal oral involvement (nonnodular disease involving the hard palate)	Tumor-associated edema or ulceration Extensive oral disease GI involvement Other nonnodal visceral involvement
Immune status	CD 4 cells at least 200/μL	CD 4 cells at least 200μL.
Systemic illness	No history of opportunistic infections, thrush No B symptoms (including diarrhea > 2 weeks) KPS at least 70%	History of opportunistic infections or thrush B symptoms KPS below 70% Other HIV-related illnesses (lymphoma, neurologic disease)

Adapted with permission from Krown SE, Metroka C, Wernz JC. Kaposi's sarcoma in the acquired immunodeficiency syndrome: a proposal for uniform evaluation, response, and staging criteria. J Clin Oncol 1989;7:1201–1207.

TREATMENTS

The indications for treatment of epidemic KS are symptomatic visceral disease, extensive cutaneous involvement, or physical disfigurement leading to emotional distress. Frequently, careful monitoring of asymptomatic cutaneous or nodal disease is warranted, as standard treatments are palliative. Similarly, available treatments are often associated with significant toxicity in these immunocompromised patients.

For localized cutaneous or mucosal disease, approaches include electrodesiccation, laser therapy, cryotherapy, photodynamic therapy, surgery, and intralesional injection of chemotherapeutic agents such as vinblastine. Radiation can also provide excellent palliation with relatively low doses (2000 cGy.).

Interferon

Interferon-α was the first approved systemic therapy for epidemic KS. Responses lasting 8 months to 2 years are seen in 20 to 50% of patients. **Interferon-α should not be used for patients with progressive or life-threatening visceral KS.** The optimal doses and schedules have yet to be identified.

Interferon-α$_{2a}$

The dose of IFN-α$_{2a}$ is 36 million IU subcutaneously or intra-muscularly daily for 8 to 12 weeks. A 4-day escalation (3 million IU, 9 million IU, 18 million IU) to desired dose of 36 million IU may reduce acute toxicity. Reduce dosing to three times a week in responders.

Interferon-α$_{2b}$

The dose of IFN-α$_{2b}$ is 30 million IU/m^2 subcutaneously or intramuscularly three times weekly.

Systemic Chemotherapy

In patients with profound immunosuppression, there are significant limitations of systemic chemotherapy in epidemic KS. Despite these concerns, chemotherapy is frequently used for patients with advanced epidemic KS. Traditional single agents have produced partial responses, usually brief. Newer liposomal anthracyclines appear to produce significantly more durable responses. While combination regimens tend to produce higher responses than single agents, any benefit to survival or quality of life remains to be determined. The variation in reported response rates may reflect patient selection rather than superiority of a single agent or regimen. Commonly used systemic treatments are listed in Table 1B.54.

AIDS-RELATED LYMPHOMA

BACKGROUND

An increase in the incidence of aggressive B-cell lymphomas in young men in the 1980s in areas of high HIV prevalence led to the recognition of non-Hodgkin's lymphoma (NHL) as an AIDS-defining illness. Since most patients with HIV-related NHL have both advanced AIDS and advanced lymphoma at diagnosis, the treatments are often poorly tolerated, and infectious complications are frequent. Thus, the prognosis remains poor. AIDS-related lymphoma causes approximately 15% of all AIDS deaths.

More recently, Hodgkin's disease has also been identified with increased frequency in HIV patients. Though it is not yet considered an AIDS-defining illness, some data suggest that HIV infection alters the natural history of Hodgkin's disease. Patients with AIDS-related Hodgkin's disease tend to present with more advanced disease, B symptoms, and extranodal sites. The staging and treatment of patients with Hodgkin's disease is reviewed in Chapter 1A. Compared with immunocompetent patients, those with HIV and Hodgkin's disease have limited tol-

Table 1B.54. Systemic Chemotherapy for AIDS-Related Kaposi's Sarcoma

Regimen	Dosing and Schedule	Response Rate (%)
Daunorubicin, liposomal	40 mg/m² IV q 2 weeks	25–73
Doxorubicin	20 mg/m² IV q 2 weeks or 15 mg/m² IV q weeks	50–60
Doxorubicin, liposomal	20 mg/m² IV q 3 weeks	63–67
Etoposide	150 mg/m² IV daily × 3 days, q 3–4 weeks	75
Oral etoposide	50 mg/day orally × 14 days; repeat q 21 days	32
Paclitaxel	100 mg/m² IV over 3 hours q 2 weeks or 135 mg/m² IV over 3 hours q 3 weeks	59
Vincristine	2 mg IV weekly	20–60
Vinblastine	0.05–0.1 mg/kg IV weekly	25–30
Vinorelbine	30 mg/m² IV q 2 weeks with or without G-CSF	47
Bleomycin, vincristine	Bleomycin 10 mg/m² IV q 2 weeks Vincristine 2 mg IV q 2 weeks	62–83
Doxorubicin, bleomycin, vincristine	Doxorubicin 10–20 mg/m² IV q 2 weeks Bleomycin 10 U/m² IV q 2 weeks Vincristine 1.4 mg/m² (max 2 mg) IV q 2 weeks	40–88

erance for standard chemotherapy regimens, with increased myelosuppression and infectious complications

EPIDEMIOLOGY

HIV-infected patients have a 60- to 100-fold increase in NHL irrespective of their risk factor groups. Although NHL can occur at any time during the course of AIDS, the incidence appears to increase with the duration and severity of immunosuppression. While lymphoma is the AIDS-defining illness in approximately 3% of patients, it has been estimated that the probability of developing a high-grade NHL approaches 20% within 3 years of beginning antiretroviral therapy. Recent data also suggest a bimodal incidence, with Burkitt's lymphoma occurring in adolescents with AIDS, while large cell and immunoblastic lymphomas occur more in middle age. More than 90% of AIDS-related NHL are intermediate- or high-grade B-cell neoplasms, and some may be oligoclonal or polyclonal. A subset of AIDS-related NHL, primary central nervous system lymphoma (PCNSL) accounts for 10 to 20% of AIDS lymphoma and is associated with severe immunosuppression.

PATHOGENESIS

The malignant proliferation of lymphocytes associated with HIV disease is believed to result from excessive antigenic stimulation by infectious agents in combination with high levels of interleukins (IL-6, IL-10), which result in B-cell proliferation. Oncogene activation and tumor suppressor gene inactivation have been described. Reactivation of EBV infection appears to play a role in the development of AIDS lymphoma, as the EBV genome has been identified in 66% of systemic lymphoma specimens and 100% of primary CNS lymphomas. Initial concerns that zidovudine (AZT) use may predispose to the development of lymphoma have been disproved.

CLINICAL MANIFESTATIONS

AIDS lymphoma is characterized by advanced extranodal involvement (75 to 90% of patients) with common sites including the CNS, oral cavity, gastrointestinal tract, bone marrow, and soft tissues. Advanced stage is common (64 to 83%), as are B-symptoms. PCNSL may cause subtle changes in personality, focal neurologic deficits, or seizures. B-symptoms are also common, yet 20% of patients may be asymptomatic. CT, which reveals a mass lesion or lesions and lumbar punctures, is rarely diagnostic.

STAGING EVALUATION

The pretreatment evaluation of an AIDS patient with NHL is similar to that of immunocompetent patients with NHL (see Chapter 1A) with a few important exceptions. CT of the brain, chest, abdomen, and pelvis; lumbar puncture for cytology; and bilateral bone marrow biopsies with aspirate are essential. An evaluation of the patient's immune status (CD4 count, history of opportunistic infections) also provides important prognostic information. The staging classification system for AIDS-related NHL is identical to that of non-HIV patients with NHL.

PROGNOSIS

In contrast to most non-HIV-infected persons with NHL, lymphoma in AIDS patients is extremely aggressive and tends to present with both advanced stage and extranodal involvement. The overall median survival for patients with AIDS-related NHL is only 5 to 6 months. Adverse prognostic features include age more than 35, a history of intravenous drug use, a history of AIDS preceding the lymphoma diagnosis, Karnofsky performance status less than 70%, stage III or IV disease, bone marrow involvement, elevated LDH, and a CD4 count less than $100/mm^3$. In some studies, histologic subtype also factors into prognosis, as patients with large cell and immunoblastic subtypes have median survivals of only 2 months. Patients with primary CNS lymphoma have a median survival of only about 6 weeks. The limited series of patients with HIV and Hodgkin's disease also suggest a more aggressive disease course with a median survival of less than a year as a result of opportunistic infections.

TREATMENTS

The treatment of patients with AIDS-related NHL is complicated by a number of factors, including impaired tolerance of therapy, opportunistic infections, comorbid illnesses, and high frequency of CNS disease. It is not surprising that the results of current treatment approaches remain disappointing. The treatments are associated with a high mortality rate from both infections (25 to 50%) and progression of disease (30%). Complete response rates are obtained in fewer than 50% of patients, and most of these individuals relapse within 6 months.

Chemotherapy regimens for AIDS-related NHL are shown in Table 1B.55. A dose-reduced regimen of m-BACOD (methotrexate, bleomycin, doxorubicin, cyclophosphamide, vincristine, dexamethasone) evaluated by the ACTG demonstrated a complete remission rate of 46%. Median survival for patients treated with low dose m-BACOD was 35 weeks, with fewer episodes of grade III or IV toxicity than seen with standard m-BACOD. This regimen is often used for patients with poor immune function (CD4 less than 100, opportunistic infections) while patients with CD4 counts above 200 and no opportunistic infections may better tolerate standard regimens such as CHOP (cyclophosphamide, doxorubicin, vincristine, prednisone). Various dose-reduced CHOP regimens have also been reported for patients with poor prognostic features. Another treatment for AIDS-related NHL include an infusional CDE (cyclophosphamide, doxorubicin, etoposide) regimen, which produced complete remissions in 62% of patients and a median survival of 18 months.

Primary CNS lymphoma is generally treated with radiation therapy alone. A 20 to 50% complete response rate can be obtained, and up to 75% of patients achieve some clinical benefit, although the median survival remains only 2 to 4 months. Studies evaluating the role of systemic chemotherapy plus radiation therapy have yielded promising preliminary results.

Table 1B.55. Chemotherapy Regimens for AIDS-Related Non-Hodgkin's Lymphoma

Regimens	Days of Cycle
Low-dose m-BACOD	
Cyclophosphamide 300 mg/m²	1
Doxorubicin 25 mg/m²	1
Vincristine 1.4 mg/m²	1
Bleomycin 4 mg/m²	1
Dexamethasone 3 mg/m²	1–5
Methotrexate 500 mg/m² with leucovorin rescue	14
IT ara-C 50 mg	1, 8, 21, 28 (first cycle only)
Infusional CDE	
Cyclophosphamide 187.5 mg/m²/day	All by continuous infusion over 96 hr
Doxorubicin 12.5 mg/m²/day	
Etoposide 60 mg/m²/day	

AIDS-RELATED CERVICAL CANCER

Cervical cancer was added to the list of AIDS-defining illnesses in 1993. Evidence to support this association comes from studies that demonstrate a higher incidence of HPV, abnormal Pap smears, and abnormal cervical cytology in women with HIV. Cervical cancer, the AIDS-defining illness in approximately 4% of women, constitutes 55% of AIDS-related malignancies in women. The causation, clinical manifestations, staging, and treatment of cervical cancer in women with HIV are similar to those for immunocompetent women (see gynecologic malignancies, earlier in this chapter).

In women with HIV, cervical cancer progresses more rapidly from premalignant CIN to invasive cancer. As a result, patients with HIV should be screened for cervical cancer every 6 months. Attempts to control CIN with cryotherapy and conization are also less effective than in the immunocompetent population. Attempts to improve local control with topical 5-FU are under investigation by the ACTG.

Similarly, invasive cervical cancer in women with AIDS tends to be poorly differentiated and clinically more aggressive, with an increased frequency of advanced disease at presentation. Median survivals are approximately half as long as in the HIV-negative population. In one study 88% of women with HIV had recurrence of cervical cancer following primary treatment. Cervical cancer was the cause of death in 95% of these same patients.

Chemotherapeutic agents such as cisplatin, bleomycin, and vincristine have been used for advanced or recurrent cervical cancer. Extra caution must be employed, however, because of the underlying immunocompromised state of the patients and comorbid conditions. Hematologic toxicities are encountered more frequently and may be aggravated by the concurrent use of antiretroviral agents.

AIDS-RELATED ANAL CANCER

The AIDS epidemic has produced a dramatic increase in the incidence of anal carcinoma. It is estimated that there is a 40- to 80-fold excess of anal cancer in the HIV-infected population. Men with a history of receptive anal intercourse, perianal herpes simplex, or condyloma are at highest risk. Also, HIV-infected persons have a higher incidence of premalignant anal lesions and HPV infections. As with cervical cancer in HIV-infected women, anal cancer tends to have a more aggressive clinical course. Vigilant screening is recommended, although no specific guidelines have been provided by the CDC. The causation, clinical presentation, diagnostic evaluation, staging, and treatment principles for anal cancer in HIV-infected persons are similar to those of immunocompetent patients as described in the gastrointestinal malignancies earlier in this chapter.

Local ablative therapies (cryoablation, laser therapy, electrocautery) are recommended for patients with anal intraepithelial neoplasia grade II or III. For patients with invasive carcinoma, combined modality treatments with chemotherapy and concurrent radiation therapy as described in the gastrointestinal malignancies earlier in this chapter should be used. Care should be taken, as these patients may have unusual amounts of local tissue damage from radiation therapy and hematologic toxicity from chemotherapy.

BIBLIOGRAPHY

Biggar RJ, Rabkin CS. Epidemiology of AIDS-related neoplasms. Hematol Oncol Clin North Am 1996;10:997–1010.

Chadha M, Rosenblatt EA, Malamud S, et al. Squamous-cell carcinoma of the anus in HIV-positive patients. Dis Colon Rectum 1994;37:861–865.

Chang Y, Cesarman E, Pessin MS, et al. Identification of herpesvirus-like DNA sequences in AIDS-associated Kaposi's sarcoma. Science 1994;266:1865–1869.

Feingold AR, Vermund SH, Burk RD, et al. Cervical cytologic abnormalities and papillomavirus in women infected with the human immunodeficiency virus. J AIDS 1990;3:896–903.

Galetto G, Levine AM. AIDS-associated primary central nervous system lymphoma. Oncology Core Committee, AIDS Clinical Trial Group. JAMA 1993;269:92–93.

Kaplan LD, Strauss DJ, Testa MA, et al. Low-dose compared with standard dose m-BACOD chemotherapy for nonHodgkin's lymphoma associated with the human immunodeficiency virus infection. N Engl J Med 1997;336:1641–1648.

Krown SE, Metroka C, Wernz JC. Kaposi's sarcoma in the acquired immunod-eficiency syndrome: a proposal for uniform evaluation, response, and staging criteria. J Clin Oncol 1989;7:1201–1207.

Levine AM. AIDS-related lymphoma. Blood 1992;80:8–20.

Maiman M. Cervical neoplasia in women with HIV infection. Oncology 1994;8:83–89.

Maiman M, Fruchter RG, Clark M, et al. Cervical cancer as an AIDS-defining illness. Obstet Gynecol 1997;89:76–80.

Maiman M. Fruchter RG, Gay L, et al. HIV infection and invasive cervical carcinoma. Cancer 1993;71, 402–406.

Melbye M, Cote TR, Kessler L, et al. High incidence of anal cancer among AIDS patients. Lancet 1994;343:636–639.

Sparano JA, Wiernik PH, Strack M, et al. Infusional cyclophosphamide, dox-orubicin, and etoposide in human immunodeficiency virus- and human T-cell leukemia virus type I-related nonHodgkin's lymphoma: a highly active regimen. Blood 1993;81:2810–2815.

2
Chemotherapy Programs

Victoria J. Dorr, John D. Wilkes,
and Deborah Morris

This chapter is a reference for the chemotherapy chapters cited elsewhere in this text and currently in use. Also included are references considered to be either historically important or potentially important as second-line chemotherapy. No attempt has been made to be encyclopedic, and the choice of regimens must therefore be considered arbitrary. The reader is cautioned to review the cited articles to confirm doses and schedules and for specifics regarding patient selection, dose adjustments, and other modifications. When available, ongoing clinical trials should always be considered for treatment. The treatments listed in this book are not intended to indicate standard versus investigational treatment and should not be used as the basis for reimbursement. Variations in dosage and frequency may have to be made according to individual patients' responses. No liability will be assumed for the use of this book, and the absence of typographical errors is not guaranteed. The reader is cautioned to refer to the original reference or to the package insert of the drug for additional information.

AIDS-RELATED MALIGNANCIES

KAPOSI'S SARCOMA

ABV

Doxorubicin (Adriamycin)	10 mg/m^2 i.v. day 1, 15
Bleomycin	15 U i.v. days 1, 15
Vincristine	1 mg i.v. days 1, 15

*Repeat every 28 days

Source: Gill PS, Wernz J, Scadden DT, et al. Randomized phase III trial of liposomal daunorubicin versus doxorubicin, bleomycin, and vincristine in AIDS-related Kaposi's sarcoma. J Clin Oncol 1996;14:2353–2364.

BV

Bleomycin	10 U/m^2 i.v. days 1, 15
Vincristine	1.4 mg/m^2 (2 mg max) i.v. days 1, 15

*Repeat every 2 weeks

Source: Ireland-Gill A, Espina BM, Akil B, Gill PS. Treatment of acquired immunodeficiency syndrome-related Kaposi's sarcoma using bleomycin-containing chemotherapy regimens. Semin Oncol 1992;19(Suppl 5);32–37.

DBV

Doxorubicin	40 mg/m^2 i.v. day 1
Bleomycin	15 U/m^2 i.v. days 1, 15
Vinblastine	6 mg/m^2 i.v. day 1

*Repeat every 28 days

Source: Laubenstein LL, Krigel RL, Odajnyk CM, et al. Treatment of epidemic Kaposi's sarcoma with etoposide or a combination of doxorubicin, bleomycin, and vinblastine. J Clin Oncol 1984;2:1115–1120.

Interferon-α

Interferon-α$_{2a}$	36 million IU s.q. or i.m., daily for 8–12 weeks; four-day escalation (3 million IU, 9 million IU, 18 million IU) to desired dose of 36 million IU may reduce acute toxicity

Source: Real FX, Oettgen HF, Krown SE. Kaposi's sarcoma and the acquired immunodeficiency syndrome: treatment with high and low doses of recombinant leukocyte A interferon. J Clin Oncol 1986;4:544–551.

Interferon-α$_{2b}$	30 million IU/m^2 s.q. or i.m., 3 times weekly

Source: Groopman JE, Gottlieb MS, Goodman J, et al. Recombinant α$_2$ interferon therapy for Kaposi's sarcoma associated with the acquired immunodeficiency syndrome. Ann Intern Med 1984;100:671–676.

Liposomal Daunorubicin

Liposomal daunorubicin	40 mg/m^2 i.v. days 1, 15

*Repeat every 28 days

Source: Gill PS, Wernz J, Scadden DT, et al. Randomized phase III trial of liposomal daunorubicin versus doxorubicin, bleomycin, and vincristine in AIDS-related Kaposi's sarcoma. J Clin Oncol 1996;14:2353–2364.

Liposomal Doxorubicin

Liposomal doxorubicin	20 mg/m^2 i.v. day 1

*Repeat every 21 days

Source: Northfelt DW, Dezube BJ, Thommes JA, et al. Efficacy of pegylated-liposomal doxorubicin in the treatment of AIDS-related Kaposi's sarcoma after failure of standard chemotherapy. J Clin Oncol 1997;15:653–659.

NON-HODGKIN'S LYMPHOMA

Low-Dose m-BACOD

Cyclophosphamide	300 mg/m^2 i.v. day 1
Doxorubicin	25 mg/m^2 i.v. day 1
Vincristine	1.4 mg/m^2 (2 mg max) i.v. day 1
Bleomycin	4 U/m^2 i.v. day 1
Methotrexate	500 mg/m^2 i.v. day 15
Dexamethasone	3 mg/m^2 p.o. days 1–5
Leucovorin	25 mg p.o. every 6 hr beginning 6 hr after methotrexate

CNS therapy (see below)

*Repeat cycle every 28 days

CNS prophylaxis employs intrathecal cytosine arabinoside 50 mg. i.t. on days 1, 8, 21, 28. For patients with known CNS lymphoma, i.t. therapy is administered every other day until CSF clears. Then, weekly i.t. treatments for 4 weeks are given followed by monthly i.t. treatments for 2 years. CNS radiation therapy and postchemotherapy HIV therapy (i.e., zidovudine) are also incorporated.

Source: Levine AM, Wernz JC, Kaplan L, et al. Low-dose chemotherapy with central nervous system prophylaxis and zidovudine maintenance in AIDS-related lymphoma: a prospective multi-institutional trial. JAMA 1991;266:84–88.

Infusional CDE

Cyclophosphamide	187.5 mg/m^2 i.v. continuous for 96 hr
Doxorubicin	12.5 mg/m^2 i.v. continuous for 96 hr
Etoposide	60 mg/m^2 i.v. continuous for 96 hr

*Repeat cycle every 28 days

CNS prophylaxis consisted of methotrexate 15 mg i.t. days 1, 4 of each cycle with leucovorin rescue. Patients with documented

CNS involvement receive i.t. methotrexate three times weekly until CSF clears, then twice weekly for 2 weeks, weekly for 4 weeks, and monthly for a year. Whole-brain radiation is administered to responding patients during the second or third cycle.

Source: Sparano JA, Wiernik PH, Strack M, et al. Infusional cyclophosphamide, doxorubicin, and etoposide in human immunodeficiency virus- and human T-cell leukemia virus type I-related non-Hodgkin's lymphoma: a highly active regimen. Blood 1993;81:2810–2815.

BREAST CARCINOMA

AC (Adjuvant)

Doxorubicin	60 mg/m^2 i.v. day 1
Cyclophosphamide	600 mg/m^2 i.v. day 1

*Repeat every 21 days for 4 cycles

Source: Fisher B, Brown AM, Dimitrov NV, et al. Two months of Adriamycin-cyclophosphamide with and without interval reinduction therapy compared with six months of cyclophosphamide, methotrexate and 5-fluorouracil in positive-node breast cancer patients with tamoxifen-nonresponsive tumors: results from NSABP B-15. J Clin Oncol 1990;8;1483–1496.

Or

Doxorubicin	30 mg/m^2 i.v. day 1
Cyclophosphamide	150 mg/m^2 p.o. days 3–6

*Repeat every 21 days

Source: Brooks RJ, Jones SE, Salmon SE, et al. Adjuvant chemotherapy of axillary node-negative carcinoma of the breast using doxorubicin and cyclophosphamide. NCI Monographs 1986;1:135–137.

CAF (Adjuvant or Metastatic)

Cyclophosphamide	500 mg/m^2 i.v. day 1
Doxorubicin	50 mg/m^2 i.v. day 1
5-Fluorouracil	500 mg/m^2 i.v. day 1

*Repeat cycle every 21 days

Source: Smalley RV, Carpenter J, Bartolucci A, et al. A comparison of cyclophosphamide, Adriamycin, 5-fluorouracil (CAF) and cyclophosphamide, methotrexate, 5-fluorouracil, vincristine, prednisone (CMFVP) in patients with metastatic breast cancer: a Southeastern Cancer Study Group project. Cancer 1977;40:625–632.

Or

Cyclophosphamide	100 mg/m^2/day p.o. days 1–14
Doxorubicin	30 mg/m^2 i.v. days 1, 8
5-Fluorouracil	500 mg/m^2 i.v. days 1, 8

*Repeat every 28 days

Source: Aisner J, Weinberg V, Perloff M, et al. Chemotherapy versus chemoimmunotherapy (CAF v CAFVP v CMF ± MER) for metastatic carcinoma of the breast: a CALGB study. J Clin Oncol 1987;5:1523–1533.

CFP (Adjuvant)

Cyclophosphamide	150 mg/m^2/day i.v. days 1–5
5-Fluorouracil	300 mg/m^2/day i.v. days 1–5
Prednisone	10 mg/m^2/day p.o. days 1–7

Source: Ingle JN, Everson LK, Wieand HS, et al. Randomized trial to evaluate the addition of tamoxifen to cyclophosphamide, 5-fluorouracil, prednisone adjuvant therapy in premenopausal women with node-positive breast cancer. Cancer 1989;63:1257–1264.

CMF (Adjuvant or Metastatic)

Below age 60:

Cyclophosphamide	100 mg/m^2/day p.o. days 1–14
Methotrexate	40 mg/m^2 i.v. days 1, 8
5-Fluorouracil	600 mg/m^2 i.v. days 1, 8

Above age 60:

Cyclophosphamide	100 mg/m^2/day p.o. days 1–14
Methotrexate	30 mg/m^2 i.v. days 1, 8
5-Fluorouracil	400 mg/m^2 i.v. days 1, 8

*Repeat every 28 days for 6 cycles

Source: Bonadonna G, Brusamolino E, Valagussa P, et al. Combination chemotherapy as an adjuvant treatment in operable breast cancer. N Engl J Med 1976;294:405–410.

CMFP (Adjuvant and Metastatic)

Cyclophosphamide	100 mg/m^2 p.o. days 1–14
Methotrexate	40 mg/m^2 i.v. days 1, 8
5-Fluorouracil	600 mg/m^2 i.v. days 1, 8
Prednisone	20 mg p.o. q.i.d. days 1–7

*Repeat every 28 days

**For women over age 65 the following substitutions are recommended:

| Methotrexate | 30 mg/m^2 i.v. days 1, 8 |
| 5-Fluorouracil | 400 mg/m^2 i.v. days 1, 8 |

Source: Marschke RF Jr, Ingle JN, Schaid DJ, et al. Randomized clinical trial of CFP versus CMFP in women with metastatic breast cancer. Cancer 1989;63:1931–1937.

CNF (Metastatic)

Cyclophosphamide	500 mg/m^2 i.v. day 1
Mitoxantrone	10 mg/m^2 i.v. day 1
5-Fluorouracil	500 mg/m^2 i.v. day 1

*Repeat every 21 days

Source: Bennett JM, Muss HB, Doroshow JH, et al. A randomized multicenter trial comparing mitoxantrone, cyclophosphamide, and fluorouracil with doxorubicin, cyclophosphamide, and fluorouracil in the therapy of metastatic breast carcinoma. J Clin Oncol 1988;6:1611–1620.

Cooper Regimen (Adjuvant)

5-Fluorouracil	12 mg/kg/week for 8 weeks i.v., then every other week for 7 months
Methotrexate	0.7 mg/kg/week for 8 weeks i.v., then every other week for 7 months
Vincristine	0.035 mg/kg/week for 5 weeks i.v., then once a month
Cyclophosphamide	2 mg/kg/day p.o. for 9 months
Prednisone	0.75 mg/kg/day p.o. for 10 days, then half that dose daily for 10 days, then a quarter of the above daily for 10 days, then 5 mg/day for 20 days, then discontinue

Source: Cooper RG, Holland JF, Glidewell O. Adjuvant therapy of breast cancer. Cancer 1979;44:793–798.

Docetaxel (Taxotere) (Metastatic)

Taxotere	100 mg/m^2 i.v. over 1 hr day 1

*Repeat every 21 days

Source: Chan S. Docetaxel vs doxorubicin in metastatic breast cancer resistant to alkylating chemotherapy. Oncology (Huntingt) 1997;11(8 Suppl 8):19–24.

DVM (Metastatic)

Doxorubicin	50 mg/m^2 i.v. days 1, 28
Vincristine	1 mg/m^2 i.v. days 1, 28
Mitomycin C	10 mg/m^2 i.v. day 1

*Repeat every 8 weeks

Source: Ingle JN, Mailliard JA, Schaid DJ, et al. Randomized trial of doxorubicin alone or combined with vincristine and mitomycin C in women with metastatic breast cancer. Am J Clin Oncol 1989;12:474–480.

FAC (Adjuvant or Metastatic)

5-Fluorouracil	500 mg/m^2 i.v. days 1, 5
Doxorubicin	50 mg/m^2 i.v. day 1 by continuous infusion over 48–96 hr
Cyclophosphamide	500 mg/m^2 i.v. day 1

*Repeat every 21 days

Source: Hortobagyi GN, Frye D, Buzdar AU, et al. Decreased cardiac toxicity of doxorubicin administered by continuous intravenous infusion in combination chemotherapy for metastatic breast carcinoma. Cancer 1989;63:37–45.

Gemcitabine

Gemcitabine	1200 mg/m^2 i.v. days 1, 8, 15

*Repeat every 28 days

Source: Blackstein M, Vogel CL, Ambinder R, et al. Phase II study of gemcitabine in patients with metastatic breast cancer. Proc Annu Meet Am Soc Clin Oncol 1996;15:A135.

Liposomal Doxorubicin

Doxil	45–60 mg/m^2 i.v. day 1

*Repeat every 3–4 weeks for a maximum of 6 cycles

Source: Ranson MR, Carmichael J, O'Byrne K, et al. Treatment of advanced breast cancer with sterically stabilized liposomal doxorubicin: results of a multicenter phase II trial. J Clin Oncol 1997;15:3185–3191.

M-VAC (Metastatic)

Methotrexate	30 mg/m^2 i.v. days 1, 15, 22
Vinblastine	3 mg/m^2 i.v. days 2, 15, 22
Doxorubicin	30 mg/m^2 i.v. day 2
Cisplatin	70 mg/m^2 i.v. day 2

*Repeat every 28 days

Source: Langer CJ, Catalano R, Weiner LM, et al. Phase II evaluation of methotrexate, vinblastine, doxorubicin, and cisplatin (M-VAC) in advanced, measurable breast carcinoma. Cancer Invest 1995;13:150–159.

NFL

Mitoxantrone (Novantrone)	12 mg/m^2 i.v. day 1
5-Fluorouracil	350 mg/m^2/day i.v. days 1–3
Leucovorin	300 mg/day i.v. days 1–3 (1 hr prior to 5-fluorouracil)

*Repeat every 21 days

Source: Hainsworth JD, Andrews MB, Johnson DH, et al. Mitoxantrone, fluorouracil, and high dose leucovorin: an effective, well-tolerated regimen for metastatic breast cancer. J Clin Oncol 1991;9:1731–1736.

Paclitaxel (Taxol) (Metastatic)

Paclitaxel	175 mg/m^2 i.v. over 3 hr day 1

*Premedicate with dexamethasone (Decadron) 20 mg p.o. 6 and 12 hr prior to paclitaxel; diphenhydramine 50 mg i.v. 30–60 min prior to paclitaxel; and cimetidine 300 mg or ranitidine 50 mg i.v. 30–60 min prior to paclitaxel

*Repeat every 21 days

Source: Gelmon K, Nabholtz JM, Bontenbal M, et al. Randomized trial of two doses of paclitaxel in metastatic breast cancer after failure of standard therapy. Ann Oncol 1994;198(Suppl 5):A493.

Or

Paclitaxel	125 mg/m^2 i.v. over 96 hr

*Repeat every 4 weeks

**Granulocyte colony–stimulating factor was given days 5–12

Source: Constenla M, Lorenzo I, Garcia-Arroyo FR, et al. Phase II trial of paclitaxel 96-hour infusion with G-CSF in anthracycline-resistant metastatic breast cancer. Proc Annu Meet Am Soc Clin Oncol 1997;16:A574.

TA

| Doxorubicin | 50 mg/m^2 i.v. day 1 |
| Docetaxel | 75 mg/m^2 i.v. day 1 |

Or

| Doxorubicin | 60 mg/m^2 i.v. day 1 |
| Docetaxel | 60 mg/m^2 i.v. day 1 |

Source: Dieras V. Review of docetaxel/doxorubicin combination in metastatic breast cancer. Oncology (Huntingt) 1997;11(8 Suppl 8):31–33.

TAC

Doxorubicin	50 mg/m^2 i.v. day 1, then
Docetaxel	75 mg/m^2 i.v. day 1
Cyclophosphamide	500 mg/m^2 i.v. day 1

*Repeat every 3 weeks

**Antibiotic prophylaxis with ciprofloxacin was used

Source: Bozec I, Nabholtz JM, Dieras V, et al. Docetaxel (D) in combination with doxorubicin (Dx) (AT) and with cyclophosphamide (CTX) (TAC) as first-line chemotherapy (CT) in metastatic breast cancer (MBC): high activity and absence of cardiotoxicity. Proc Annu Meet Am Soc Clin Oncol 1997; 16:A566 (abstract).

VAM (Metastatic)

Vinblastine	6 mg/m^2 i.v. days 1, 28
Adriamycin	30 mg/m^2 i.v. days 1, 28
Mitomycin C	10 mg/m^2 i.v. day 1

*Repeat every 8 weeks

Source: Shipp SK, Muss HB, Westrick MA, et al. Vincristine, doxorubicin and mitomycin (VAM) in patients with advanced breast cancer previously treated with cyclophosphamide, methotrexate and fluorouracil (CMF): a clinical trial of the Piedmont Oncology Association (POA). Cancer Chemother Pharmacol 1983;11:130–133.

VATH (Metastatic)

Vinblastine	4.5 mg/m^2 i.v. day 1
Doxorubicin	45 mg/m^2 i.v. day 1
Thiotepa	12 mg/m^2 i.v. day 1
Fluoxymesterone (Halotestin)	10 mg/m^2 p.o. t.i.d.

*Repeat every 21–28 days

Source: Hart RD, Perloff M, Holland JF. One day VATH (vinblastine, Adriamycin, thiotepa, and Halotestin) therapy for advanced breast cancer refractory to prior chemotherapy. Cancer 1981;48:1522–1527.

VC

Vinorelbine	30 mg/m^2 i.v. days 1, 8
Cisplatin	75 mg/m^2 i.v. day 1

*Repeat every 21 days

Source: Hochster H, Wasserheit C, Siddiqui N, et al. Vinorelbine/cisplatin therapy of locally advanced and metastatic breast cancer: an active regimen. Proc Annu Meet Am Soc Clin Oncol 1997;16:A606.

VD (Metastatic)

Vinorelbine (Navelbine)	25 mg/m^2 i.v. days 1, 8
Doxorubicin	50 mg/m^2 i.v. day 1

*Repeat every 21 days

Source: Hochster HS. Combined doxorubicin/vinorelbine (Navelbine) therapy in the treatment advanced breast cancer. Semin Oncol 1995;22(2 Suppl 5):55–59; discussion 59–60.

Vinblastine and Mitomycin C (Metastatic)

First 2 cycles:	
Mitomycin C	10 mg/m^2 i.v. days 1, 28
Vinblastine	5 mg/m^2 i.v. days 1, 14, 28, 42
Subsequent cycles:	
Mitomycin C	10 mg/m^2 i.v. day 1
Vinblastine	5 mg/m^2 i.v. days 1, 21

*Repeat every 6 to 8 weeks

Source: Garewal HS, Brooks RJ, Jones SE, Miller TP. Treatment of advanced breast cancer with mitomycin C combined with vinblastine or vindesine. J Clin Oncol 1983;1:772–775.

Vinorelbine (Navelbine) (Metastatic)

Vinorelbine	30 mg/m^2 i.v. days 1, 8, 15, 22

*Repeat every 28 days

Source: Fumoleau P, Delozier T, Extra JM, et al. Vinorelbine (Navelbine) in the treatment of breast cancer: the European experience. Semin Oncol 1995;22(2 Suppl 5):22–28; discussion 28–29.

CARCINOMA OF UNKNOWN PRIMARY SITE

BEP

Cisplatin	20 mg/m^2/day i.v.p.b. days 1–5
Etoposide	100 mg/m^2/day i.v.p.b. days 1–5
Bleomycin	30 U i.v. day 1

*Repeat cycle every 21 days

p.b. = piggy back. Source: Hainsworth JD, Johnson DH, Grecco FA. Cisplatin-based combination chemotherapy in the treatment of poorly differentiated carcinoma and poorly differentiated adenocarcinoma of unknown primary site. Results of a 12-year experience. J Clin Oncol 1992;10:912–922.

ICE (mini)

Ifosfamide	1000 mg/m^2 i.v. day 1, hr 0–1
Mesna	333 mg/m^2 i.v. day 1, 30 min before ifosfamide, then 4 and 8 hr after ifosfamide
Etoposide	150 mg/m^2 i.v. over 11 hr, day 1, hr 1–11
Carboplatin	200 mg/m^2 i.v. day 1, hr 11–12
Etoposide	150 mg/m^2 i.v. over 11 hr, day 1, hr 12–24

*Entire 24-hr cycle is repeated on day 2 for total administration time of 48 hr

**This 48-hr cycle is repeated every 28 days

Source: Fields KK, Zorsky PE, Hiemenz JW, et al. Ifosfamide, carboplatin, and etoposide: a new regimen with a broad spectrum of activity. J Clin Oncol 1994;12:544–552.

PCE

Paclitaxel	200 mg/m^2 i.v. over 1 hr day 1
Carboplatin	Area under the curve (AUC) 6 i.v. day 1
Etoposide	50 mg alternating with 100 mg p.o. days 1–10

*Repeat cycle every 21 days

Source: Hainsworth JD, Erland JB, Kalman LA, et al. Carcinoma of unknown primary site: treatment with 1-hour paclitaxel, carboplatin, and extended-schedule etoposide. J Clin Oncol 1997;15:2385–2393.

Taxol-Carboplatin

Paclitaxel	175 mg/m^2 i.v. over 3 hr
Carboplatin	to an AUC of 7 to 7.5

*Paclitaxel is administered prior to carboplatin

**Cycles repeat every 21 days

Source: Coleman RL, Bagnell KG, Townley PM. Carboplatin and short-infusion paclitaxel in high-risk and advanced-stage ovarian carcinoma. Cancer J Sci Am 1997;3:246–253.

ENDOCRINE TUMORS

ADRENAL GLAND NEOPLASM

Cisplatin and Etoposide

Cisplatin	25 mg/m^2/day i.v. days 1–3
Etoposide	100 mg/m^2/day i.v. days 1–3

*Repeat every 21–28 days

Source: Burgess MA, Legha SS, Sellin RV. Chemotherapy with cisplatin and etoposide (VP-16) for patients with advanced adrenal cortical-carcinoma. Proc Annu Meet Am Soc Clin Oncol 1993;12:A544.

Mitotane (o,p′-DDD)

Mitotane	2–10 g/day p.o. in three or four divided doses

*Recommend glucocorticoid and mineralocorticoid replacement

Source: Luton JP, Cerdas S, Billaud L, et al. Clinical features of adrenocortical carcinoma, prognostic factors, and the effect of mitotane therapy. N Engl J Med 1990;322:1195–1201.

PHEOCHROMOCYTOMA

CVD

Cyclophosphamide	750 mg/m^2 i.v. day 1
Vincristine	1.4 mg/m^2 i.v. day 1
Dacarbazine	600 mg/m^2 i.v. days 1, 2

*Repeat every 21 days

Source: Averbuch SD, Steakley CS, Young RC, et al. Malignant pheochromocytoma: effective treatment with a combination of cyclophosphamide, vincristine, and dacarbazine. Ann Intern Med 1988;109:267–273.

PITUITARY ADENOMAS

Octreotide

Octreotide	50–100 µg s.q., b.i.d. or t.i.d. (titrate dose)

Source: Chanson P, Weintraub BD, Harris AG. Octreotide therapy for thyroid-stimulating hormone-secreting pituitary adenomas: a follow-up of 52 patients. Ann Intern Med 1993;119:236–240.

THYROID CANCER

Doxorubicin

Doxorubicin	60 mg/m^2 i.v. day 1

*Repeat every 21 days

Source: Shimaoka K, Schoenfeld DA, DeWys WD, et al. A randomized trial of doxorubicin versus doxorubicin plus cisplatin in patients with advanced thyroid carcinoma. Cancer 1985;566:2155–2160.

Doxorubicin and Cisplatin

Doxorubicin	60 mg/m^2 i.v. day 1
Cisplatin	40 mg/m^2 i.v. day 1

*Repeat every 21 days

Source: Shimaoka K, Schoenfeld DA, DeWys WD, et al. A randomized trial of doxorubicin versus doxorubicin plus cisplatin in patients with advanced thyroid carcinoma. Cancer 1985;566:2155–2160.

GASTROINTESTINAL NEOPLASMS

ANAL CANCER

CF (Metastatic)

Cisplatin	100 mg/m^2 i.v. day 1 or 2
5-Fluorouracil	1000 mg/m^2 CI i.v. days 1–5

*Repeat cycle every 3–4 weeks

Source: Mahjoubi M. Sadek H, Francois E, et al. Epidermoid anal canal carcinoma (EACC): activity of cisplatin (P) and continuous 5 fluorouracil (5FU) in metastatic (M) and/or local recurrent (LR) disease. Proc Am Soc Clin Oncol 1990;9:114 (abstract).

5-FU-MMC-RT (Wayne State)

5-Fluorouracil	1000 mg/m^2 CI i.v. days 1–4, 29–32
Mitomycin	15 mg/m^2 i.v. push day 1
Radiation therapy	3000 cGy (200 cGy/day) days 1–5, 8–12, 15–19

Source: Nigro ND, Seydel HG, Considine B, et al. Combined preoperative radiation and chemotherapy for squamous cell carcinoma of the anal canal. Cancer 1983;51:1826–1829.

5-FU-MMC-RT (EORTC)

5-Fluorouracil	750 mg/m^2/day i.v. days 1–5, 29–33
Mitomycin C	15 mg/m^2 i.v. day 1
Radiation therapy	45 Gy over 5 weeks (1.8 Gy/day)

*After a rest period of 6 weeks a boost of 15–20 Gy was given if partial or complete response

**Surgical resection was performed in the case of residual disease or no response

Source: Roelofsen F, Bosset JF, Eschwege F, et al. Concomitant radiotherapy and chemotherapy is superior to radiotherapy alone in the treatment of locally advanced anal cancer: results of a phase III randomized trial of the European Organization for Research and Treatment of Cancer Radiotherapy and Gastrointestinal Cooperative Groups. J Clin Oncol 1997;15:2040–2049.

5-FU-MMC-RT (RTOG/ECOG)

5-Fluorouracil	1000 mg/m^2/day CI i.v. days 1–4, 29–32 (96-hr infusion)
Mitomycin C	10 mg/m^2 (max 20 mg) i.v. days 1, 29
Radiation therapy	45 Gy over 5 weeks (1.8 Gy/day)

*Patients with residual tumor at biopsy 6 weeks after treatment received salvage CT-RT including

5-Fluorouracil	1000 mg/m^2/day CI i.v. for 96 hr
Cisplatin	100 mg/m^2 i.v. on 2nd day of 5-fluorouracil infusion
Radiation therapy boost	9 Gy over 5 days (1.8 Gy/day)

Source: Flam MS, John M, Pajak T, et al. Role of mitomycin in combination with fluorouracil and radiotherapy, and of salvage chemoradiation in the definitive nonsurgical treatment of epidermoid carcinoma of the anal canal: results of a phase III randomized intergroup study. J Clin Oncol 1996;14:2527–2539.

BILE DUCT CANCER
FAM

5-Fluorouracil	600 mg/m^2 i.v. push days 1, 8, 29, 36
Doxorubicin	30 mg/m^2 i.v. push days 1, 29
Mitomycin	10 mg/m^2 i.v. push day 1

*Repeat cycle every 8 weeks

Source: Harvey JH, Smith FP, Schein PS. 5-Fluorouracil, mitomycin, and doxorubicin (FAM) in carcinoma of the biliary tract. J Clin Oncol 1984;2:1245–1248.

COLORECTAL CANCER
Adjuvant Therapy
5-FU-Levamisole

5-Fluorouracil	450 mg/m^2/day i.v. push days 1–5, then 450 mg/m^2 weekly for 48 weeks beginning day 29
Levamisole	50 mg p.o. t.i.d days 1–3, then 3 consecutive days every 2 weeks for a year

Source: Moertel CG, Fleming TR, MacDonald JS, et al. Levamisole and fluorouracil for adjuvant therapy of resected colon carcinoma. N Engl J Med 1990;322:352–358.

Low-Dose Leucovorin/5-FU

5-Fluorouracil	425 mg/m^2/day i.v. days 1–5
Leucovorin	20 mg/m^2/day i.v. days 1–5

*Repeat every 4–5 weeks for 6 months; leucovorin administered prior to 5-fluorouracil

Source: O'Connell MJ, Mailliard JA, Kahn MJ, et al. Controlled trial of fluorouracil and low-dose leucovorin given for 6 months as postoperative adjuvant therapy for colon cancer. J Clin Oncol 1997;15:246–250.

Weekly Fluorouracil plus High-Dose Leucovorin

5-Fluorouracil	500 mg/m^2 i.v. day 1, weeks 1–6
Leucovorin	500 mg/m^2 i.v. day 1, weeks 1–6

*Repeat every 8 weeks for 6 cycles (1 year); leucovorin administered prior to 5-fluorouracil

Source: Wolmark N, Rockette H, Fisher B, et al. The benefit of leucovorin-modulated fluorouracil as postoperative adjuvant therapy for primary colon cancer: results from the National Surgical Adjuvant Breast and Bowel Project protocol C-03. J Clin Oncol 1993;11:1879–1887.

5-FU-RT (Rectal)

5-Fluorouracil	500 mg/m^2/day i.v. days 1–5, 36–40
	225 mg/m^2 CI i.v. days 56–96
	450 mg/m^2/day i.v. days 120–124, 134–138, 169–173
Radiation therapy	4500 cGy in 180 cGy fractions daily for 6 weeks, start day 56

Source: O'Connell MJ, Martensen JA, Wieand US, et al. Improved adjuvant therapy for rectal cancer by combining protracted infusion fluorouracil with radiation therapy after curative surgery. N Engl J Med 1994;331:502–507.

Metastatic Disease
FUCI

| 5-Fluorouracil | 300 mg/m^2/day CI i.v. |

*Continued until progression or toxicity

Source: Lokich JA, Ahlgren JD, Gullo JJ, et al. A prospective randomized comparison of continuous infusion fluorouracil with a conventional bolus schedule in metastatic colorectal carcinoma: a Mid-Atlantic Oncology Program study. J Clin Oncol 1989;7:425–432.

5-FU-Leucovorin (Mayo Clinic Schedule)

| 5-Fluorouracil | 425 mg/m^2 i.v. daily for 5 days |
| Leucovorin | 20 mg/m^2 i.v. daily for 5 days |

*Repeat cycle every 4 to 5 weeks; administer leucovorin before 5-fluorouracil

Source: Buroker TR, O'Connell MJ, Wieand HS, et al. Randomized comparison of two schedules of fluorouracil and leucovorin in the treatment of advanced colorectal cancer. J Clin Oncol 1994;12:14–20.

5-FU-Leucovorin (Roswell Park-GITSG)

| 5-Fluorouracil | 600 mg/m^2 i.v. day 1 weekly × 6 |
| Leucovorin | 500 mg/m^2 i.v. day 1 weekly × 6 |

*Repeat cycle following 2-week rest period; administer 5-fluorouracil 1 hr after initiating leucovorin

Source: Petrelli N, Douglass HO, Herrera L, et al. The modulation of fluorouracil with leucovorin in metastatic colorectal carcinoma: a prospective randomized phase III trial. J Clin Oncol 1989;7:1419–1426.

Intra-arterial FUDR/5-FU-Leucovorin

FUDR	0.2 mg/kg/day via hepatic artery catheter days 1–14
5-Fluorouracil	425 mg/m^2/day i.v. days 22–26
Leucovorin	20 mg/m^2/day i.v. days 22–26

*Repeat every 5 weeks

Source: O'Connell M, Mailliard J, Nagorney D, et al. Sequential intrahepatic 5-fluorodeoxyuridine (FUDR) and systemic 5-fluorouracil (5FU) + leucovorin (LV) in patients with metastatic colorectal cancer (CRC) confined to the liver. Proc Annu Meet Am Soc Clin Oncol 1994;13:A662 (abstract).

Intra-arterial FUDR-Leucovorin-Dexamethasone (MSKCC)

Floxuridine (FUDR)	0.3 mg/kg/day via hepatic artery pump days 1–14
Leucovorin	15 mg/m^2/day via hepatic artery pump days 1–14
Decadron	20 mg total via hepatic artery pump days 1–14
Heparin	10,000 U via hepatic artery pump days 1–14

*Repeat cycle every 28 days; fill pump with saline during 14 days off chemotherapy each cycle

Source: Kemeny N, Conti JA, Cohen A, et al. Phase II study of hepatic arterial floxuridine, leucovorin, and dexamethasone for unresectable liver metastases from colorectal carcinoma. J Clin Oncol 1994;12:2288–2295.

Irinotecan

Irinotecan (CPT-11)	125 mg/m^2 i.v. weekly for 4 weeks

*Repeat cycle after a 2-week rest

Source: Pitot HC, Wender DB, O'Connell MJ, et al. Phase II trial of irinotecan in patients with metastatic colorectal carcinoma. J Clin Oncol 1997;15: 2910–2919.

MFL

Methotrexate	250 mg/m^2 i.v. day 1 hr 0–2
5-Fluorouracil	500 mg/m^2 i.v. day 1 hr 3 and 23
Leucovorin	15 mg/m^2 i.v. push for 1 on hr 24, then 15 mg/m^2 p.o. every 6 hr × 7 doses.

*Alkalinize urine to pH of 8 prior to administration of methotrexate

**Repeat every 2 weeks × 8, every 3 weeks × 2, every 4 weeks × 2

Source: Glimelius B. Biochemical modulation of 5-fluorouracil: a randomized comparison of sequential methotrexate, 5-fluorouracil and leucovorin versus sequential 5-fluorouracil and leucovorin in patients with advanced symptomatic colorectal cancer. Nordic Gastrointestinal Adjuvant Tumor Therapy Group. Ann Oncol 1993;4:235–240.

ESOPHAGEAL CANCER

Concurrent Chemoradiotherapy Regimens

5-FU-MMC

Radiation therapy	200 cGy/day (maximum 6000 cGy over 6 to 7 weeks) start day 1
Fluorouracil	1000 mg/m^2/day CI i.v. days 2–5
Mitomycin	10 mg/m^2 i.v. day 2

Source: Coia LR, Paul AR, Engstrom PF. Combined radiation and chemotherapy as primary management of adenocarcinoma of the esophagus and gastroesophageal junction. Cancer 1988;61:643–649.

FU-PT-XRT (Johns Hopkins)

Fluorouracil	300 mg/m^2 CI i.v. days 1–30
Cisplatin	26 mg/m^2 CI i.v. days 1–5, 26–30
Radiation therapy	44 Gy in 2 Gy fractions days 1–30

Source: Forastiere AA, Heitmiller RF, Lee DJ, et al. Intensive chemoradiation followed by esophagectomy for squamous cell and adenocarcinoma of the esophagus. Cancer J Sci Am 1997;3:144–152.

FU-PT-XRT (North Carolina)

5-Fluorouracil	1000 mg/m^2 i.v. days 1–4, 29–32 (96 hr continuous infusion)
Cisplatin	100 mg/m^2 i.v. day 1 only
Radiation therapy	45 Gy over 5 weeks

Source: Bates BA, Detterbeck FC, Bernard SA, et al. Concurrent radiation and chemotherapy followed by esophagectomy for localized esophageal carcinoma. J Clin Oncol 1996;14:156–163.

FU-PT-XRT (Wayne State)

Fluorouracil	1000 mg/m^2 CI i.v. days 1–4
Cisplatin	75 mg/m^2 i.v. day 1
Radiation therapy	50 Gy over 5 weeks

*Chemotherapy given weeks 1, 5, 8, 11

Source: Herskovic A, Martz K, al-Sarraf M, et al. Combined chemotherapy and radiotherapy compared with radiotherapy alone in patients with cancer of the esophagus. N Engl J Med 1992;326:1593–1598.

Ireland Regimen

5-Fluorouracil	15 mg/kg CI i.v. over 16 hr, days 1–5
Cisplatin	75 mg/m^2 CI i.v. over 8 hr, day 7
*Radiation therapy	40 Gy in 15 fractions; begin day 1

**Repeat cycle in week 6

Source: Walsh TN, Noonan N, Hollywood D, et al. A comparison of multimodal therapy and surgery for esophageal adenocarcinoma. N Engl J Med 1996;335:462–467.

Michigan Regimen

Vinblastine	1 mg/m^2 i.v. days 1–4, 17–20
5-Fluorouracil	300 mg/m^2 CI i.v. days 1–21
Cisplatin	20 mg/m^2 CI i.v. days 1–5, 17–21
*Radiation therapy	45 Gy in 15 fractions (bid); begin day 1

Source: Forastiere AA, Orringer MB, Perez-Tamayo C, et al. Preoperative chemoradiotherapy followed by transhiatal esophagectomy for carcinoma of the esophagus: final report. J Clin Oncol 1993;11:1118–1123.

Chemotherapy Regimens for Advanced Disease

Cisplatin-Bleomycin

Cisplatin	35 mg/m² i.v. days 1–3
Bleomycin	15 mg i.v. as an 18 hr infusion days 1–3

*Repeat cycle every 21–28 days

Source: Marcuello E, Alba E, Gomez de Segura G, et al. Cisplatin and intravenous continuous infusion of bleomycin in advanced and metastatic esophageal cancer. Eur J Cancer Clin Oncol 1988;24:633–635.

Cisplatin-Methotrexate

Cisplatin	20 mg/m² i.v. days 1–5
Methotrexate	200 mg/m² i.v. day 1

*Repeat cycle every 2 weeks for 2 cycles

Source: Saikia TK, Advani S, Ramakrishnan G, et al. Intermediate-dose methotrexate and cisplatin in the treatment of advanced epidermoid esophageal carcinoma: response rate and disease-free survival. Cancer 1989;64:371–373.

Etoposide-Adriamycin-Cisplatin

Etoposide	80 mg/m² i.v. days 1–3
Doxorubicin	20 mg/m² i.v. days 1, 8
Cisplatin	40 mg/m² i.v. days 2, 8

*Repeat cycle every 28 days

Source: Wright C, Mathisen D, Wain J, et al. Adenocarcinoma of the esophagus: results of a pilot study of neoadjuvant chemotherapy with surgical resection. Proc Annu Meet Am Soc Clin Oncol 1994;13:A671 (abstract).

FAP

5-Fluorouracil	600 mg/m² i.v. days 1, 8
Doxorubicin	30 mg/m² i.v. day 1
Cisplatin	75 mg/m² i.v. day 1

*Repeat cycle every 4 weeks

Source: Gisselbrecht C, Calvo F, Mignot L, et al. Fluorouracil (F), Adriamycin (A), and cisplatin (P)(FAP): combination chemotherapy of advanced esophageal carcinoma. Cancer 1983;52:974–977.

FLEP

5-Fluorouracil	500 mg/m^2 i.v. days 1–3
Leucovorin	300 mg/m^2 i.v. days 1–3
Etoposide	100 mg/m^2 i.v. days 1–3
Cisplatin	30 mg/m^2 i.v. days 1–3

*Repeat cycle every 21–28 days

Source: Stahl M, Wilke H, Meyer HJ, et al. 5-Fluorouracil, folinic acid, etoposide and cisplatin chemotherapy for locally advanced or metastatic carcinoma of the oesophagus. Eur J Cancer 1994;30A;325–328.

MBC

Methotrexate	40 mg/m^2 i.v. days 1, 14
Bleomycin	10 U i.m. days 1, 8, 15
Cisplatin	50 mg/m^2 i.v. day 4

*Repeat cycle every 21 days

Source: Vogl SE, Greenwald E, Kaplan BH, et al. Effective chemotherapy for esophageal carcinoma with methotrexate, bleomycin, and cis-diamminedichloroplatinum II. Cancer 1981;48:2555–2558.

Paclitaxel

Paclitaxel (Taxol)	250mg/m^2 i.v. over 24 hr day 1

*Repeat every 21 days

**Granulocyte colony-stimulating factor was used to prevent neutropenia

Source: Ajani JA, Ilson DH, Daugherty K, Kelsen DP. Paclitaxel in the treatment of carcinoma of the esophagus. Semin Oncol 1995;22(3 Suppl 6):35–40.

PF

Cisplatin	100 mg/m^2 i.v. day 1
5-Fluorouracil	1000 mg/m^2/day days 1–5 CI i.v.

*Repeat cycle every 21–28 days

Source: Kies MS, Rosen ST, Tsang TK, et al. Cisplatin and 5-fluorouracil in the primary management of squamous esophageal cancer. Cancer 1987;60: 2156–2160.

TCF

Paclitaxel (Taxol)	175 mg/m^2 i.v. over 3 hr day 1
Cisplatin	20 mg/m^2/day i.v. days 1–5
5-Fluorouracil	750 mg/m^2/day i.v. days 1–5

*Repeat every 28 days

Source: Ajani JA, Ilson D, Bhalla K, et al. Taxol, cisplatin, and 5-fluorouracil (TCF): a multi-institutional phase II study in patients with carcinoma of the esophagus. Proc Annu Meet Am Soc Clin Oncol 1995;14:A489.

Gastric Cancer

EAP

Etoposide	120 mg/m^2 i.v. days 4–6
Doxorubicin	20 mg/m^2 i.v. push days 1 and 7
Cisplatin	40 mg/m^2 i.v. days 2 and 8

*Repeat cycle every 3 to 4 weeks

Source: Wilke M, Preusser P, Fink U, et al. Preoperative chemotherapy in locally advanced and nonresectable gastric cancer: a phase II study with etoposide, doxorubicin, and cisplatin. J Clin Oncol 1989;7:1318–1326.

ELF

Etoposide	120 mg/m^2/day i.v. days 1–3
Leucovorin	300 mg/m^2 i.v. days 1–3
5-Fluorouracil	500 mg/m^2 i.v. push days 1–3

*Repeat every 21 days

Source: Wilke H, Preusser P, Stahl M, et al. Etoposide, folinic acid, and 5-fluorouracil in carboplatin-pretreated patients with advanced gastric cancer. Cancer Chemother Pharm 1991;29:83–84.

FAM

5-Fluorouracil	600 mg/m^2 i.v. push days 1, 8, 29, 36
Doxorubicin	30 mg/m^2 i.v. push days 1, 29
Mitomycin	10 mg/m^2 i.v. push day 1

*Repeat cycle every 8 weeks

Source: MacDonald JS, Schein PS, Woolley PV, et al. 5-Fluorouracil, doxorubicin, and mitomycin (FAM) combination chemotherapy for advanced gastric cancer. Ann Intern Med 1980;93:533–536.

FAMTX

5-Fluorouracil	1500 mg/m^2 i.v. day 1 (1 hr after MTX)
Doxorubicin	30 mg/m^2 i.v. day 15
Methotrexate (MTX)	1500 mg/m^2 i.v. day 1
Leucovorin	15 mg/m^2 p.o. every 6 hr for 12 (start 24 hr after MTX)

*Hydrate and alkalinize urine prior to MTX

**Repeat every 28 days

Source: Wils JA, Klein HO, Wagener DJ, et al. Sequential high-dose methotrexate and fluorouracil combined with doxorubicin: a step ahead in the treatment of advanced gastric cancer: a trial of the European Organization for Research and Treatment of Cancer Gastrointestinal Tract Cooperative Group. J Clin Oncol 1991;9:827–831.

FAP

5-Fluorouracil	300 mg/m^2 i.v. push days 1–5
Doxorubicin	40 mg/m^2 i.v. push day 1
Cisplatin	60 mg/m^2 i.v. day 1

*Cycle repeated every 5 weeks

Source: Cullinan, SA, Moertel CG, Wieand HS, et al. Controlled evaluation of three drug combination regimens versus fluorouracil alone for the therapy of advanced gastric cancer. North Central Cancer Treatment Group. J Clin Oncol 1994;12:412–416.

5-FU

5-Fluorouracil	500 mg/m^2/day i.v. days 1–5

*Repeat every 28 days

Source: Cullinan, SA, Moertel CG, Wieand HS, et al. Controlled evaluation of three drug combination regimens versus fluorouracil alone for the therapy of advanced gastric cancer. North Central Cancer Treatment Group. J Clin Oncol 1994;12:412–416.

Carcinoid Tumors

Interferon

interferon-α	6 × 10^6 IU i.m. daily for 8 weeks, then 6 × 10^6 IU i.m. 3 times weekly

Source: Bajetta E, Zilembo N, di Bartolomeo M, et al. Treatment of metastatic carcinoids and other neuroendocrine tumors with recombinant interferon-α2a. A study by the Italian Trials in Medical Oncology group. Cancer 1993;72: 3099–3105.

Octreotide

Octreotide	150–500 μg s.q. t.i.d. (titrate dose)

Source: Moertel CG. An odyssey in the land of small tumors. J Clin Oncol 1987;5:1503–1522.

Streptozocin and 5-Fluorouracil

Streptozocin	500 mg/m² /day i.v. days 1–5
5-Fluorouracil	400 mg/m² /day i.v. days 1–5

*Repeat every 6 weeks

Source: Moertel CG, Hanley JA, Johnson LA. Streptozocin alone compared with streptozocin plus fluorouracil in the treatment of advanced islet-cell carcinoma. N Engl J Med 1980;303:1189–1194.

PANCREATIC CANCER

FAM

5-Fluorouracil	600 mg/m² i.v. push days 1, 8, 29, and 36
Doxorubicin	30 mg/m² i.v. push days 1 and 29
Mitomycin	10 mg/m² i.v. push day 1

*Repeat cycle every 8 weeks

Source: Leonard RC, Cull A, Stewart ME, et al. Chemotherapy for pancreatic cancer significantly prolongs survival and quality of life is unimpaired. Br J Cancer 1992;65:8.

FAP

5-Fluorouracil	300 mg/m² i.v. days 1–5
Doxorubicin	40 mg/m² i.v. day 1
Cisplatin	60 mg/m² i.v. day 1

*Repeat cycle every 5 weeks

Source: Moertel CG, Rubin J, O'Connell MJ, et al. A phase II study of combined 5-fluorouracil, doxorubicin, and cisplatin in the treatment of advanced upper gastrointestinal adenocarcinomas. J Clin Oncol 1986;4:1053–1057.

5-FU-RT (Adjuvant-GITSG)

5-Fluorouracil	500 mg/m^2 i.v. days 1–3, 29–31, then weekly for 2 years beginning day 71
Radiation therapy	20 Gy over 2 weeks followed by a 2-week break; repeat 20 Gy over 2 weeks (40 Gy total)

Source: Gastrointestinal Study Group. Comparative therapeutic trial of radiation with or without chemotherapy in pancreatic carcinoma. Int J Radiat Oncol Biol Phys 1979;5:1643–1647.

5-FU-MMC-RT (Fox Chase/ECOG-Preoperative)

5-Fluorouracil	1000 mg/m^2 CI i.v. days 2–5, 29–32
Mitomycin C	10 mg/m^2 i.v. day 2
Radiation therapy	5040 cGy total in 28 fractions

Source: Hoffman JP, Weese JL, Solin JL, et al. A pilot study of preoperative chemoradiation for patients with localized adenocarcinoma of the pancreas. Am J Surg 1995;169:71–77.

5-FU-RT (M. D. Anderson-Preoperative)

5-Fluorouracil	300 mg/m^2 CI i.v.
Radiation therapy	50.4 Gy total over 28 fractions

*Chemotherapy administered by continuous infusion Monday morning through Friday afternoon for the duration of radiation therapy

Source: Spitz FR, Abbruzzese JL, Lee JE, et al. Preoperative and postoperative chemoradiation strategies in patients treated with pancreaticoduodenectomy for adenocarcinoma of the pancreas. J Clin Oncol 1997;15:928–937.

Gemcitabine

Gemcitabine	1000 mg/m^2 i.v. weekly for up to 7 weeks, then 1 week rest, then 1000 mg/m^2 i.v. weekly for 3 weeks, then 1-week rest

*Repeat 3-week cycle every 28 days

Source: Rothenberg ML, Burris HA 3rd, Andersen JS, et al. Gemcitabine: effective palliative therapy for pancreas cancer patients failing 5-fluorouracil. Proc Annu Meet Am Soc Clin Oncol 1995;14:A470 (abstract).

SMF

Streptozocin	1000 mg/m^2 i.v. days 1, 8, 29, 36
5-Fluorouracil	600 mg/m^2 i.v. push days 1, 8, 29, 36
Mitomycin C	10 mg/m^2 i.v. push day 1

Source: Bukowsi RM, Balcerzak SP, O'Bryan RM, et al. Randomized trial of 5-fluorouracil and mitomycin C with or without streptozocin for advanced pancreatic cancer: a Southwest Oncology Group study. Cancer 1983;52:1577–1582.

UCLA Regimen

5-Fluorouracil	200 mg/m^2/day CI i.v.
Leucovorin	30 mg/m^2 i.v. weekly
Mitomycin C	10 mg/m^2 (15 mg max) i.v. every 6 weeks
Dipyridamole	75 mg p.o. q.i.d.

Source: Isacoff WH, Reber H, Tompkins R, et al. Continuous infusion (CI) 5-fluorouracil (5-FU), calcium leucovorin (LV), mitomycin-C (mito C), and dipyridamole (D) treatment for patients with locally advanced pancreatic cancer. Proc Annu Meet Am Soc Clin Oncol 195;14:A471 (abstract).

PANCREATIC ISLET CELL TUMORS

Interferon

interferon-α	6 × 10^6 IU i.m. daily for 8 weeks, then 6 × 10^6 IU i.m. 3 times weekly

Source: Bajetta E, Zilembo N, di Bartolomeo M, et al. Treatment of metastatic carcinoids and other neuroendocrine tumors with recombinant interferon-α-2a: a study by the Italian Trials in Medical Oncology group. Cancer 1993;72: 3099–3105.

Octreotide

Octreotide	50 μg s.q. initial test dose day 1; then 150–250 μg s.q. t.i.d.

Source: Saltz L, Trochanowski B, Buckley M, et al. Octreotide as an antineoplastic agent in the treatment of functional and nonfunctional neuroendocrine tumors. Cancer 1993;72:244–248.

Streptozocin and Doxorubicin

Streptozocin	500 mg/m^2/day i.v. days 1–5
Doxorubicin	50 mg/m^2 i.v. days 1, 22

*Repeat every 6 weeks

Source: Moertel CG, Lefkopulo M, Lipsitz S, et al. Streptozocin-doxorubicin, streptozocin-fluorouracil or chlorozotocin in the treatment of advanced islet-cell carcinoma. N Engl J Med 1992;326:519–523.

Streptozocin and 5-Fluorouracil

Streptozocin	500 mg/m^2/day i.v. days 1–5
5-Fluorouracil	400 mg/m^2/day i.v. days 1–5

*Repeat every 6 weeks

Source: Moertel CG, Hanley JA, Johnson LA. Streptozocin alone compared with streptozocin plus fluorouracil in the treatment of advanced islet-cell carcinoma. N Engl J Med 1980;303:1189–1194.

GENITOURINARY CANCERS
BLADDER CANCER

CAP

Cyclophosphamide	400 mg/m^2 i.v. day 1
Doxorubicin	40 mg/m^2 i.v. day 1
Cisplatin	50 mg/m^2 i.v. day 1

*Repeat every 21 days

Source: Campbell M, Baker LH, Opipari M, Al-Sarraf M. Phase II trial with cisplatin, doxorubicin, and cyclophosphamide (CAP) in the treatment of urothelial transitional cell carcinoma. Cancer Treat Rep 1981;65:897–899.

CAP-M

Cyclophosphamide	500 mg/m^2 i.v. days 1, 21
Doxorubicin	40 mg/m^2 i.v. days 1, 21
Cisplatin	40 mg/m^2 i.v. days 2, 22
Methotrexate	40 mg/m^2 i.v. days 42, 49, 56, 63, 70, 77, 84

*Repeat every 15 weeks

Source: Citrin DL, Hogan TF, Davis TE. A study of cyclophosphamide, Adriamycin, cis-platinum and methotrexate in advanced transitional cell carcinoma of the urinary tract. Cancer 1983;51:1–4.

CISCA

Cyclophosphamide	650 mg/m^2 i.v. day 1
Doxorubicin	50 mg/m^2 i.v. day 1
Cisplatin	100 mg/m^2 i.v. day 2

*Repeat every 21–28 days

Source: Sternberg JJ, Bracken RB, Handel PB, et al. Combination chemotherapy (Cisca) for advanced urinary tract carcinoma: a preliminary report. JAMA 1977;238:2282–2287.

CMV

Cisplatin	100 mg/m² i.v. day 2 (give 12 hr after MTX)
Methotrexate (MTX)	30 mg/m² i.v. days 1, 8
Vinblastine	4 mg/m² i.v. days 1, 8

*Repeat every 21 days

Source: Harker WG, Meyers FJ, Freiha FS, et al. Cisplatin, methotrexate, and vinblastine (CMV): an effective chemotherapy regimen for metastatic transitional cell carcinoma of the urinary tract: a Northern California Oncology Group study. J Clin Oncol 1985;3:1463–1470.

CF

| Carboplatin | 100–125 mg/m² i.v. days 1–3 |
| 5-fluorouracil | 500–625 mg/m² i.v. days 1–3 |

*Repeat every 21 days

Source: Arena MG, Sternberg CN, Zeuli M, et al. Carboplatin and 5-fluorouracil in poor performance status patients with advanced urothelial cancer. Ann Oncol 1993;4:241–244.

CP

| Carboplatin | AUC 5 i.v. day 1 |
| Paclitaxel | 175 mg/m² i.v. day 1 |

*Repeat every 21 days

Source: Schnack B, Grbovic M, Brodowicz T, et al. High efficacy of a combination of Taxol with carboplatin in the treatment of metastatic urothelial cancer. Proc Annu Meet Am Soc Clin Oncol 1997;16:A1159.

Gemcitabine

| Gemcitabine | 1200 mg/m²/day i.v. days 1, 8, 15 |

*Repeat every 28 days

Source: Moore MJ, Tannock IF, Ernst DS, et al. Gemcitabine: a promising new agent in the treatment of advanced urothelial cancer. J Clin Oncol 1997;15: 3441–3445.

MVAC

Methotrexate	30 mg/m^2 i.v. days 1, 15, 22
Vinblastine	3 mg/m^2 i.v. days 2, 15, 22
Doxorubicin	30 mg/m^2 i.v. day 2
Cisplatin	70 mg/m^2 i.v. day 2

*Repeat every 28 days

Source: Sternberg CH, Yagoda A, Scher HI, et al. Preliminary results of M-VAC (methotrexate, vinblastine, doxorubicin, and cisplatin) for transitional cell carcinoma of the urothelium. J Urol 1985;133:403–407.

Paclitaxel

Paclitaxel (Taxol)	250 mg/m^2 i.v. over 24 hr day 1

*Repeat every 21 days

**Recombinant human granulocyte colony-stimulating factor (rhG-CSF) was given at 5 μg/kg/day s.q. for at least 10 days each cycle

Source: Roth BJ, Dreicer R, Einhorn LH, et al. Significant activity of paclitaxel in advanced transitional-cell carcinoma of the urothelium: a phase II trial of the Eastern Cooperative Oncology Group. J Clin Oncol 1994;12:2264–2270.

Piritrexim

Piritrexim	25–50 mg t.i.d. days 1–5, 8–12, 15–19

*Repeat every 28 days

Source: Khorsand M, Lange J, Feun L, et al. Phase II trial of oral piritrexim in advanced, previously treated transitional cell cancer of bladder. Invest New Drugs 1997;15:157–163.

VIG

Vinblastine	0.11 mg/kg/day i.v. days 1, 2
Ifosfamide	1200 mg/m^2/day i.v. days 1–5
Gallium nitrate	300 mg/m^2/day i.v. CI days 1–5
Calcitriol	0.5 μg/day p.o. days 3–5

*Repeat every 21 days

**Recombinant human granulocyte colony-stimulating factor (rhG-CSF) was given at 5 μg/kg/day s.q. days 7–16

Source: Einhorn LH, Roth BJ, Ansari R, et al. Phase II trial of vinblastine, ifosfamide, and gallium combination chemotherapy in metastatic urothelial carcinoma. J Clin Oncol 1994;12:2271–2276.

PENILE CANCER

CF

Cisplatin	100 mg/m² i.v. day 1
5-Fluorouracil	1000 mg/m² i.v. days 1–5

*Repeat every 21 days

Source: Shammas FV, Ous S, Fossa SD. Cisplatin and 5-fluorouracil in advanced cancer of the penis. J Urol 1992;147:630–632.

MF (Adjuvant)

Mitomycin C	10 mg/m² i.v. day 1
5- Fluorouracil	1000 mg/m²/day i.v. CI for 96 hr

*Chemotherapy cycle given days 1, 28 of radiation

Source: Oberfield RA, Zinman LN, Leibenhaut M, et al. Management of invasive squamous cell carcinoma of the bulbomembranous male urethra with co-ordinated chemo-radiation therapy and genital preservation. Br J Urol 1996; 78:573–578.

VBM

Vincristine	1 mg i.v. day 1
Bleomycin	15 mg i.m. days 1, 2
Methotrexate	30 mg p.o. day 3

*Each cycle is repeated weekly for up to 15 courses

Source: Bandieramonte G, Lepera P, Moglia D, et al. Neoadjuvant chemotherapy and conservative surgery for exophytic T1N0 carcinoma of the penis. Fourth International Congress on Anti-Cancer Chemotherapy, Paris. February 2–5, 1993;102.

PROSTATE CANCER

Cyclophosphamide (Oral)

Cyclophosphamide	150 mg p.o. days 1–14

*Repeat every 28 days

Source: Raghavan D, Cox K, Pearson BS, et al. Oral cyclophosphamide for the management of hormone-refractory prostate cancer. Br J Urol 1993;72:625–628.

DOX/CY

Doxorubicin	40 mg/m^2 i.v. day 1
Cyclophosphamide	1200 mg/m^2 i.v. day 1

*Repeat every 21 days

**G-CSF support recommended

Source: Small EJ, Apodaca D, Baron A. Second-line chemotherapy with doxorubicin/cyclophosphamide (DOX/CY) for hormone refractory prostate cancer (HRPC). Proc Annu Meet Am Soc Clin Oncol 1997; 16:A1227.

Estramustine

Estramustine	14 mg/kg/day p.o. in 3 or 4 divided doses

Source: Murphy GP, Slack NH, Mittelman A. Use of estramustine phosphate in prostate cancer by the National Prostatic Cancer Project and by Roswell Park Memorial Institute. Urology 1984;23(Suppl):54–63.

Estramustine plus Vinblastine

Estramustine phosphate	600 mg/m^2/day p.o. days 1–42
Vinblastine	4 mg/m^2/week i.v. weekly for 6 weeks

*Repeat every 8 weeks

Source: Hudes G, Greenburg R, Krigel RL, et al. Phase II study of estramustine and vinblastine, two microtubule inhibitors, in hormone-refractory prostate cancer. J Clin Oncol 1992;11:1754–1761.

MP

Mitoxantrone	12 mg/m^2 i.v. day 1
Prednisone	5 mg p.o. b.i.d.

*Repeat every 21 days

Source: Tannock I, Osaha D, Ernst S, et al. Chemotherapy with mitoxantrone (M) and prednisone (P) palliates patients with hormone-resistant prostate cancer (HRPC): results of a randomized Canadian trial. Proc Am Soc Oncol 1995;14:245 A653.

Hormone Therapy

DES

Diethylstilbestrol	1–3 mg p.o. daily

Source: Bailar JC 3d, Byar DP. Estrogen treatment for cancer of the prostate: early results with 3 doses of diethylstilbestrol and placebo. Cancer 1970;26:257–261.

Leuprolide

| Leuprolide | 1 mg s.q. daily |

Source: Leuprolide Study Group. Leuprolide versus diethylstilbestrol for metastatic prostate cancer. N Engl J Med 1984;311:1281–1286.

Or

| Leuprolide | 7.5 mg depot i.m. day 1 |

*Repeat every 28 days

Source: Leuprolide Study Group. Leuprolide versus diethylstilbestrol for metastatic prostate cancer. N Engl J Med 1984;311:1281–1286.

Or

| Leuprolide | 22.5 mg depot i.m. day 1 |

*Repeat every 3 months

Source: Sharifi R, Bruskewitz RC, Gittleman MC, et al. Leuprolide acetate 22.5 mg 12-week depot formulation in the treatment of patients with advanced prostate cancer. Clin Ther 1996;18:647–657.

Zoladex

| Goserlin acetate | 3.6 mg depot s.q. day 1 |

*Repeat every 28 days

Source: Soloway MS, Chodak G, Vogelzang NJ, et al. Zoladex versus orchiectomy in treatment of advanced prostate cancer: a randomized trial. Zoladex Prostate Study Group. Urology 1991;37:46–51.

Or

| Goserlin acetate | 10.8 mg depot s.q. day 1 |

Source: Dijkman GA, Debruyne FM, Fernandez del Moral P, et al. A randomised trial comparing the safety and efficacy of the Zoladex 10.8-mg depot, administered every 12 weeks, to that of the Zoladex 3.6-mg depot, administered every 4 weeks, in patients with advanced prostate cancer. Dutch South East Cooperative Urological Group. Eur Urol 1995;27:43–46.

Casodex

| Biclutamide | 50 mg p.o. daily |

Source: Schellhammer P, Sharifi R, Block N, et al. A controlled trial of bicalutamide versus flutamide, each in combination with luteinizing hormone-releasing hormone analogue therapy, in patients with advanced prostate cancer. Casodex Combination Study Group Urology 1995;45:745–752.

Flutamide

| Flutamide | 250 mg p.o. t.i.d. |

Source: McLeod DG, Benson RC Jr., Eisenberger MA, et al. The use of flutamide in hormone-refractory metastatic prostate cancer. Cancer 1993;72:3870–3873.

Nilandron

Nilutamide	300 mg p.o. daily for 30 days; then
	150 mg p.o. daily

Source: Janknegt R, Abbou CC, Bartoletti R, et al. Orchiectomy and nilutamide or placebo as treatment of metastatic prostatic cancer in a multinational double-blind randomized trial. J Urology 1993;72:77–83.

RENAL CELL CARCINOMA

Alpha Interferon

Interferon-α	$5–15 \times 10^6$ IU s.q. or i.m. daily or 3–5 times a week

Source: Tsavaris N, Mylonakis N, Bacoyiannis C, et al. Treatment of renal cell carcinoma with escalating doses of interferon-α. Chemotherapy 1993;39: 361–366.

Circadian or Constant Infusion FUDR

Floxuridine (FUDR)	0.15 mg/kg/day CI i.v.
Or	
	0.25 mg/kg/day via hepatic artery catheter days 1–14

*For circadian: 68% of dose between 3 P.M. and 9 P.M. plus 15% between 9 P.M. and 3 A.M. plus 2% between 3 A.M. and 9 A.M. plus 15% between 9 A.M. and 3 P.M.

**Repeat every 28 days

Source: Hrushesky WJM, von Roemling R, Lanning RM, et al. Circadian-shaped infusions of floxuridine for progressive metastatic renal cell carcinoma. J Clin Oncol 1990;8:1504–1513.

High-Dose IL-2

Interleukin-2	600,000 or 720,000 IU/kg i.v. every 8 hr to 14 doses or toxicity

*Repeat cycle in 7–10 days; this course can be repeated every 12 weeks

**Discontinue therapy for hypotension requiring pressor support, oliguria unresponsive to fluid and diuretics, respiratory distress, cardiac arrhythmias, mental confusion

Source: Parkinson DR, Sznol M. High-dose Interleukin-2 in the therapy of metastatic renal-cell carcinoma. Semin Oncol 1195:22:61–66.

Low-Dose IL-2

Interleukin-2	3×10^6 IU s.q. b.i.d. days 1–5 for 6 weeks

Source: Stadler WM, Vogelzang NJ. Low-dose Interleukin-2 in the treatment of metastatic renal-cell carcinoma. Semin Oncol 1995;22:67–73.

IL-2/αIFN/5-FU

Interleukin-2	20×10^6 IU/m^2 s.q. 3 days 1, 3, 5 weeks 1, 4
	5×10^6 IU/m^2 s.q. 3 days 1, 3, 5 weeks 2, 3
Interferon-α	6×10^6 IU/m^2 s.q. day 1 weeks 1, 4
	5×10^6 IU/m^2 s.q. days 1, 3, 5 weeks 2, 3
	9×10^6 IU/m^2 s.q. days 1, 3, 5 weeks 5–8
5-Fluorouracil	750 mg/m^2 i.v. day 1 weeks 5–8

*Repeat every 2 months

Source: Atzpodien J, Kirchner H, Hanninen EL, et al. Interleukin-2 in combination with interferon-α and 5-fluorouracil for metastatic renal cell cancer. Eur J Cancer 1993;29A (Suppl 5):6–8.

IFN/IL-2

interferon-α	9×10^6 IU s.q. days 1, 4, weeks 1–4
Interleukin-2	12×10^6 IU/day s.q. days 1–4, weeks 1–4

*Repeat every 6 weeks

Source: Voglezang NJ, Lipton A, Figlin RA. Subcutaneous interleukin-2 plus interferon-α-2a in metastatic renal cancer: an outpatient multicenter trial. J Clin Oncol 1993;11:1809–1816.

TESTICULAR CANCER

BEP

Bleomycin	30 U i.v. days 2, 9, 16
Etoposide	100 mg/m^2/day i.v. days 1–5
Cisplatin	20 mg/m^2/day i.v. days 1–5

*Repeat every 21 days

Source: Williams SD, Birch R, Einhorn LH, et al. Disseminated germ cell tumors: chemotherapy with cisplatin plus bleomycin plus either vinblastine or etoposide: a trial of the Southeastern Cancer Study Group. N Engl J Med 1987;316:1435–1440.

EP

| Cisplatin | 20 mg/m^2/day i.v. days 1–5 |
| Etoposide | 100 mg/m^2/day i.v. days 1–5 |

*Repeat every 21 days

Source: Motzer RJ, Sheinfeld J, Mazumdar M, et al. Etoposide and cisplatin adjuvant therapy for patients with pathologic stage II germ cell tumors. J Clin Oncol 1995;13:2700–2704.

PVB

Cisplatin	20 mg/m^2/day i.v. days 1–5
Vinblastine	0.15 mg/kg i.v. days 1, 2
Bleomycin	30 U i.v. days 2, 9, 16

*Repeat every 21 days

Source: Einhorn LH, Donohue J. Cis-dichlorodiammineplatinum, vinblastine and bleomycin combination chemotherapy in disseminated testicular cancer. Ann Intern Med 1977;87:293–298.

VAB-6

Vinblastine	4 mg/m^2 i.v. day 1
Dactinomycin	1 mg/m^2 i.v. day 1
Bleomycin	30 U i.v. Push day 1, then 20 U/m^2/day i.v. CI days 1–3
Cisplatin	120 mg/m^2 i.v. day 4
Cyclophosphamide	600 mg/m^2 i.v. day 1

*Repeat every 21 days

Source: Vugrin D, Herr HW, Whitmore WF, et al. VAB-6 combination chemotherapy in disseminated cancer of the testis. Ann Intern Med 1981;95:59–61.

VeIP (Salvage)

Vinblastine	0.11 mg/kg i.v. days 1, 2
Ifosfamide	1200 mg/m^2/day i.v. days 1–5
Cisplatin	20 mg/m^2/day i.v. days 1–5

*Repeat every 21 days

Source: Motzer RJ, Geller NL, Tan CCY, et al. Salvage chemotherapy for patients with germ cell tumors: the Memorial Sloan Kettering Cancer Center experience (1979–1989). Cancer 1991;67:1305–1310.

VIP (Salvage)

Etoposide (VP-16)	100 mg/m^2/day i.v. days 1–5
Ifosfamide	1200 mg/m^2/day i.v. days 1–5
Cisplatin	20 mg/m^2/day i.v. days 1–5

*Repeat every 21 days

Source: Harstrick A, Schmall HJ, Wilke H, et al. Cisplatin, etoposide, and ifosfamide salvage therapy for refractory or relapsing germ cell carcinoma. J Clin Oncol 1991;9:1549–1555.

GYNECOLOGICAL CANCERS
CERVICAL CANCER

BIP

Bleomycin	30 U i.v. over 24 hr, day 1
Ifosfamide	5000 mg/m^2 i.v. over 24 hr, day 2
Mesna	6000 mg/m^2 i.v. over 36 hr, day 2
Cisplatin	50 mg/m^2 i.v. day 2

*Repeat every 21 days

Source: Buxton EJ, Meanwell CA, Hilton C, et al. Combination bleomycin, ifosfamide, and cisplatin chemotherapy in cervical cancer. J Natl Cancer Inst 1989;81:359–361.

BOMP

Bleomycin	10 U i.m. days 1, 8, 15, 22
Vincristine	1 mg/m^2 i.v. days 1, 8, 22, 29
Mitomycin C	10 mg/m^2 i.v. day 1
Cisplatin	50 mg/m^2 i.v. days 1, 22

*Repeat every 6 weeks

Source: Vogl SE, Moukhtar M, Calony A, et al. Chemotherapy for advanced cervical cancer with bleomycin, vincristine, mitomycin-C, and cis-platinum (BOMP). Cancer Treat Rep 1980;64:1005–1007.

Docetaxel

Docetaxel	100 mg/m^2 i.v. day 1

*Repeat every 21 days

Source: Levy T, Kudelka AP, Verschraegen CF, et al. Advanced squamous cell cancer (SCC) of the cervix: a phase II study of docetaxel (Taxotere) 100 mg/m^2 intravenously (iv) over 1 hr every 21 days: a preliminary report. Proc Annu Meet Am Soc Clin Oncol 1996;15:A800.

Adjuvant Hydroxyurea

Hydroxyurea	80 mg/kg p.o. twice weekly with XRT

Source: Stehman FB. Experience with hydroxyurea as a radiosensitizer in carcinoma of the cervix. Semin Oncol 1992;19(3 Suppl 9):48–52.

Paclitaxel

Paclitaxel	175–250 mg/m^2 i.v. day 1

*Repeat every 21 days

Source: Thigpen T, Vance R, Khansur T, Malamud F. The role of paclitaxel in the management of patients with carcinoma of the cervix. Semin Oncol 1997;24(1 Suppl 2):S41–46.

ENDOMETRIAL CANCER

AC

Doxorubicin	60 mg/m^2 i.v. day 1
Cyclophosphamide	500 mg/m^2 i.v. day 1

*Repeat every 21 days

Source: Thigpen JT, Blessing JA, DiSaia PJ, et al. A randomized comparison of doxorubicin alone versus doxorubicin plus cyclophosphamide in the management of advanced recurrent endometrial carcinoma: a Gynecological Oncology Group study. J Clin Oncol 1994;12:1408–1414.

MCA

Megestrol	80 mg p.o. t.i.d.
Doxorubicin	40 mg/m^2 i.v. day 1
Cyclophosphamide	400 mg/m^2 i.v. day 1

*Repeat every 28 days

Source: Horton J, Elson P, Gordon P, et al. Combination chemotherapy for advanced endometrial cancer: an evaluation of three regimens. Cancer 1982;49:2441–2445.

MVAC

Methotrexate	30 mg/m^2 i.v. days 1, 15, 22
Vinblastine	3 mg/m^2 i.v. days 2, 15, 22
Doxorubicin	30 mg/m^2 i.v. day 2
Cisplatin	70 mg/m^2 i.v. day 2

*Repeat every 28 days

Source: Long HJ 3rd, Langdon RM Jr, Cha SS, et al. Phase II trial of methotrexate, vinblastine, doxorubicin, and cisplatin in advanced/recurrent endometrial carcinoma. Gynecol Oncol 1995;58:240–243.

PA

| Cisplatin | 50 mg/m² i.v. day 1 |
| Doxorubicin | 50 mg/m² i.v. day 1 |

*Repeat every 21 days

Source: Deppe G, Malviya VK, Malone JM, et al. Treatment of recurrent and metastatic endometrial carcinoma with cisplatin and doxorubicin. Eur J Gynaecol Oncol 1994;15:263–266.

PAC

Cisplatin	50 mg/m² i.v. day 1
Doxorubicin	50 mg/m² i.v. day 1
Cyclophosphamide	500 mg/m² i.v. day 1

*Repeat every 28 days

Source: Burke TW, Gershenson DM, Morris M, et al. Postoperative adjuvant cisplatin, doxorubicin, and cyclophosphamide (PAC) chemotherapy in women with high-risk endometrial carcinoma. Gynecol Oncol 1994;55:47–50.

VFP

Etoposide (VP-16)	80 mg/m²/day i.v. days 1–3
5-Fluorouracil	600 mg/m²/day i.v. days 1–3
Cisplatin	35 mg/m²/day i.v. days 1–3

*Repeat every 28 days

Source: Paraiso D, Dorval T, Boufessa F, et al. Phase ii study of VP-16–213(VP), 5-fluorouracil (5FU) and cisplatin (CDDP) for patients (PTS) with metastatic endometrial carcinoma. Proc Annu Meet Am Soc Clin Oncol 1992;11:A711.

GESTATIONAL TROPHOBLASTIC NEOPLASM

EMA/CO (High-Risk Disease)

Etoposide (VP-16)	100 mg/m²/day i.v. days 1, 2
Methotrexate	100 mg/m² i.v. bolus day 1, then
	200 mg/m² i.v. by 12-hr infusion
Leucovorin	15 mg p.o. every 12 hr days 2, 3 (Start 24 hr after methotrexate started)

Actinomycin-D	0.5 mg/day i.v. days 1, 2
Cyclophosphamide	600 mg/m^2 i.v. day 8
Vincristine	1 mg/m^2 i.v. day 8 (max 2 mg)
Methotrexate	12.5 mg intrathecal day 8

*Intrathecal methotrexate is given with alternating courses

**Repeat every 14 days

Source: Newlands ES, Bagshawe KD, Begent RH, et al. Results with the EMA/CA (etoposide, methotrexate, actinomycin D, cyclophosphamide, vincristine) regimen in high risk gestational trophoblastic tumors, 1979 to 1989. Br J Ob Gyn 1991;98:550–557.

Methotrexate (Low-Risk Disease)

| Methotrexate | 1 mg/kg/day i.m. days 1, 3, 5, 7 |
| Leucovorin | 0.1 mg/kg/day i.m. or p.o. days 2, 4, 6, 8 |

*Repeat every 14 days until serum HCG ≤ 5 million IU/mL, then give one additional cycle

**If HCG does not fall by 1 log at day 14, increase doses by 50%. If no response after 2 cycles, the patient should be switched to

| Actinomycin D | 12–15 μg/kg/day i.v. days 1–5 |

*Repeat every 2 weeks

Source: Berkowitz RS, Goldstein DP, Bernstein MR. Ten year's experience with methotrexate and folinic acid as primary therapy for gestational trophoblastic disease. Gynecol Oncol 1986;23:111–118.

Weekly Methotrexate (Low-Risk Disease)

| Methotrexate | 40–60 mg/m^2 i.m. day 1 |

*Repeat every 7 days until 3 normal consecutive weekly serum HCG

Source: Gleeson NC, Finan MA, Fiorica JV, et al. Nonmetastatic gestational trophoblastic disease: weekly methotrexate compared with 8-day methotrexate-folinic acid. Eur J Gynaecol Oncol 1993;14:461–465.

MAC III (High-Risk Disease)

Methotrexate	1 mg/kg/day i.m. days 1, 3, 5, 7
Leucovorin	0.1 mg/kg/day i.m. or p.o. days 2, 4, 6, 8
Actinomycin-D	12 µg/kg/day i.v. days 1–5
Cyclophosphamide	3 mg/kg/day i.v. days 1–5

*Repeat every 21 days

Source: Berkowitz RS, Goldstein DP, Bernstein MR. Modified triple chemotherapy in the management of high-risk metastatic gestational trophoblastic tumors. Gynecol Oncol 1984;19:173–181.

Paclitaxel

Paclitaxel	250 mg/m^2 i.v. over 24 hr day 1

*Repeat every 21 days

Source: Termrungruanglert W, Kudelka AP, Piamsomboon S, et al. Remission of refractory gestational trophoblastic disease with high-dose paclitaxel. Anticancer Drugs 1996;7:503–506.

PVB

Cisplatin	20 mg/m^2/day i.v. days 1–5
Vinblastine	0.15 mg/kg/day i.v. days 1, 2
Bleomycin	30 U i.v. days 2, 9, 16

*Repeat every 21 days

Source: Hainsworth JD, Burnett LS, Jones HW, et al. Resistant gestational choriocarcinoma: successful treatment with vinblastine, bleomycin, and cisplatin (VBP). Cancer Treat Rep 1983; 67:393–395.

GERM CELL OVARIAN CANCER

BEP (Germ Cell Tumor)

Bleomycin	30 U i.v. days 2, 9, 16
Etoposide	100 mg/m^2/day i.v. days 1–5
Cisplatin	20 mg/m^2/day i.v. days 1–5

*Repeat every 21 days

Source: Williams SD. Treatment of germ cell tumors of the ovary. Semin Oncol 1991;18:292–296.

OVARIAN CANCER

CarboC

| Carboplatin | 300 mg/m^2 i.v. day 1 |
| Cyclophosphamide | 600 mg/m^2 i.v. day 1 |

*Repeat every 21 days

Source: Swerenton K, Jeffrey J, Stuart G, et al. Cisplatin-cyclophosphamide versus carboplatin-cyclophosphamide in advanced ovarian cancer: a randomized phase III study of the National Cancer Institute of Canada Clinical Trials Group. J Clin Oncol 1992;10:718–726.

CAP

Hexamethylmelamine	150 mg/m^2/day p.o. days 1–14
Cyclophosphamide	350 mg/m^2 i.v. days 1, 8
Doxorubicin	20 mg/m^2 i.v. days 1, 8
Cisplatin	60 mg/m^2 i.v. days 1, 8

*Repeat every 4 weeks

Source: Grecco FA, Johnson DH, Hainsworth JD. A comparison of hexamethylmelamine (Altretamine), cyclophosphamide, doxorubicin and cisplatin (H-CAP) Vs cyclophosphamide, doxorubicin and cisplatin (CAP) in advanced ovarian cancer. Cancer Treat Rev 1991;18(Suppl A):47–55.

CC

| Cisplatin | 75 mg/m^2 i.v. day 1 |
| Cyclophosphamide | 600 mg/m^2 i.v. day 1 |

*Repeat every 21 days

Source: Swerenton K, Jeffrey J, Stuart G, et al. Cisplatin-cyclophosphamide versus carboplatin-cyclophosphamide in advanced ovarian cancer: a randomized phase III study of the National Cancer Institute of Canada Clinical Trials Group. J Clin Oncol 1992;10:718–726.

CIS/TAX

| Cisplatin | 75 mg/m^2 i.v. day 2 |
| Paclitaxel | 135 mg/m^2 i.v. over 24 hr day 1 |

*Repeat every 21 days

**Premedicate with dexamethasone 20 mg p.o. every 6 and 12 hr prior to paclitaxel; diphenhydramine 50 mg i.v. and cimetidine 300 mg i.v. or ranitidine 50 mg i.v. 30–60 min prior to paclitaxel

Source: McGuire WP, Hoskins WJ, Brady MF, et al. Cyclophosphamide and cisplatin compared with paclitaxel and cisplatin in patients stage III and stage IV ovarian carcinoma. N Engl J Med 1996;334:1–6.

CIS/TAX (PT)

Cisplatin	75 mg/m^2 i.v. day 1
Paclitaxel	175 mg/m^2 i.v. day 1 over 3 hr

*Repeat every 21 days

**Premedicate with dexamethasone 20 mg p.o. every 6 and 12 hr prior to paclitaxel; diphenhydramine 50 mg i.v. and cimetidine 300 mg i.v. or ranitidine 50 mg i.v. 30–60 min prior to paclitaxel

Source: Piccart MJ, Bertelsen K, Stuart G, et al. Is cisplatin-paclitaxel (P-T) the standard in first-line treatment of advanced ovarian cancer (Ov Ca)? The EORTC-GCCG, NOCOVA, NCI-C and Scottish intergroup experience. Proc Annu Meet Am Soc Clin Oncol 1997; 16:A1258.

Docetaxel

Docetaxel	100 mg/m^2 i.v. day 1

*Repeat every 21 days

Source: Verschraegen C, Kudelka A, Steger M, et al. Randomized phase II study of two dose levels of docetaxel in patients with advanced epithelial ovarian cancer who have failed paclitaxel chemotherapy. Proc Annu Meet Am Soc Clin Oncol 1997;16:A1355.

Doxil

Liposomal doxorubicin	50 mg/m^2 i.v. day 1

*Repeat every 21 days

Source: Muggia F, Hainsworth J, Jeffers S, et al. Liposomal doxorubicin (Doxil) is active against refractory ovarian cancer. Proc Annu Meet Am Soc Clin Oncol 1996;15:A781.

Gemcitabine

Gemcitabine	800 mg/m^2 i.v. days 1, 15, 22

*Repeat every 28 days

Source: Lund B, Hansen OP, Theilade K, et al. Phase II study of Gemcitabine (2',2'-difluorodeoxycytidine) in previously treated ovarian cancer patients. J Natl Cancer Inst 1994;86:1530–1533.

Hexa-CAF

Hexamethylmelamine	150 mg/m^2/day p.o. days 1–14
Cyclophosphamide	150 mg/m^2/day p.o. days 1–14

| Methotrexate | 40 mg/m^2 i.v. days 1, 8 |
| 5-Fluorouracil | 600 mg/m^2 i.v. days 1, 8 |

*Repeat every 28 days

Source: Young RC, Chabner BA, Hubbard SP. Advanced ovarian adenocarcinoma: a prospective clinical trial of melphalan (L-PAM) versus combination chemotherapy. N Engl J Med 1978;299:1261–1266.

Hexalen

| Hexamethylmelamine | 65 mg/m^2/day p.o. q.i.d. days 1–14 |

*Repeat every 28 days

Source: Rustin G, Crawford M, Lambert J, et al. Phase 2 trial of oral Hexalen inpatients with ovarian carcinoma relapsing in more than 6 months after initial chemotherapy. Br J Cancer 1994;69(Suppl 21):13.

Ifos/Cis

| Ifosfamide | 1500 mg/m^2 i.v. bolus days 1–5 or 5000 mg/m^2 i.v. CI over 18 hr day 1 |
| Cisplatin | 100 mg/m^2 i.v. day 1 |

*Repeat every 21 days

Source: Vallejos C, Solidoro A, Gomez H, et al. Ifosfamide plus cisplatin as primary chemotherapy of advanced ovarian cancer. Gynecol Oncol 1997;67:168–171.

Oral Etoposide

| Etoposide | 50 mg p.o. days 1–7 |

*Repeat every 21 days

**Dose may be escalated to 10–14 days' duration

Source: de Jong RS, Hofstra LS, Willemse PH, et al. Effect of low-dose oral etoposide on serum CA-125 in patients with advanced epithelial ovarian cancer. Gynecol Oncol 1997;66:197–201.

PAC-I

Cisplatin (platinum)	50 mg/m^2 i.v. day 1
Doxorubicin (Adriamycin)	50 mg/m^2 i.v. day 1
Cyclophosphamide	750 mg/m^2 i.v. day 1

*Repeat every 3 weeks

Source: Ehrlich CE, Einhorn L, Williams SD, Moorage J. Chemotherapy for Stage III-IV epithelial ovarian cancer with cis-dichlorodiammineplatinum (II), Adriamycin, and cyclophosphamide: a preliminary report. Cancer Treat Rep 1979;63:281–288.

Taxol

Paclitaxel (Taxol)	175 mg/m^2 i.v. over 3 hr day 1

*Repeat every 21 days

*Source: Eisenhauer EA, ten Bokkel Huinink WW, Swenerton KD, et al. Euro-
pean-Canadian randomized trial of paclitaxel in relapsed ovarian cancer: high-
dose versus low-dose and long versus short infusion. J Clin Oncol
1994;12:2654–2666.*

Topotecan

Topotecan	1.5 mg/m^2 i.v. days 1–5

*Repeat every 21 days

*Source: Gordon A, ten Bokkel Huinink W, Gore M, et al. Pooled analysis of pa-
tients (pts) with recurrent ovarian cancer (ROC) who were treated with topotecan (T) after progression or failure on first- or second-line platinum (PLAT) and
paclitaxel (P). Proc Annu Meet Am Soc Clin Oncol 1997;16:A1319.*

Weekly Paclitaxel

Paclitaxel	80 mg/m^2 i.v. weekly

*Source: Abu-Rustum NR, Aghajanian C, Barakat RR, et al. Salvage weekly pa-
clitaxel in recurrent ovarian cancer. Semin Oncol 1997;24(5 Suppl 15):
S62–S67.*

HEAD AND NECK CANCERS

Docetaxel

Taxotere (Docetaxel)	100 mg/m^2 i.v. over 1 hr day 1

*Repeat every 21 days

*Source: Dreyfuss A, Posner M, Clark J, et al. Docetaxel (TXTR): an active drug
against squamous cell carcinoma of the head and neck (SCCHN). Proc Annu
Meet Am Soc Clin Oncol 1995;14:A875 (abstract).*

Methotrexate

Methotrexate	40–60 mg/m^2 i.v. or i.m. weekly

*Source: Taylor SG, McGuire WP, Hauck WW, et al. A randomized comparison
of high-dose infusion methotrexate versus standard-dose weekly therapy in head
and neck squamous cancer. J Clin Oncol 1984;2:1006–1011.*

Paclitaxel

Taxol (paclitaxel)	250 mg/m^2 i.v. day 1 over 24 hr

*Repeat every 21 days

**Granulocyte colony-stimulating factor used to prevent neutropenia

***Premedicate with dexamethasone 20 mg p.o. 6 and 12 hr prior to paclitaxel; diphenhydramine 50 mg i.v. 30–60 min prior to paclitaxel; cimetidine 300 mg or ranitidine 50 mg i.v. 30–60 min prior to paclitaxel

Source: Forastiere AA. Current and future trials of Taxol (paclitaxel) in head and neck cancer. Ann Oncol 1994;5(Suppl 6);S51–S54.

Paclitaxel and Carboplatin

Paclitaxel	200 mg/m^2 i.v. over 3 hr day 1
Carboplatin	To AUC of 7 i.v. day 1
G-CSF	5 mg/kg/day s.q. days 2–12

*Cycles repeated every 28 days

Source: Fountzilas G, Athanassiadis A, Samantas E, et al. Paclitaxel and carboplatin in recurrent or metastatic head and neck cancer: a phase II study. Semin Oncol 1997;24(1 Suppl 2);65–67.

Paclitaxel-Cisplatin

Paclitaxel	200 mg/m^2 i.v. over 3 hr day 1
Cisplatin	75 mg/m^2 i.v. day 2
G-CSF	5 mg/kg/day s.q. days 4–10

*Cycles repeated every 21 days

Source: Hitt R, Hornedo J, Colomer R, et al. A phase I/II study of paclitaxel plus cisplatin as first-line therapy for head and neck cancers: preliminary results. Semin Oncol 1995;22(Suppl 15);50–54.

PF-Larynx Preservation

Cisplatin	100 mg/m^2 i.v. day 1
Fluorouracil	1000 mg/m^2/day days 1–5 CI i.v.
Radiation therapy	66–76 Gy in 180–200 cGy fractions

*Repeat every 21–28 days for 3 cycles

Source: The Department of Veterans Affairs Laryngeal Cancer Study Group. Induction chemotherapy plus radiation compared with surgery plus radiation in patients with advanced laryngeal cancer. N Engl J Med 1991;324:1685–1690.

PF (Wayne State)

Cisplatin	100 mg/m^2 i.v. day 1
Fluorouracil	1000 mg/m^2/day, days 1–4 CI i.v.

*Repeat every 21–28 days

Source: Kish JA, Weaver A, Jacobs J, et al. Cisplatin and 5-fluorouracil infusion in patients with recurrent and disseminated epidermoid cancer of the head and neck. Cancer 1984;53:1819–1824.

PFL

Cisplatin	100 mg/m^2 i.v. day 1
Fluorouracil	800 mg/m^2/day CI i.v. days 1–5
Leucovorin	50 mg/m^2/day p.o. every 6 hr days 1–5

*Repeat every 21 days

Source: Vokes EE, Schilsky RL, Weichselbaum RR, et al. Cisplatin, 5-fluorouracil, and high-dose oral leucovorin for advanced head and neck cancer. Cancer 1989;63(6 Suppl):1048–1053.

VP

Navelbine (vinorelbine)	25 mg/m^2 i.v. days 1, 8
Cisplatin	80 mg/m^2 i.v. day 1

*Repeat every 3 weeks

Source: Gebbia V, Testa A, Di Gregorio C, et al. Vinorelbine plus cisplatin in recurrent or previously untreated unresectable squamous cell carcinoma of the head and neck. Am J Clin Oncol 1995;18:293–296.

LEUKEMIA
ACUTE LYMPHOCYTIC LEUKEMIA
Childhood, Standard Risk

Induction

VP

Vincristine	1.5 mg/m^2 i.v. days 1, 8, 15, 22 (max 2 mg/day)
Prednisone	40 mg/m^2 p.o. daily days 1–29 (max 60 mg/day)
L-Asparaginase	6000 IU/m^2/day 3 for weekly for 6 doses

CNS Therapy

Triple Intrathecal Therapy

Methotrexate	15 mg i.t.
Hydrocortisone	50 mg i.t.
Cytarabine	50 mg i.t.

*Given days 0, 22, 29, 35 then every 2 months

Consolidation

6-Mercaptopurine	75 mg/m^2/day p.o. days 29–43

Continuation

Methotrexate	1000 mg/m^2 i.v. over 24 hr on week 7; at 12 hr start Ara-C 20 mg/m^2 i.m. weekly on weeks 10–17; 22–29; 34–41; 46–53; 58–65; 70–156
Cytarabine	1000 mg/m^2 i.v. over 24 hr on weeks 7, 19, 31, 43, 55, 67
6-Mercaptopurine	75 mg/m^2 p.o. daily on weeks 10–17; 22–29; 34–41; 46–53; 58–65; 70–156
Vincristine	1.5 mg/m^2 i.v. days 1, 8 of weeks 8, 17, 25, 41, 57 (max 2 mg/day)
Prednisone	40 mg/m^2 p.o. days 1–7 of weeks 8, 17, 25, 41, 57 (max 60 mg/day)

Source: Land VJ, Shuster JJ, Crist WM, et al. Comparison of two schedules of intermediate-dose methotrexate and cytarabine consolidation therapy for childhood B-precursor cell acute lymphoblastic leukemia: a Pediatric Oncology Group study. J Clin Oncol 1995;12:1939–1945.

Adult

L-10

Prednisone	60 mg/m^2 p.o. daily for 35 days, then taper
Vincristine	1.5–2 mg/m^2 i.v. days 1, 7, 14, 21, 28
Cyclophosphamide	600–1000 mg/m^2 i.v. day 1 (optional)
Adriamycin	20 mg/m^2 i.v. days 15, 16, 17

Methotrexate	6 mg/m^2 i.v. days 3, 4, 9, 10, 34, 35
Cyclophosphamide	600 mg/m^2 i.v. day 35
Doxorubicin	30 mg/m^2 i.v. day 35

Source: Schauer P, Arlin ZA, Mertelsmann R, et al. Treatment of acute lymphoblastic leukemia in adults: result of the L-10 and L-10m protocols. J Clin Oncol 1983;1:462–470.

Linker Regimen

Induction Therapy

Daunorubicin	50 mg/m^2 i.v. days 1–3
Vincristine	2 mg/m^2 days 1, 8, 15, 22
Prednisone	60 mg/m^2 p.o. days 1–28 (divided into 3 doses)
L-Asparaginase	6000 U/m^2 i.m. days 17–28

If bone marrow on day 14 has residual leukemia:

| Daunorubicin | 50 mg/m^2, day 15 |

If bone marrow on day 28 has residual leukemia:

Daunorubicin	50 mg/m^2 i.v. days 29, 30
Vincristine	2 mg i.v. days 29 and 36
Prednisone	60 mg/m^2 p.o. days 29–42 (divided into 3 doses)
L-Asparaginase	6000 U/m^2 i.m. days 29–35

CNS Prophylaxis

Initiated within 1 week of CR:

| Cranial irradiation | 1800 rad in 10 fractions over 12–14 days |
| Methotrexate | 12 mg i.t. weekly for 6 weeks |

Patients with CNS involvement at diagnosis: begin weekly intrathecal methotrexate during induction chemotherapy:

| Methotrexate | 12 mg i.t. weekly for 10 doses |
| Radiation therapy | 2800 rad |

Consolidation Therapy

Treatment A (cycles 1, 3, 5, and 7)

Daunorubicin	50 mg/m^2 i.v. days 1, 2
Vincristine	2 mg i.v. days 1, 8
Prednisone	60 mg/m^2 p.o. days 1–14
L-Asparaginase	12,000 U i.m. days 2, 4, 7, 9, 11, 14

Treatment B (cycles 2, 4, 6, 8)

Teniposide	165 mg/m² i.v. days 1, 4, 8, 11
Ara-C	300 mg/m² i.v. days 1, 4, 8, 11

Treatment C (cycle 9)

Methotrexate	690 mg/m² i.v. over 42 hr
Leucovorin	15 mg/m² i.v. q 6 hr for 12 doses beginning at 42 hr

Maintenance Therapy

Methotrexate	20 mg/m² p.o. weekly
6-Mercaptopurine	75 mg/m² p.o. daily

*Continue for 30 months of complete response

Source: Linker CA, Levitt LJ, O'Donnell M, et al. Treatment of adult acute lymphoblastic leukemia with intensive cyclical chemotherapy: a follow-up report. Blood 78:2814–2822.

Larson Regimen

Induction Therapy

Course I: Induction (4 weeks)

Cyclophosphamide	1200 mg/m² i.v. day 1
Daunorubicin*	45 mg/m²/day i.v. days 1, 2, 3
Vincristine	2 mg i.v. days 1, 8, 15, 22
Prednisone*	60 mg/m²/day p.o. or i.v. days 1–21
L-Asparaginase	6000 IU/m² s.q. days 5, 8, 11, 15, 18, 22

*For patients aged 60 years or older:

Cyclophosphamide	800 mg/m² i.v. day 1
Daunorubicin	30 mg/m² i.v. days 1, 2, 3
Prednisone	60 mg/m²/day p.o. or i.v. days 1–7

Course II: Early intensification (4 weeks, repeat once)

Intrathecal methotrexate	15 mg i.t. day 1
Cyclophosphamide	1000 mg/m² i.v. day 1
6-Mercaptopurine	60 mg/m²/day p.o. days 1–14
Cytarabine	75 mg/m²/day s.q. days 1–4, 8–11
Vincristine	2 mg i.v. days 15, 22
L-asparaginase	6000 IU/m² s.q. days 15, 18, 22, 25

Course III: CNS prophylaxis and interim maintenance (12 weeks)

Cranial irradiation	2400 cGy days 1–12
Intrathecal methotrexate	15 mg i.t. days 1, 8, 15, 22, 29

| 6-Mercaptopurine | 60 mg/m^2/day p.o. days 1–70 |
| Methotrexate | 20 mg/m^2 p.o. days 36, 43, 50, 57, 64 |

Course IV: Late intensification (8 weeks)

Doxorubicin	30 mg/m^2 i.v. days 1, 8, 15
Vincristine	2 mg i.v. days 1, 8, 15
Dexamethasone	10 mg/m^2/day p.o. days 1–14
Cyclophosphamide	1000 mg/m^2 i.v. day 29
6-Thioguanine	60 mg/m^2/day p.o. days 29–42
Cytarabine	75 mg/m^2/day s.q. days 29–32, 36–39

Course V: Prolonged maintenance (until 24 mo from diagnosis)

Vincristine	2 mg i.v. day 1 of every 4 wk
Prednisone	60 mg/m^2/day p.o. days 1–5 every 4 weeks
Methotrexate	20 mg/m^2 p.o. days 1, 8, 15, 22
6-Mercaptopurine	60 mg/m^2/day p.o. days 1–28

Source: Larson RA, Dodge RK, Burns CP, et al. A five-drug regimen with intensive consolidation for adults with acute lymphoblastic leukemia: Cancer and Leukemia Group B study 8811. Blood 85:2025–2037.

B-CELL ALL/L3

Induction

| Cyclophosphamide | 200 mg/m^2 i.v. days 1–5 |
| Prednisone | 20 mg/m^2 p.o. t.i.d. days 1–5 |

Course A

Vincristine	2 mg i.v. day 1
Methotrexate	1500 mg/m^2 i.v. over 24 hr
Ifosfamide	800 mg/m^2 i.v. days 1–5
VM-26	100 mg/m^2 i.v. days 4, 5
Ara-C	150 mg/m^2 i.v. every 12 hr days 4, 5 (4 doses total)
Dexamethasone	10 mg/m^2 p.o. continued through course B
Leucovorin rescue	30 mg/m^2 i.v. at 36 hr
	30 mg/m^2 p.o. at 42 hr
	15 mg/m^2 p.o. at 48 hr
	5 mg/m^2 p.o. at 54, 68, and 78 hr
TIT (see CNS prophylaxis)	days 1, 5

*Measure methotrexate level at 42 and 68 hr; if elevated, increase the leucovorin rescue dose

**Alternate Course A with Course B every 21 days for a total of 6 cycles

Course B

Vincristine	2 mg i.v. day 1
Methotrexate	1500 mg/m^2 i.v. over 24 hr
Cyclophosphamide	200 mg/m^2 i.v. 200 mg/m^2 i.v. days 1–5
Doxorubicin	25 mg/m^2 i.v. days 4, 5 over 15 min
Dexamethasone	10 mg/m^2 p.o. continued through course A
Leucovorin rescue	30 mg/m^2 i.v. at 36 hr 30 mg/m^2 p.o. at 42 hr 15 mg/m^2 p.o. at 48 hr 5 mg/m^2 p.o. at 54, 68, and 78 hr
TIT (see CNS Prophylaxis)	day 1

CNS Prophylaxis (Triple Intrathecal Therapy)

Methotrexate	15 mg i.t.
Ara-C	40 mg i.t.
Dexamethasone	4 mg i.t.
CNS irradiation	24 Gy if CNS negative; 30 Gy if CNS positive after first completion of course A and B

*Each cycle was alternated for a total of 6 cycles

Source: Hoelzer D, Ludwig WD, Thiel E, et al. Improved outcome in adult B-cell acute lymphoblastic leukemia. Blood 1996;87:495–508.

ACUTE MYELOGENOUS LEUKEMIA

7 + 3 (Ara-C/Dauno) (Induction)

| Cytarabine | 100 mg/m^2 i.v. infusion over 24 hr for 7 days |
| Daunorubicin | 45 mg/m^2 i.v. days 1, 2, and 3 |

*Begin consolidation when ANC is greater than 1500 and platelets are above 100,000

Source: Yates JW, Wallace HJ Jr, Ellison RR, Holland JF. Cytosine arabinoside and daunorubicin therapy in acute nonlymphocytic leukemia. Cancer Chemother Rep 1973;57:485–488.

5 + 2 (Ara-C/Dauno) (Consolidation)

Cytarabine	100 mg/m^2 i.v. infusion over 24 hr for 5 days
Daunorubicin	45 mg/m^2 i.v. days 1, 2

Source: Yates JW, Wallace HJ Jr, Ellison RR, et al. Cytosine arabinoside and daunorubicin therapy in acute nonlymphocytic leukemia. Cancer Chemother Rep, 1973;57:485–488.

7 + 3 + 3 (Ara-C/Dauno) (Induction and Consolidation)

Induction

Cytarabine	100 mg/m^2 i.v. infusion over 24 hr for 7 days; then 2000 mg/m^2 i.v. every 12 hr days 8–10
Daunorubicin	45 mg/m^2 i.v. days 1, 2, 3

Consolidation

Cycles 1 and 3

Cytarabine	200 mg/m^2 i.v. infusion over 24 hr for 5 days
Daunorubicin	60 mg/m^2 i.v. days 1, 2

Cycle 2

Cytarabine	2000 mg/m^2 i.v. every 12 hr days 1, 2, 3
Etoposide	100 mg/m^2 i.v. days 4, 5

*Patients were offered autologous or allogeneic transplant in first remission

Source: Mitus J, Miller KB, Schenkein DP, et al. Improved survival for patients with acute myelogenous leukemia. J Clin Oncol 1995;13:560–569.

Ara-C/Dox

Induction

Cytarabine	100 mg/m^2 i.v. infusion over 24 hr for 7 days
Doxorubicin	30 mg/m^2 i.v. days 1, 2, 3

Source: Preisler HD, Bjornsson S, Henderson ES. Adriamycin-cytosine arabinoside therapy for adult acute myelocytic leukemia. Cancer Treat Rep 1977;61:89–92.

Ara-C/Ida (Induction and Consolidation)

Induction

Cytarabine	100 mg/m^2 i.v. infusion over 24 hr × 7 days
Idarubicin	12 mg/m^2 i.v. days 1, 2, 3

*Repeat if leukemia present on day 14 bone marrow

Consolidation

Cytarabine	100 mg/m^2 i.v. every 12 hr days 1–5
Idarubicin	15 mg/m^2 i.v. day 1
Thioguanine	100 mg/m^2 p.o. every 12 hr days 1–5

**Repeat every 21–28 days

Maintenance

Cytarabine	100 mg/m^2 i.v. days 1–5
Idarubicin	12 mg/m^2 i.v. days 1, 2

***Repeat every 13 weeks for 4 cycles

Source: Vogler WR, Velez-Garcia E, Omura G, Remey M. A phase three trial comparing daunorubicin or idarubicin combined with cytosine arabinoside in acute myelogenous leukemia. Semin Oncol 1989;16(Suppl 2):21–24.

Ara-C/Mito for Elderly

Cytarabine	3000 mg/m^2 i.v. days 1–5
Mitoxantrone	12 mg/m^2 i.v. over 30 min days 1–3

*No consolidation was given

Source: Feldman EJ, Seiter K, Damon L, et al. A randomized trial of high- vs standard-dose mitoxantrone with cytarabine in elderly patients with acute myeloid leukemia. Leukemia 1997;11:485–489.

Ara-C/Thioguanine (Induction)

Cytarabine	100 mg/m^2 i.v. every 12 hr for 10 days
6-Thioguanine	100 mg/m^2 i.v. every 12 hr p.o. for 10 days

*Repeat every 30 days until remission

Source: Bodey GP, Freireich EJ, McCredie KB, et al. Combinations of arabinosyl cytosine and 6-thioguanine for treatment of adults with acute leukemia. Med Pediatr Oncol 1975;1:149–158.

Ara-C-Thioguanine (Maintenance)

Cytarabine	100 mg/m² i.v. every 12 hr for 5 days
6-Thioguanine	100 mg/m² i.v. every 12 hr p.o. for 5 days

*Repeat every 28 days

Source: Armitage JO, Burns CP. Maintenance of remission in adult acute non-lymphoblastic leukemia using intermittent courses of cytosine arabinoside (NSC-63878) and 6-thioguanine (NSC-752). Cancer Treat Rep 1976;60:585–589.

ATRA (APL only)

All *trans* retinoic acid	22.5 mg/m² p.o. every 12 hr until CR or for 90 days
Then	
Cytarabine	200 mg/m² i.v. infusion over 24 hr for 7 days
Daunorubicin	60 mg/m² i.v. days, 1, 2, and 3
Consolidation	
Cytarabine	1000 mg/m² i.v. every 12 hr days 1–4
Daunorubicin	45 mg/m² i.v. days 1–3

Source: Fenaux P, DeLey MC, Castaigne S, et al. Effect of all trans retinoic acid in newly diagnosed acute promyelocytic leukemia: results of a multicenter randomized trial. European APL 91 Group. Blood 1993;82:3241–249.

DAT

Induction

Daunorubicin	60 mg/m² i.v. days 5, 6, 7
Cytarabine (Ara-C)	100 mg/m² i.v. over 30 min b.i.d. for 7 days
6-Thioguanine	100 mg/m² p.o. every 12 hr for 7 days

Consolidation Therapy

Two cycles of cytarabine (Ara-C) and thioguanine every 12 hr for 5 days followed by a single injection of daunorubicin. Consolidation cycles were given at 21-day intervals.

CNS Therapy

Prophylactic 2400-rad cranial irradiation; cytarabine 100 mg/m² i.t. divided into 5 doses.

Maintenance therapy

Monthly 5-day cycles of cytarabine-thioguanine alternating with a single dose of daunorubicin

Source: Gale RP, Cline MJ. High remission-induction rate in acute myeloid leukemia. Lancet 1977;1:497–499.

HiDAC Consolidation

Cytarabine	3000 mg/m² i.v. every 12 hr days 1, 3, 5

*Initial chemo with 7 + 3

**Repeat every 28 days for 4 cycles

Source: Mayer RJ, Davis RB, Schiffer CA, et al. Intensive postremission chemotherapy in adults with acute myelogenous leukemia. Cancer and Leukemia Group B. N Engl J Med 1994;331:896–903.

Mito/VP-16

Induction

Mitoxantrone	10 mg/m² i.v. days 1–5
Etoposide	100 mg/m² i.v. days 1–3

Consolidation

Mitoxantrone	8 mg/m² i.v. days 1–5
Etoposide	75 mg/m² i.v. days 1–5
Cytarabine	75 mg/m² i.v. every 12 hr days 1–5

Source: Ho AD, Lipp T, Ehninger G, et al. Combination therapy with mitoxantrone and etoposide in refractory acute myelogenous leukemia. Cancer Treat Rep 1986;70:1025–1027.

Plicamycin/Hydrea

Plicamycin	25 µg/kg i.v. q.o.d. for 21 days
Hydroxyurea	4 g/day p.o. for WBC >100,000
	3g/day p.o. for WBC > 75,000
	2g/day p.o. for WBC > 50,000
	1.5 g/day p.o. for WBC > 30,000
	1g/day p.o. for WBC > 15,000
	0.5 g/day p.o. for WBC >7500
	Hold if WBC < 7500

Source: Koller CA, Miller DM. Preliminary observations on the therapy of the myeloid blast phase of chronic granulocytic leukemia with plicamycin and hydroxyurea. N Engl J Med 1986;315:1433–1438.

CHRONIC LYMPHOCYTIC LEUKEMIA

2-CDA

Cladaribine	0.09 mg/kg/day i.v. CI days 1–7

Source: Saven A, Lemon RH, Kotsy M, et al. 2-Chlorodeoxyadenosine activity in patients with untreated chronic lymphocytic leukemia. J Clin Oncol 1995;13:590–594.

Pulse CP

Chlorambucil	30 mg/m^2 p.o. day 1
Prednisone	80 mg p.o. days 1–5

*Repeat every 4 weeks

Source: Raphael B, Andersen JW, Silber R, et al. Comparison of chlorambucil and prednisone versus cyclophosphamide, vincristine, and prednisone as initial treatment of chronic lymphocytic leukemia: long-term follow-up of an Eastern Cooperative Oncology Group randomized clinical trial. J Clin Oncol 1991;9:770–776.

CVP

Cyclophosphamide	400 mg/m^2 p.o. days 1–5
Vincristine	1.4 mg/m^2 i.v. day 1 (max 2 mg)
Prednisone	100 mg/m^2 p.o. days 1–5; then taper

*Repeat every 21 days

Source: Raphael B, Andersen JW, Silber R, et al. Comparison of chlorambucil and prednisone versus cyclophosphamide, vincristine, and prednisone as initial treatment of chronic lymphocytic leukemia: long-term follow-up of an Eastern Cooperative Oncology Group randomized clinical trial. J Clin Oncol 1991;9:770–776.

Fludarabine and Prednisone

Fludarabine	30 mg/m^2 i.v. days 1–5
Prednisone	30 mg/m^2 i.v. days 1–5

*Repeat every 4 weeks

Source: O'Brien S, Kantarjian H, Beron M, et al. Results of fludarabine and prednisone therapy in 264 patients with chronic lymphocytic leukemia with multivariate analysis-derived prognostic model for response to treatment. Blood 1993;82:1695–1700.

CHRONIC MYELOGENOUS LEUKEMIA
Hydrea

Hydrea	40 mg/kg/day p.o. daily

Source: Hehlmann R, Heimpel H, Hasford J, et al. Randomized comparison of interferon-α with busulfan and hydrea in chronic myelogenous leukemia. Blood 1994;12:4064–4077.

Interferon

Interferon-α	5×10^6 IU/m^2 s.q. daily

*Treatment was given at maximal tolerated dose to maintain WBC of 2×10^9 to 4×10^9/L and to reach hematologic remission

Source: Hehlmann R, Heimpel H, Hasford J, et al. Randomized comparison of interferon-α with busulfan and hydrea in chronic myelogenous leukemia. Blood 1994;84:382a.

HAIRY CELL LEUKEMIA
2-CdA

Cladaribine	0.09 mg/kg/day CI i.v. days 1–7

Source: Tallman MS, Hakimian D, Variakojis D, et al. A single cycle of 2-chlorodeoxyadenosine results in complete remission in the majority of patients with hairy cell leukemia. Blood 1992;80:2203–2209.

LUNG CANCERS
NON-SMALL CELL LUNG CANCER
CaN

Carboplatin	300 mg/m^2 i.v. day 1
Navelbine (vinorelbine)	25 mg/m^2 i.v. day 1

*Repeat every 28 days

Source: Masotti A, Borzellino G, Zannini G, et al. Efficacy and toxicity of vinorelbine-carboplatin combination in the treatment of advanced adenocarcinoma or large-cell carcinoma of the lung. Tumori 1995;81:112–116.

CAP

Cyclophosphamide	400 mg/m^2 i.v. day 2
Doxorubicin (Adriamycin)	40 mg/m^2 i.v. day 1
Platinum (cisplatin)	60 mg/m^2 i.v. day 1

*Repeat every 28 days

Source: Eagan RT, Frytak S, Creagan ET, et al. Phase II study of cyclophosphamide, Adriamycin, and cis-dichlorodiammineplatinum (II) by infusion in patients with adenocarcinoma and large cell carcinoma of the lung. Cancer Treat Rep 1979;63:1589–1591.

CaT

Carboplatin	7.5 AUC i.v. day 1 after Taxol
Taxol (Paclitaxel)	175 mg/m^2 i.v. over 1 hr day 1

*Repeat every 21 days

**Granulocyte colony-stimulating support was used

***If absolute neutrophil count > 500 and platelet > 50,000, paclitaxel was increased by 35 mg/m^2/cycle to a max dose of 280 mg/m^2

Source: Langer CJ, Leighton JC, Comis RL, et al. Paclitaxel by 24- or 1-hr infusion in combination with carboplatin in advanced non-small cell lung cancer: the Fox Chase Cancer Center experience. Semin Oncol 1995;22(4 Suppl 9):18–29.

Or

Carboplatin	7 AUC i.v. day 1
Taxol (Paclitaxel)	175 mg/m^2 i.v. day 1 over 3 hr

*Repeat every 21 days

Source: Kosmidis PA, Mylonakis N, Fountzilas G, et al. Paclitaxel and carboplatin in inoperable non-small-cell lung cancer: a phase II study. Ann Oncol 1997; 8:697–679.

CT

Cisplatin	75 mg/m^2 i.v. after Taxol day 2
Taxol (Paclitaxel)	135 mg/m^2 i.v. day 1 over 24 hr

*Repeat every 21 days

Or

Cisplatin	75 mg/m^2 i.v. after Taxol day 2
Taxol (paclitaxel)	250 mg/m^2 i.v. day 1 over 24 hr

*Granulocyte colony-stimulating factor was used

**Repeat every 3 weeks

Source: Rowinsky EK, Bonomi P, Jiroutek M, et al. Pharmacodynamic (PD) studies of paclitaxel (T) in ECOG 5592: a phase III trial comparing etoposide (E) plus cisplatin (C) Vs low-dose paclitaxel plus cisplatin Vs high-dose paclitaxel plus cisplatin plus G-CSF in advanced non-small cell lung cancer (NSCLC). Proc Annu Meet Am Soc Clin Oncol 1997;16:A1618.

Or

| Cisplatin | 80 mg/m^2 i.v. day 1 after Taxol |
| Taxol (paclitaxel) | 175 mg/m^2 i.v. day 1 over 3 hr |

*Repeat every 3 weeks

Source: Giaccone G, Postmus PE, Splinter TA, et al. Cisplatin/paclitaxel Vs cisplatin/teniposide for advanced non-small-cell lung cancer: the EORTC Lung Cancer Cooperative Group. The European Organization for Research and Treatment of Cancer. Oncology (Huntingt) 1997;11(4 Suppl 3):11–14.

Docetaxel

| Docetaxel | 100 mg/m^2 i.v. day 1 |

*Repeat every 21 days

Source: Gandara DR, Vokes E, Green M, et al. Docetaxel (Taxotere) in platinum-treated non-small cell lung cancer (NSCLC): confirmation of prolonged survival in a multicenter trial. Proc Annu Meet Am Soc Clin Oncol 1997;16:A1632.

Doxorubicin and Cisplatin

| Doxorubicin | 60 mg/m^2 i.v. day 1 |
| Cisplatin | 60 mg/m^2 i.v. day 1 |

*Repeat every 21 days

Source: Morris RW, Brubaker LH, Kardinal CG, et al. Adriamycin and cis-dichlorodiammineplatinum in nonresectable and metastatic carcinoma of the lung. Cancer Clin Trials 1979;2(1):37–41.

Gemcitabine

| Gemcitabine | 1000 mg/m^2 i.v. days 1, 8, 15 |

*Repeat every 28 days

Source: Dornoff W, Drings P, Kellokumpu-Lehtinen P, et al. Single-agent gemcitabine versus cisplatin-etoposide: early results of a randomized phase II study in locally advanced or metastatic non-small-cell lung cancer. Ann Oncol 1997;8:525–529.

Gemcitabine and Cisplatin

| Gemcitabine | 1000 mg/m^2 i.v. days 1, 8, 15 |
| Cisplatin | 100 mg/m^2 i.v. day 15 |

*Repeat every 21 days

Source: Einhorn LH. Phase II trial of gemcitabine plus cisplatin in non-small cell lung cancer: a Hoosier Oncology Group study. Semin Oncol 1997;24(3 Suppl 8):S24–S26.

Gemcitabine and Docetaxel

Gemcitabine	900 mg/m^2 i.v. days 1, 8
Docetaxel	100 mg/m^2 i.v. day 8

*Repeat every 21 days

*Colony-stimulating support used

Source: Georgoulias V, Kourousis C, Androulakis N, et al. Docetaxel (Taxotere) and gemcitabine in the treatment of non-small cell lung cancer: preliminary results. Semin Oncol 1997;24(4 Suppl 14):S22–S25.

Gemcitabine and Paclitaxel

Gemcitabine	900 mg/m^2 i.v. days 1, 8
Paclitaxel	175 mg/m^2 i.v. day 8

*Repeat every 21 days

**Colony-stimulating support used

Source: Georgoulias V, Kourousis C, Kakolyris S, et al. Second-line treatment of advanced non-small cell lung cancer with paclitaxel and gemcitabine: a preliminary report on an active regimen. Semin Oncol 1997;24(4 Suppl 12): S61–S66.

MVP

Mitomycin C	8 mg/m^2 i.v. days 1
Vinblastine	6 mg/m^2 i.v. days 1, 22
Cisplatin	50 mg/m^2 i.v. days 1, 22

*Repeat every 6 weeks

Source: Ellis PA, Nicolson MC, Tait D, Smith IE. MVP with moderate dose cisplatin: a pragmatic and effective chemotherapy for symptom relief in non-small cell lung cancer. Br J Cancer 1994;69(Suppl 21):14.

Navelbine (Vinorelbine)

Vinorelbine	25 mg/m^2 i.v. day 1 weekly

Source: Furuse K, Fukuoka M, Kuba M, et al. Randomized study of vinorelbine (VRB) versus vindesine (VDS) in previously untreated stage IIIB or IV non-small-cell lung cancer (NSCLC): the Japan Vinorelbine Lung Cancer Cooperative Study Group. Ann Oncol 1996;7:815–820.

Navelbine and Cisplatin

Cisplatin	100 mg/m^2 i.v. days 1, 29 and every 6 weeks
Navelbine	35 mg/m^2 i.v. days 1, 15, 29; 17.5 mg/m^2 i.v. days 8, 22; then 35 mg/m^2 i.v. every 2 weeks

Source: Brooks BJ, Gralla RJ, McGaw HJ, et al. Cisplatin + vinorelbine (Navelbine) combination chemotherapy for advanced non-small cell lung cancer: testing the efficacy of a regimen designed to reduce toxicity and increase dose-intensity. Proc Annu Meet Am Soc Clin Oncol 1994; 13:A1162.

Paclitaxel

Paclitaxel	100 mg/m^2 i.v. day 1

*Repeat every 21 days

Source: Tester WJ, Jin PY, Reardon DH, et al. Phase II study of patients with metastatic nonsmall cell carcinoma of the lung treated with paclitaxel by 3-hr infusion. Cancer 1997;79:724–729.

SMALL CELL CARCINOMA

ACE

Doxorubicin	45 mg/m^2 i.v. day 1
Cyclophosphamide	1000 mg/m^2 i.v. day 1
Etoposide	50 mg/m^2 i.v. day 1

*Repeat every 21–28 days

Source: Aisner J, Whitacre M, Abrams J, et al. Doxorubicin, cyclophosphamide, etoposide and platinum, doxorubicin, cyclophosphamide and etoposide for small-cell carcinoma of the lung. Semin Oncol 1986;13(3 Suppl 3):54–62.

PEC

Paclitaxel	200 mg/m^2 i.v. day 1
Etoposide	50 mg p.o. days 1, 3, 5, 7, 9; 100 mg p.o. days 2, 4, 6, 8, 10
Carboplatin	AUC 6 i.v. day 1

*Repeat every 21 days for 4 cycles

**Radiation therapy with cycles 3 and 4

Source: Hainsworth JD, Gray JR, Stroup SL, et al. Paclitaxel, carboplatin, and extended-schedule etoposide in the treatment of small-cell lung cancer: comparison of sequential phase II trials using different dose-intensities. J Clin Oncol 1997;15:3464–70.

CAV

Cyclophosphamide	1000 mg/m^2 i.v. day 1
Doxorubicin (Adriamycin)	50 mg/m^2 i.v. day 1
Vincristine	1.4 mg/m^2 (maximum dose 2 mg) i.v.

*Repeat every 21 days

Source: Comis RL. Clinical trials of cyclophosphamide, etoposide, and vincristine in the treatment of small-cell lung cancer. Semin Oncol 1986;13(3 Suppl 3):40–44.

CAVE

Cyclophosphamide	1,000 mg/m^2 i.v. day 1
Doxorubicin	50 mg/m^2 i.v. day 1
Vincristine	1.4 mg/m^2 i.v. day 1
	(maximum 2 mg)
Etoposide	100 mg/m^2 i.v. day 1

*Repeat every 21 days

Source: Tummarello D, Graziano F, Mari D, et al. Small cell lung cancer (SCLC): a randomized trial of cyclophosphamide, Adriamycin, vincristine plus etoposide (CAV-E) or teniposide (CAV-T) as induction treatment, followed in complete responders by interferon-α or no treatment, as maintenance therapy. Anticancer Res 1994;14:2221–2227.

CAV/PE

PE	
Cisplatin	60 mg/m^2 i.v. day 1
Etoposide	120 mg/m^2 i.v. days 1–3
CAV	
Cyclophosphamide	600 mg/m^2 i.v. day 1
Doxorubicin	50 mg/m^2 i.v. day 1
Vincristine	2 mg IVP day 1

*Alternate PE and CAV every 21 days for a total of 6 courses

**Radiation therapy 5000 Gy in 25 fractions over 5 weeks

Source: Souhami RL, Rudd R, Ruiz de Elvira MC, et al. Randomized trial comparing weekly versus 3-week chemotherapy in small-cell lung cancer: a Cancer Research Campaign trial. J Clin Oncol 1994;12:1806–1813.

CEV

Cyclophosphamide	1000 mg/m^2 i.v. day 1
Etoposide	50 mg/m^2 i.v. day 1; 100 mg/m^2 p.o. days 2–5
Vincristine	1.4 mg/m^2 i.v. day 1 (maximum dose 2 mg)

*Repeat every 21 days

Source: Comis RL. Clinical trials of cyclophosphamide, etoposide, and vincristine in the treatment of small-cell lung cancer. Semin Oncol 1986;13(3 Suppl 3):40–44.

PACE

Cisplatin	20 mg/m^2 i.v. days 1–5
Doxorubicin	45 mg/m^2 i.v. day 1
Cyclophosphamide	50 mg/m^2 i.v. day 1

*Repeat every 21–28 days

Source: Aisner J, Whitacre M, Abrams J, et al. Doxorubicin, cyclophosphamide, etoposide and platinum, doxorubicin, cyclophosphamide and etoposide for small-cell carcinoma of the lung. Semin Oncol 1986;13(3 Suppl 3):54–62.

Topotecan

Topotecan	1.5 mg/m^2 i.v. days 1–5

*Repeat every 21 days

Source: Ardizzoni A, Hansen H, Dombernowsky P, et al. Topotecan, a new active drug in the second-line treatment of small-cell lung cancer: a phase II study in patients with refractory and sensitive disease. The European Organization for Research and Treatment of Cancer Early Clinical Studies Group and New Drug Development Office, and the Lung Cancer Cooperative Group. J Clin Oncol 1997;15:2090–2096.

VP16/DDP

Cisplatin	25 mg/m^2 i.v. days 1–3
Etoposide	100 mg/m^2 i.v. days 1–3

*Repeat every 21 days

Source: Loehrer PJ Sr, Einhorn LH, Greco FA. Cisplatin plus etoposide in small cell lung cancer. Semin Oncol 1988;15(3 Suppl 3):2–8.

LYMPHOMA

HODGKIN'S DISEASE

ABVD

Doxorubicin	25 mg/m^2 i.v. days 1, 15
Bleomycin	10 U/m^2 i.v. days 1, 15
Vinblastine	6 mg/m^2 i.v. days 1, 15
Dacarbazine (DTIC)**	150 mg/m^2/day i.v. days 1–5

*Repeat every 28 days

**Dacarbazine can also be given as 375 mg/m^2 i.v. days 1, 15

Source: Bonadonna G, Zucali R, Monfardini S, et al. Combination chemotherapy of Hodgkin's disease with Adriamycin, bleomycin, vinblastine, and imidazole carboxamide vs MOPP. Cancer 1975;36:252–259.

B-CAVe

Bleomycin	5 U/m^2 i.v. days 1, 28, 35
Lomustine (CCNU)	100 mg/m^2 p.o. days 1, 28
Doxorubicin	60 mg/m^2 i.v. days 1, 28
Vinblastine	5 mg/m^2 i.v. days 1, 28

*Repeat every 8 weeks

Source: Harker GW, Kushlan P, Rosenberg SA. Combination chemotherapy for advanced Hodgkin's disease after failure of MOPP: ABVD and B-CAVe. Ann Intern Med 1984;101:440–446.

BVCPP

BCNU	100 mg/m^2 i.v. day 1
Cyclophosphamide	600 mg/m^2 i.v. day 1
Vinblastine	5 mg/m^2 i.v. day 1
Procarbazine	50 mg/m^2 day 1 p.o.
	100 mg/m^2 p.o. days 2–10
Prednisone	60 mg/m^2 p.o. days 1–10

*Repeat every 28 days

Source: Bakemeier RF, Anderson JR, Castello WM, et. al. BCVPP chemotherapy for advanced Hodgkin's disease: evidence for greater duration of complete remission, greater survival and less toxicity than with a MOPP regimen. Ann Intern Med 1984;101:447–456.

ChlVPP

Chlorambucil	6 mg/m^2 p.o. days 1–14 (max 10 mg per dose)
Vinblastine	6 mg/m^2 i.v. days 1–8 (max 10 mg per dose)
Procarbazine	100 mg/m^2 p.o. days 1–14 (max 150 mg/day)
Prednisone	40 mg p.o. days 1–14

*Repeat every 28 days

Source: Selby P, Milan PS, Meldrum M, et al. Chl/VPP combination chemotherapy for Hodgkin's disease: long term results. Br J Cancer 1990;62:279–285.

C-MOPP

Cyclophosphamide	650 mg/m^2 i.v. days 1, 8
Vincristine (Oncovin)	1.4 mg/m^2 i.v. days 1, 8
Procarbazine	100 mg/m^2 p.o. days 1–14
Prednisone	40 mg/m^2 p.o. days 1–14

*Prednisone is used only in first and fourth courses

**Repeat every 28 days

Source: DeVita VT Jr., Serpick AA, Carbone PP. Combination chemotherapy in the treatment of advanced Hodgkin's disease. Ann Intern Med 1970;73:881–895.

MOPP

Nitrogen mustard	6 mg/m^2 i.v. days 1, 8
Vincristine (Oncovin)	1.4 mg/m^2 i.v. days 1, 8
Procarbazine	100 mg/m^2 p.o. days 1–14
Prednisone	40 mg/m^2 p.o. days 1–14

*Prednisone in the original report was given only in cycles 1 and 4; it is now given with all cycles

**Repeat every 28 days

Source: DeVita VT Jr., Serpick AA, Carbone PP. Combination chemotherapy in the treatment of advanced Hodgkin's disease. Ann Intern Med 1970; 73:881–895.

MOPP/ABV Hybrid

Mechlorethamine	6 mg/m^2 i.v. day 1
Vincristine	1.4 mg/m^2 i.v. day 1 (maximum dose 2 mg)
Procarbazine	100 mg/m^2 p.o. days 1–7
Prednisone	40 mg/m^2 p.o. days 1–14
Doxorubicin	35 mg/m^2 i.v. day 8
Bleomycin	10 U/m^2 i.v. day 8, preceded by
Hydrocortisone	100 mg i.v.
Vinblastine	6 mg/m^2 i.v. day 8

*Repeat every 28 days

*If intractable chemical phlebitis develops 600 mg/m^2 of i.v. cyclophosphamide is substituted

Source: Conners JM, Klimo P. MOPP/ABV hybrid chemotherapy for advanced Hodgkin's disease. Semin Hematol 1987;24:35–40.

MVPP

Nitrogen mustard	6 mg/m^2 i.v. days 1, 8
Vinblastine	6 mg/m^2 i.v. days 1, 8
Procarbazine	100 mg/m^2 p.o. days 1, 14
Prednisone	40 mg/m^2 p.o. days 1–14

*Repeat every 28 days

Source: Nicholson WM, Beard MEJ, Crowther D, et. al. Combination chemotherapy in generalized Hodgkin's disease. Br Med J 1970;3:7–10.

MVVPP

Nitrogen mustard	0.4 mg/m^2 i.v. day 1
Vincristine	1.4 mg/m^2 i.v. days 1, 8, 15
Vinblastine	6 mg/m^2 i.v. days 22, 29, 36
Procarbazine	100 mg/m^2 days 22–43
Prednisone	40 mg/m^2 p.o. days 1–21, then taper off over 2 weeks, omit from course 2 and 4

*Repeat every 56 days for 3 courses

Source: Prosnitz LR, Farber LR, Fischer JJ, et al. Long-term remissions with combined modality therapy for advanced Hodgkin's disease. Cancer 1976;37:2826–2833.

Stanford V

Doxorubicin	25 mg/m^2 i.v. days 1, 15
Vinblastine	6 mg/m^2 i.v. days 1, 15
Mechlorethamine	6 mg/m^2 i.v. day 1
Vincristine	1.4 mg/m^2 i.v. days 8, 22 (2 mg max)
Bleomycin	5 U/m^2 i.v. days 8, 22
Etoposide	60 mg/m^2 i.v. days 15, 16
Prednisone	40 mg/m^2 p.o. q.o.d.

*Repeat cycles every 28 days for a total of 3 cycles

**Vincristine and vinblastine doses reduced for patients > 50 years of age

***Prednisone tapered beginning week 10

Source: Bartlett NL, Rosenberg SA, Hoppe RT, et al. Brief chemotherapy, Stanford V, and adjuvant radiotherapy for bulky or advanced-stage Hodgkin's disease: a preliminary report. J Clin Oncol 1995;13:1080–1088.

Salvage Treatments

ABDIC

Doxorubicin	45 mg/m^2 i.v. day 1
Bleomycin	5 U/m^2 i.v. days 1, 5
Dacarbazine (DTIC)	200 mg/m^2 i.v. days 1–5
CCNU	50 mg/m^2 p.o. day 1
Prednisone	40 mg/m^2 p.o. days 1–5

*Repeat every 28 days

Source: Tannie N, Hagemeister F, Velasquez W, et al. Long-term follow-up with ABDIC salvage chemotherapy of MOPP-resistant Hodgkin's disease. J Clin Oncol 1983;1:432–439.

Dexa-BEAM

Dexamethasone	8 mg every 8 hr p.o. days 1–10
Carmustine	60 mg/m^2 i.v. day 2
Etoposide	75 mg/m^2/day i.v. days 4–7
Cytarabine	100 mg/m^2/day i.v. every 12 hr days 4–7
Melphalan	20 mg/m^2 i.v. day 3

*Repeat every 28 days

Source: Pfrundschuh MG, Rueffer U, Lathan B, et al. Dexa-BEAM in patients with Hodgkin's disease refractory to multi-drug chemotherapy regimens: a trial of the German Hodgkin's Disease Study Group. J Clin Oncol 1994;12:580–586.

Mini-BEAM

BCNU	60 mg/m^2 i.v. day 1
Etoposide	75 mg/m^2 i.v. days 2–5
Ara-C	100 mg/m^2 i.v. every 12 hr days 2–5
Melphalan	30 mg/m^2 i.v. on day 6

*Repeat every 4–6 weeks

Source: Colwill R, Crump M, Couture F, et al. Mini BEAM as salvage therapy for relapsed or refractory Hodgkin's disease before intensive therapy and autologous bone marrow transplant. J Clin Oncol 1995;13:396–402.

CBVD

CCNU	120 mg/m^2 p.o. day 1
Bleomycin	15 U i.v. days 1, 22
Vinblastine	6 mg/m^2 i.v. days 1, 22
Dexamethasone	3 mg/m^2 p.o. days 1–21

*Repeat every 6 weeks

Source: Weiss J, Van Roemeling R, Peters HD, et al. Chemotherapy in pretreated Hodgkin's disease with lomustine, bleomycin, vinblastine, and dexamethasone. Deutsch Med Wochenschr 1983;108:1428–1432.

CEP

CCNU	80 mg/m^2 p.o. day 1
Etoposide (VP-16)	100 mg/m^2/day p.o. days 1–5
Prednimustine	60 mg/m^2/day p.o. days 1–5

*Repeat every 28 days

Source: Santoro A, Viviani S, Valaqussa P, et al. CCNU, etoposide, and prednimustine (EP) in refractory Hodgkin's disease. Semin Oncol 1986;13:23–26.

CEVD

CCNU	80 mg/m^2 p.o. day 1
Etoposide (VP-16)	120 mg/m^2/day p.o. days 1–5, 22–26
	Or
	60 mg/m^2 i.v. days 1–5
Vindesine	3 mg/m^2 p.o. days 1, 22
Dexamethasone	3 mg/m^2/day p.o. days 1–8
	1.5 mg/m^2/day p.o. days 9–26

*Repeat every 42 days

Source: Pfreundschuh MG, Schoppe WD, Fuchs R, et al. Lomustine, etoposide, vindesine, and dexamethasone (LEVD) in Hodgkin's lymphoma refractory to cyclophosphamide, vincristine, procarbazine, and prednisone (COPP) and doxorubicin, bleomycin, vinblastine, and dacarbazine (ABVD): a multicenter trial of the German Hodgkin's Study Group cancer treatment reports 1987;71:1203–1207.

EVA

Etoposide (VP-16)	200 mg/m^2/day p.o. days 1–5
Vincristine	2 mg i.v. day 1
Adriamycin	50 mg/m^2 i.v. day 1

*Repeat every 21–28 days

Source: Richards MA, Waxman JH, Man T, et al. EVA treatment for recurrent or unresponsive Hodgkin's disease. Cancer Chemother Pharmacol 1986;18: 51–53.

EVAP

Etoposide	120 mg/m^2 i.v. days 1, 8, 15
Vinblastine	4 mg/m^2 i.v. days 1, 8, 15
Cytarabine (Ara-C)	30 mg/m^2 i.v. days 1, 8, 15
Cisplatin	40 mg/m^2 i.v. days 1, 8, 15

*Repeat every 4 weeks

Source: Longo DL. The use of chemotherapy in the treatment of Hodgkin's disease. Semin Oncol 1990;17:716–735.

PCVP

Vinblastine	3 mg/m^2 i.v. day 1 every 2 weeks
Procarbazine	70 mg/m^2 p.o. every other day
Cyclophosphamide	70 mg/m^2 p.o. every other day
Prednisone	8 mg/m^2 p.o. every other day

*Therapy lasts for 1 year

Source: Mandelli F, Cimino G, Mauro FR, et al. Prognosis and management of patients affected by multi pre-treated Hodgkin's disease. 1986 Haematologia 71:205–208.

VABCD

Vinblastine	6 mg/m^2 i.v. days 1, 22
Doxorubicin	400 mg/m^2 i.v. days 1, 22
Dacarbazine	800 mg/m^2 i.v. days 1, 22
CCNU	80 mg/m^2 p.o. day 1 every 6 weeks
Bleomycin	15 U i.v. days 1, 8, 15, 22, 29, 35

*Repeat every 6 weeks

Source: Einhorn LH, Williams SD, Stevens EE, et al. Treatment of MOPP-refractory Hodgkin's disease with vinblastine, doxorubicin, bleomycin, CCNU, and dacarbazine. Cancer 1983;51:1348–1352.

NON-HODGKIN'S LYMPHOMA

BACOP

Bleomycin	5 U/m^2 i.v. days 15, 22
Doxorubicin	25 mg/m^2 i.v. days 1, 8
Cyclophosphamide	650 mg/m^2 i.v. days 1, 8
Vincristine (Oncovin)	1.4 mg/m^2 i.v. days 1, 8
Prednisone	60 mg/m^2/day p.o. days 15–28

*Repeat every 28 days

Sources: Schein PS, DeVita VT Jr, Hubbard S. Bleomycin, Adriamycin, cyclophosphamide, vincristine, and prednisone (BACOP) combination chemotherapy in the treatment of advanced histiocytic lymphoma. Ann Intern Med 1976; 85:417–422.

CEPP(B)

| Cyclophosphamide | 600 mg/m^2 i.v. days 1, 8 |
| Etoposide | 70 mg/m^2 i.v. days 1–3 |

Procarbazine	60 mg/m^2 p.o. days 1–10
Prednisone	60 mg/m^2 p.o. days 1–10
*(Bleomycin)	(15 U/m^2 i.v. days 1, 15)

*Response to this regimen does not seem to be significantly different without bleomycin

**Repeat every 28 days

Source: Chao NJ, Rosenberg SA, Horning SJ. CEPP(B): an effective and well-tolerated regimen in poor risk, aggressive non-Hodgkin's lymphoma. Blood 1990;76:1293–1298.

CHOP

Cyclophosphamide (Cytoxan)	750 mg/m^2 i.v. day 1
Doxorubicin	50 mg/m^2 i.v. day 1
Vincristine (Oncovin)	1.4 mg/m^2 i.v. day 1
	(maximum 2 mg)
Prednisone	100 mg p.o. days 1–5

*Repeat every 21 days

Source: McKelvey EM, Gottlieb JA, Wilson HE. Hydroxydaunomycin (Adriamycin) combination chemotherapy in malignant lymphoma. Cancer 1976;38:1484–1493.

CHOP-BLEO

Cyclophosphamide	750 mg/m^2 i.v. day 1
Doxorubicin	50 mg/m^2 i.v. day 1
Vincristine (Oncovin)	2 mg i.v. days 1, 5
Prednisone	100 mg p.o. days 1–5
Bleomycin	15 U i.v. days 1–5

*Repeat every 21 or 28 days

Source: Rodriguez V, Cabanillas F, Burgess M. Combination chemotherapy (CHOP-bleo) in advanced (non-Hodgkin's) malignant lymphoma. Blood 1977;49:325–333.

C-MOPP

Cyclophosphamide	650 mg/m^2 i.v. days 1, 8
Vincristine (Oncovin)	1.4 mg/m^2 i.v. days 1, 8
Procarbazine	100 mg/m^2 p.o. days 1–14
Prednisone	40 mg/m^2 p.o. days 1–14

*Repeat every 28 days

**Note: Prednisone is used only in the first and fourth cycle

Source: DeVita VT Jr, Canellos GP, Chabner B, et al. Advanced diffuse histiocytic lymphoma, a potentially curable disease: results with combination chemotherapy. Lancet 1975;1:248–250.

CNOP

Cyclophosphamide (Cytoxan)	750 mg/m^2 i.v. day 1
Mitoxantrone	10 mg/m^2 i.v. day 1
Vincristine (Oncovin)	1.4 mg/m^2 i.v. day 1 (max 2 mg)
Prednisone	100 mg p.o. days 1–5

*Repeat every 21 days

Source: Sonneveld P, de Ridder M, van der Lelie, et al. Comparison of doxorubicin and mitoxantrone in the treatment of elderly patients with advanced diffuse non-Hodgkin's lymphoma using CHOP versus CNOP chemotherapy. J Clin Oncol 1995;13:2530–2539.

COD-BLAM IV

Cyclophosphamide	350 mg/m^2 i.v. day 1 (escalate 50 mg per cycle)
Adriamycin	35 mg/m^2 i.v. day 1(escalate 5 mg per cycle)
Vincristine	1 mg/m^2 i.v. (max dose 2 mg) CI days 1, 2
Bleomycin	4 U/m^2 i.v. bolus day 1 Then 4 U/m^2 CI i.v. for 5 days
Dexamethasone	10 mg/m^2 i.v. daily for 5 days
Procarbazine	100 mg/m^2 daily p.o. for 5 days

*Repeat every 21 days for 4 cycles

Cycle 5

Adriamycin	90 mg/m^2 i.v. day 1
Vincristine	1 mg/m^2 (maximum dose 2 mg) i.v. day 1
Dexamethasone	10 mg/m^2 p.o. for 5 days

Cycles 7 through 12 (MACE)

Methotrexate	120 mg/m^2 i.v. day 1 then citrovorum factor
Cytarabine	250 mg/m^2 i.v. day 1
Citrovorum factor	25 mg/m^2/day every 6 hr for 4 doses, start 24 hr after methotrexate
Etoposide	100 mg/m^2 i.v. day 1

Source: Coleman M, Armitage JO, Gaynor M, et al. The COP-BLAM programs: evolving chemo-therapy concepts in large cell lymphoma. Semin Hematol 1988;25(Suppl 2):23–33.

COMLA

Cyclophosphamide	1500 mg/m^2 i.v. day 1
Vincristine (Oncovin)	1.4 mg/m^2 i.v. days 1, 8, 15
Methotrexate	120 mg/m^2 i.v. days 22, 29, 36, 43, 50, 57, 64, 71
Leucovorin	25 mg/m^2 p.o. every 6 hr for 4 doses; start 24 hr after methotrexate
Cytarabine (Ara-C)	300 mg/m^2 i.v. days 22, 29, 36, 43, 50, 57, 64, 71

*Repeat every 85 days

Source: Berd D, Cornog J, DeConti RC, et al. Long-term remission in diffuse histiocytic lymphoma treated with combination sequential chemotherapy. Cancer 1975;35:1050–1054.

COP

Cyclophosphamide	800 mg/m^2 i.v. day 1
Vincristine	2 mg i.v. day 1
Prednisone	60 mg/m^2/day p.o. days 1–5, taper over 3 days

*Repeat day 14

Source: Luce JK, Gamble JF, Wilson HE. Combined cyclophosphamide, vincristine, and prednisone therapy of malignant lymphoma. Cancer 1971; 28:306–317.

COPP

Cyclophosphamide	600 mg/m^2 i.v. days 1, 8
Vincristine (Oncovin)	1.4 mg/m^2 i.v. days 1, 8
Procarbazine	100 mg/m^2 i.v. days 1–10
Prednisone	40 mg/m^2 i.v. days 1–14

*Repeat every 28 days

Source: Stein RS, Moran EM, Desser RK. Combination chemotherapy of lymphomas other than Hodgkin's disease. Ann Intern Med 1974; 81:601–609.

CVP

Cyclophosphamide	400 mg/m^2 p.o. days 1–5
Vincristine	1.4 mg/m^2 i.v. day 1
Prednisone	100 mg/m^2 p.o. days 1–5

*Repeat every 21 days

Source: Bagley CM Jr, DeVita VT Jr, Berard CW, et al. Advanced lymphosarcoma: intensive cyclical combination chemotherapy with cyclophosphamide, vincristine, and prednisone. Ann Intern Med 1972;76:227–234.

DHAP

Dexamethasone	40 mg/day i.v. days 1–4
Cytarabine (Ara-C)	2000 mg/m^2 every 12 hr for 2 day 2
Cisplatin	100 mg/m^2 i.v. CI day 1

*Repeat every 21 days

Source: Cabanillas F, Velasquez WS, McLaughlin P. Results of recent salvage chemotherapy regimens for lymphoma and Hodgkin's disease. Semin Hematol 1988;25(Suppl 2):47–50.

DICE

Dexamethasone	10 mg i.v. every 6 hr days 1–14
Ifosfamide	1000 mg/m^2 (max 1750 mg) i.v. days 1–14
Cisplatin	25 mg/m^2 i.v. days 1–4
Etoposide	100 mg/m^2 i.v. days 1–4
Mesna	200 mg/m^2 i.v. 1 hr prior to ifosfamide 900 mg/m^2 24 hr i.v., continue 12 hr after last dose of ifosfamide

*Repeat every 21 days

Source: Goss PE, Shepherd FA, Scott JG, et al. Dexamethasone/ifosfamide/cis-platin/etoposide (DICE) as therapy for patients with advanced refractory non-Hodgkin's lymphoma: preliminary report of a phase II study. Ann Oncol 1991;2 Suppl 1:43–46.

ESHAP

Etoposide	40 mg/m^2/day i.v. days 1–4
Methyl prednisone	500 mg/day i.v. days 1–5
High-dose cytarabine	2000 mg/m^2 i.v. day 5 after cisplatin
Cisplatin	25 mg/m^2/day CI i.v. days 1–4

*Repeat every 21 days

Source: Velasquez WS, McLaughlin P, Tucker S, et al. ESHAP: an effective chemotherapy regimen in refractory and relapsing lymphoma: a 4-year follow-up study. J Clin Oncol 1994;12:1169–1176.

FND

Fludarabine	25 mg/m^2 i.v. days 1–3
Mitoxantrone	10 mg/m^2 i.v. day 1
Dexamethasone	20 mg/m^2 p.o. days 1–5

*Repeat every 21–28 days

Source: McLaughlin P, Hagemeister FB, Romaguera JE, et al. Fludarabine, mitoxantrone, and dexamethasone: an effective new regimen for indolent lymphoma. J Clin Oncol 1996;14:1262–1268.

HOP

Hydroxydaunorubicin (Adriamycin)	80 mg/m^2 i.v. day 1
Vincristine	1.4 mg/m^2 i.v. day 1 (max 2 mg)
Prednisone	100 mg p.o. days 1–5

*Repeat every 21 days

Source: McKelvey EM, Gottlieb JA, Wilson HE. Hydroxydaunomycin (Adriamycin) combination chemotherapy in malignant lymphoma. Cancer, 1976;38:1484–1493.

ICE

Ifosfamide	1000 mg/m^2 over 1 hr days 1, 2 (hr 0–1)
Etoposide	150 mg/m^2 i.v. over 11 hr days 1, 2 (hr 1–11)
Carboplatin	200 mg/m^2 i.v. over 1 hr days 1, 2 (hr 11–12)
Etoposide	150 mg/m^2 i.v. over 11 hr days 1, 2 (hr 12–24)
Mesna	333 mg/m^2 i.v. 30 min prior to ifosfamide; repeat 4 and 8 hr post each dose of ifosfamide

*Repeat every 28 days

Source: Fields KK, Zorsky PE, Hiemenz JW, et al. Ifosfamide, carboplatin, and etoposide: a new regimen with a broad spectrum of activity. J Clin Oncol 1994;12:544–552.

IMVP-16

Ifosfamide	1000 mg/m^2 CI i.v., days 1–5
Mesna uroprotection	200 mg/m^2 bolus i.v. prior to ifosfamide

Then
1000 mg/m^2 CI with ifosfamide
Then
200 mg/m^2 i.v. over 12 hr after
ifosfamide

Methotrexate	30 mg/m^2 i.v. days 3, 10
Etoposide	100 mg/m^2 i.v. days 1–3

*Repeat every 21–28 days

Source: Cabanillas F, Burgess MA, Bodey GP, et al. Sequential chemotherapy and late intensification for malignant lymphomas of aggressive histologic type. Am J Med 1983;74:382–388.

MACOP-B

Methotrexate	400 mg/m^2 i.v. day 1 weeks 2, 6, 10
Leucovorin rescue	15 mg p.o. every 6 hr for 6 (24 hr after methotrexate)
Doxorubicin	50 mg/m^2 i.v. day 1 weeks 1, 3, 5, 7, 9, 11
Cyclophosphamide	350 mg/m^2 i.v. day 1 weeks 1, 3, 5, 7, 9, 11
Vincristine	1.4 mg/m^2 i.v. day 1 weeks 2, 4, 6, 8, 10, 12
Bleomycin	10 U/m^2 i.v. day 1 weeks 4, 8, 12
Prednisone	75 mg p.o. daily; taper dose over last 15 days
TMP/SMX	2 tablets p.o. twice daily throughout
Ketoconazole	200 mg p.o. once daily throughout

Source: Connors JM, Klimo P. MACOP-B chemotherapy for the treatment of diffuse large cell lymphoma: 1985 update. In: Skarin AT, ed. Update on treatment for diffuse large cell lymphoma. New York: Wiley, 1986;37–43.

Magrath Protocol (Burkitt's Lymphoma)

Cyclophosphamide (Cytoxan)	1,200 mg/m^2 i.v. day 1
Doxorubicin	40 mg/m^2 i.v. day 1
Vincristine (Oncovin)	1.4 mg/m^2 i.v. day 1 (max 2 mg)
Prednisone	40 mg/m^2 p.o. days 1–5
Methotrexate	300 mg/m^2 i.v. day 10* hr 1
	60 mg/m^2 i.v. day 10–11* hr 2–42 followed by leucovorin rescue
Intrathecal Ara-C	30 mg/m^2 i.t. day 7 cycle 1 only
	45 mg/m^2 i.t. day 7 cycle 2–6

Intrathecal methotrexate   12.5 mg i.t. day 10 cycle 1–6 only

*High-dose methotrexate infusions begin on day 10 for the first 6 cycles; then begin on day 14 for remaining cycles

**Cycles repeated as soon as ANC > 1500 (cycles 1–6), then every 28 days cycles 7–15

Source: Magrath IT, Janus C, Edwards BK, et al. An effective therapy for both undifferentiated (including Burkitt's) lymphomas and lymphoblastic lymphomas in children and young adults. Blood 1984;5:1102–1111.

m-BACOD

Methotrexate	200 mg/m^2 i.v. days 8, 15
Calcium leucovorin rescue	10 mg/m^2 p.o. every 6 hr for 8 doses, begin 24 hr after each methotrexate dose
Bleomycin	4 U/m^2 i.v. day 1
Doxorubicin	45 mg/m^2 i.v. day 1
Cyclophosphamide	600 mg/m^2 i.v. day 1
Vincristine	1 mg/m^2 i.v. day 1 (max 2 mg)
Dexamethasone	6 mg/m^2 p.o. days 1–5

*Repeat every 21 days

Source: Shipp MA, Harrington DP, Klatt MM, et al. Identification of major prognostic subgroups of patients with large cell lymphoma treated with m-BACOD or M-BACOD. Ann Intern Med 1986;104:757–765.

M-BACOD

Methotrexate	3000 mg/m^2 i.v. days 8, 15
Calcium leucovorin rescue	10 mg/m^2 p.o. every 6 hr for 8 doses beginning 24 hr after each methotrexate dose
Bleomycin	4 U/m^2 i.v. day 1
Doxorubicin	45 mg/m^2 i.v. day 1
Cyclophosphamide	600 mg/m^2 i.v. day 1
Vincristine	1 mg/m^2 i.v. day 1
Dexamethasone	6 mg/m^2 p.o. days 1–5

*Repeat every 21 days

Source: Shipp MA, Harrington DP, Klatt MM, et al. Identification of major prognostic subgroups of patients with large cell lymphoma treated with m-BACOD or M-BACOD. Ann Intern Med 1986;104:757–765.

MIME

Mesna	1330 mg/m^2/day i.v. on days 1–3
	500 mg p.o. 4 hr after ifos days 1–3
Ifosfamide	1330 mg/m^2/day i.v. days 1–3
Mitoxantrone	8 mg/m^2 i.v. day 1
Etoposide	65 mg/m^2/day i.v. days 1–3

*Repeat every 3 weeks for 6 courses; then start ESHAP regime

Source: Cabinillas F. Experience with salvage regimens at M. D. Anderson Hospital. Ann Oncol 1991;2 Suppl 1:31–32.

ProMACE-CytaBOM

Cyclophosphamide	650 mg/m^2 i.v. push day 1
Doxorubicin	25 mg/m^2 i.v. push day 1
Etoposide (VP-16)	120 mg/m^2 i.v. infused over 60 min, day 1
Prednisone	60 mg/m^2 p.o. days 1–14
Cytarabine	300 mg/m^2 i.v. push day 8
Bleomycin	5 U/m^2 i.v. push day 8
Vincristine	1.4 mg/m^2 i.v. push day 8
Methotrexate	120 mg/m^2 i.v. push day 8
Leucovorin rescue	25 mg/m^2 p.o. every 6 hr for 6 doses on day 9
TMP/SMX DS	1 tab p.o. b.i.d. days 1–21

*Repeat every 21 days

**Regimen is administered for a minimum of six cycles and should be given for two additional cycles after a clinical complete remission; no therapy is given on day 15; cycle restarts on day 22

Source: Fisher RI, DeVita VT Jr, Hubbard SM, et al. Randomized trial of Pro-MACE-MOPP vs ProMACE-CytaBOM in previously untreated, advanced stage, diffuse aggressive lymphomas. Proc Am Soc Clin Oncol 1984;3:242.

Stanford Regimen (Small Non-Cleaved Cell/Burkitt's)

Cyclophosphamide (Cytoxan)	1200 mg/m^2 i.v. day 1
Doxorubicin	40 mg/m^2 i.v. day 1
Vincristine (Oncovin)	1.4 mg/m^2 i.v. day 1 (max 2 mg)
Prednisone	40 mg/m^2 p.o. days 1–5
High-dose methotrexate	3 g/m^2 i.v. over 6 hr day 10 (cycles 1–5 only)

| Leucovorin rescue | 25 mg/m^2 i.v. or p.o. every 6 hr for 12 doses |
| Intrathecal methotrexate | 12 mg i.t. days 1, 10 (cycle 1–5 only) |

*Cycles repeated every 21 days

**6–9 cycles of therapy planned based on extent of disease

***All patients received allopurinol prior to initiation of therapy

Source: Bernstein JI, Coleman N, Strickler JG, et al. Combined modality therapy for adults with small noncleaved lymphoma (Burkitt's and non-Burkitt's types). J Clin Oncol 1986;4:847–858.

MELANOMA

Adjuvant IFN

| Interferon α_{2b} | 20 × 10^6 U/m^2 i.v. 5 times weekly for 4 weeks
Then
10 × 10^6 U/m^2 s.q. 3 times weekly for 48 weeks |

Source: Kirkwood JM, Strawdeman MH, Ernstoff MS, et al. Interferon alfa-2b adjuvant therapy of high risk resected cutaneous melanoma: the Eastern Cooperative Group Trial EST 1684. J Clin Oncol 1996;14:7–17.

CVD

Vinblastine	1.6 mg/m^2/day i.v. days 1–5
Dacarbazine	800 mg/m^2 i.v. day 1
Cisplatin	20 mg/m^2/day i.v. days 2–5

*Repeat every 21–28 days

Source: Legha SS, Ring S, Papadopoulos N, et al. A prospective evaluation of a triple-drug regimen containing cisplatin, vinblastine, and dacarbazine (CVD) for metastatic melanoma. Cancer 1989;64:2024–2029.

Dartmouth Regimen

Dacarbazine	220 mg/m^2/day i.v. days 1–3, and 22–24
Cisplatin	25 mg/m^2/day i.v. days 1–3, 22–24
Carmustine (BCNU)	150 mg/m^2 i.v. day 1
Tamoxifen	10 mg p.o. b.i.d. starting day 4

*Repeat every 6 weeks

Source: Del Prete SA, Maurer LH, O'Donnell J, et al. Combination chemotherapy with cisplatin, carmustine, dacarbazine, and tamoxifen in metastatic melanoma. Cancer Treat Rep 1987;68:1403–1405.

DTIC

Dacarbazine (DTIC)	250 mg/m^2 i.v. days 1–5

*Repeat cycle every 3 weeks

Source: Luce JK, Thurman WG, Isaacs BL, Talley RW. Clinical trials with the antitumor agent 5-(3,3-dimethyl-1-triazeno)imidazole-4-carboxamide(NSC-45388). Cancer Chemother Rep—Part 1. 1970;54:119–124.

Or

Dacarbazine (DTIC)	2–4.5 mg/kg i.v. days 1–10

*Repeat cycles every 4 weeks

Source: Nathanson L, Wolter J, Horton J, et al. Characteristics of prognosis and response to an imidazole carboxamide in malignant melanoma. Clin Pharmacol Ther 1971;12:955–962.

Or

Dacarbazine (DTIC)	850 mg/m^2 i.v. day 1

*Repeat cycle every 3–6 weeks

Source: Pritchard KI, Quirt IC, Cowan DH, et al. DTIC therapy in metastatic malignant melanoma: a simplified dose schedule. Cancer Treat Rep 1980;64:1123–1126.

IFN/IL-2

Interferon	6 × 10^6 U/m^2 s.q. day 1, 4
IL-2	7.8 × 10^6 U/m^2 CI i.v. days 1–4

*Repeat every 14 days

Source: Kruit WH, Goey SH, Calabresi F, et al. Final report of a phase II study of interleukin 2 and interferon α inpatients with metastatic melanoma. Br J Cancer 1995;71:1319–1321.

VBD

Vinblastine	6 mg/m^2 i.v. days 1, 2
Bleomycin	15 U/m^2 i.v. CI days 1–5
Cisplatin	50 mg/m^2 i.v. day 5

*Repeat every 28 days

Source: Luikart SD, Kennealey GT, Kirkwood JM. Randomized phase III trial of vinblastine, bleomycin, and cis-dichlorodiammine-platinum versus dacarbazine in malignant melanoma. J Clin Oncol 1984;2:164–168.

MULTIPLE MYELOMA

ABCM

Adriamycin	30 mg/m² i.v. day 1
Carmustine (BCNU)	30 mg/m² i.v. day 1
Cyclophosphamide	100 mg/m²/day p.o. days 22–25
Melphalan	6 mg/m²/day p.o. days 22–25

*Repeat every 6 weeks

Source: MacLennan ICM, Chapman C, Dunn J, et al. Combined chemotherapy with ABCM versus melphalan for treatment of myelomatosis. Lancet 1992;339:200–205.

BCAP

Carmustine (BCNU)	50 mg/m² i.v. day 1
Cyclophosphamide	200 mg/m² i.v. day 1
Doxorubicin (Adriamycin)	20 mg/m² i.v. day 2
Prednisone	60 mg/day p.o. days 1–5

*Repeat every 28 days

Source: Presant CA, Klahr C. Adriamycin, I, 3-bis (2-chloroethyl)-1-nitrosurea (BCNU, NSC #409962), cyclophosphamide plus prednisone (ABC-P) in melphalan resistant multiple myeloma. Cancer 1978;42:1222–1227.

Cyclophosphamide and Prednisone

Cyclophosphamide	150–250 mg/m² (500 mg max) i.v. or p.o. weekly
Prednisone	100 mg p.o. alternate days

Source: Wilson K, Shelley W, Belch A, et al. Weekly cyclophosphamide and alternate-day prednisone: an effective secondary therapy in multiple myeloma. Cancer Treat Rep 1987;71:981–982.

Dexamethasone (High Dose)

Dexamethasone	40 mg p.o. days 1–4, 9–12, 17–20

*Repeat every 28 days

Source: Alexanian R, Barlogie B, Dixon D. High-dose glucocorticoid treatment of resistant myeloma. Ann Intern Med 1986;105:8–11.

M2 (VBMCP)

Vincristine	0.03 mg/kg i.v. day 1
Carmustine (BCNU)	0.5 mg/kg i.v. day 1
Cyclophosphamide	10 mg/kg i.v. day 1
Melphalan	0.25/kg p.o. for 4 days or 0.1 mg/kg for 7–10 days

| Prednisone | 1 mg/kg/day p.o. for 7 days; taper after first week; discontinue on day 21 |

*Repeat every 35 days

Source: Case DC Jr, Lee BJ III, Clarkson BD. Improved survival times in multiple myeloma treated with melphalan, prednisone, cyclophosphamide, vincristine, and BCNU: M-2 protocol. Am J Med 1977;63:897–903.

Melphalan and Prednisone

| Melphalan | 9 mg/m^2 p.o. days 1–4 |
| Prednisone | 40 mg/m^2 p.o. t.i.d. days 1–4 |

*Repeat every 4 weeks

Source: Durie BGM, Dixon B, Carter S, et al. Improved survival duration with combination chemotherapy induction for multiple myeloma: a Southwest Oncology Group study. J Clin Oncol 1986;4:1127–1137.

VAD

Vincristine	0.4 mg/day CI i.v. days 1–4
Adriamycin	9 mg/m^2/day CI i.v. days 1–4
Dexamethasone	40 mg p.o. days 1–4, 9–12, 17–20

*Repeat every 28 days

Source: Barlogie B, Smith L, Alexanian R. Effective treatment of advanced multiple myeloma refractory to alkylating agents. N Engl J Med 1984;310:1353–1356.

VMCP-VCAP

VMCP

Vincristine	1 mg/m^2 i.v. day 1 (max dose 1.5 mg)
Melphalan	6 mg/m^2/day p.o. days 1–4
Cyclophosphamide	125 mg/m^2/day p.o. days 1–4
Prednisone	60 mg/m^2/day p.o. days 1–4

VCAP

Vincristine	1 mg/m^2 i.v. day 1 (max dose 1.5 mg)
Cyclophosphamide	123 mg/m^2/day p.o. days 1–4
Adriamycin	30 mg/m^2/day i.v. day 1
Prednisone	60 mg/m^2/day p.o. days 1–4

*Alternate VMCP with VCAP every 3 weeks for 6–12 months

Source: Salmon SE, Haut A, Bonnet JD, et al. Alternating combination chemotherapy and levamisole improves survival in multiple myeloma: a Southwest Oncology Group Study. J Clin Oncol 1983;1:453–461.

VMCP-VBAP

VMCP	
Vincristine	1 mg/m^2 i.v. day 1
	(max dose 1.5 mg)
Melphalan	6 mg/m^2/day p.o. days 1–4
Cyclophosphamide	125 mg/m^2/day p.o. days 1–4
Prednisone	60 mg/m^2/day p.o. days 1–4
VBAP	
Vincristine	1 mg/m^2 i.v. day 1
	(max dose 1.5 mg)
Carmustine (BCNU)	30 mg/m^2 i.v. day 1
Doxorubicin	30 mg/m^2 i.v. day 1
Prednisone	60 mg/m^2 p.o. days 1–4

*Repeat VMCP every 3 weeks for 3 cycles followed by VBAP for 3 cycles

Source: Salmon SE, Haut A, Bonnet JD, et al. Alternating combination chemotherapy and levamisole improves survival in multiple myeloma: a Southwest Oncology Group study. J Clin Oncol 1983;1:453–461.

MYELODYSPLASIA

5-Azacytidine

5-Azacytidine	75 mg/m^2/day CI i.v. days 1–7

*Repeat every 4 weeks

Source: Silverman LR, Davis RB, Holland JF, et al. 5-Azacytidine (AZ) as a low dose continuous infusion is an effective therapy for patients with myelodysplastic syndrome. Proc Am Soc Clin Oncol 1989;8:768A.

ADULT CENTRAL NERVOUS SYSTEM TUMORS

BCNU

Carmustine (BCNU)	200 mg/m^2 i.v. day 1

*Repeat every 6–8 weeks

Source: Levin VA, Silver P, Hannigan J, et al. Superiority of post-radiotherapy adjuvant chemotherapy with CCNU, procarbazine, and vincristine (PCV) over BCNU for anaplastic gliomas: NGOG 6g61 final report. Int J Radiat Oncol Biol Phys 1990;18:321–324.

PCV

Procarbazine	60 mg/m^2/day p.o. days 1–14
CCNU	110 mg/m^2 p.o. day 1
Vincristine	1.4 mg/m^2 i.v. days 8, 29 (max dose 2 mg)

*Repeat every 6–8 weeks

Source: Levin VA, Silver P, Hannigan J, et al. Superiority of post-radiotherapy adjuvant chemotherapy with CCNU, procarbazine, and vincristine (PCV) over BCNU for anaplastic gliomas: NGOG 6g61 final report. Int J Radiat Oncol Biol Phys 1990;18:321–324.

PEDIATRIC SOLID TUMORS

EWING'S SARCOMA

Alternating Cycles of VAdCA + I/E

VAdCA	
Vincristine	1.5 mg/m^2 i.v. day 1
Adriamycin (doxorubicin)	75 mg/m^2 i.v. day 1 (**stop** at a cumulative dose of 375 mg/m^2 and substitute actinomycin)
Actinomycin (after max doxorubicin)	1.25 mg/m^2 i.v. day 1
Cyclophosphamide	1200 mg/m^2 i.v. day 1
Mesna	360 mg/m^2 i.v. with Cytoxan, then at hr 1–4 by CI i.v., then at hr 4, 7, 10
I/E	
Ifosfamide	1800 mg/m^2/day i.v. days 1–5
Etoposide	100 mg/m^2/day i.v. days 1–5
Mesna	400 mg/m^2/day with ifosfamide, immediately after, and then every 2 hr for 7 doses

*Repeat alternate cycles of VAdCA and IE every 3 weeks

Source: Grier H, Krailo M, Link M, et al. Improved outcome in nonmetastatic Ewing's sarcoma (EWS) and PNET of bone with the addition of ifosfamide (I) and etoposide (E) to vincristine (V), Adriamycin (Ad), cyclophosphamide (C), and actinomycin (A): a Children's Cancer Group (CCG) and Pediatric Oncology Group (POG) report. Proc Annu Meet Am Soc Clin Oncol 1994;13:A1443 (abstract).

NEUROBLASTOMA

AC

| Doxorubicin (Adriamycin) | 35 mg/m^2 i.v. day 8 |
| Cyclophosphamide | 150 mg/m^2/day p.o. days 1–7 |

*Repeat every 21–28 days for 5 courses

Source: Nitschke R, Smith EI, Altshuler G, et al. Postoperative treatment of nonmetastatic visible residual neuroblastoma: a Pediatric Oncology Group study. J Clin Oncol 1991;9:1181–1188.

Cisplatin and Tenoposide

| Cisplatin | 90 mg/m^2 i.v. day 1 |
| Tenoposide | 100 mg/m^2 i.v. day 3 |

*Repeat every 21–28 days

Source: Castleberry RP, Schuster JJ, Altshuler G, et al. Infants with neuroblastoma and regional lymph ode metastases have a favorable outlook after limited postoperative chemotherapy: a Pediatric Oncology Group study. J Clin Oncol 1992;10:1299–1304.

WILM'S TUMOR

Carbo/VP-16

| Carboplatin | 500 mg/m^2 i.v. day 1 |
| Etoposide | 150 mg/m^2 i.v. days 1, 2 |

*Repeat every 4 weeks for 6 cycles

Source: Greenwald MJ. Strauss LC. Treatment of intraocular retinoblastoma with carboplatin and etoposide chemotherapy. Ophthalmology 1996;103: 1989–1997.

SARCOMA

OSTEOSARCOMA

T-10

Preoperative

| Methotrexate | 8–12 g/m^2 i.v. weekly × 4 |
| Calcium leucovorin rescue | 15 mg/m^2 i.v. or p.o. every 6 hr for at least 10 doses beginning 24 hr after MTX |

Monitor MTX levels
Postresection BCD

Bleomycin	15 U/m^2 i.v. days 1, 2
Cyclophosphamide	600 mg/m^2 i.v. days 1, 2
Actinomycin-D	600 µg/m^2 i.v. days 1, 2

Then
Methotrexate   8–12 g/m^2 i.v. day 1 at weeks 9, 10, 14, 15

Calcium leucovorin rescue   15 mg/m^2 i.v. or p.o. every 6 hr for at least 10 doses beginning 24 hr after MTX

Monitor MTX levels
Doxorubicin   30 mg/m^2 i.v. days 1, 2 week 11

Maintenance (3 weeks later)

Grade 1–2 with Response
Doxorubicin   30 mg/m^2 i.v. days 1, 22
Cisplatin   120 mg/m^2 i.v. days 1, 22
BCD as above   Day 42

*Repeat maintenance cycle for total of 3 courses

Grade 3–4
Bleomycin   15 U/m^2 i.v. days 1, 2
Cyclophosphamide   600 mg/m^2 i.v. days 1, 2
Actinomycin-D   600 μg/m^2 i.v. days 1, 2
Then
Methotrexate   8–12 g/m^2 i.v. day 1 at weeks 9, 10, 14, 15

Calcium leucovorin rescue   15 mg/m^2 i.v. or p.o. every 6 hr for at least 10 doses beginning 24 hr after MTX

Monitor MTX levels
Doxorubicin   30 mg/m^2 i.v. days 1, 2 week 11

*Repeat maintenance for 4 courses

Source: Rosen G, Caparros B, Huvos A, et al. Preoperative chemotherapy for osteogenic sarcoma: selection of postoperative adjuvant chemotherapy based on the response of the primary tumor to preoperative chemotherapy. Cancer 1982;49:1221–1230.

Weekly High-Dose Methotrexate and Doxorubicin

HDMTX
Vincristine   2.0 mg/m^2 i.v. (2 mg maximum) day 1
Methotrexate   7500 mg/m^2 i.v. day 1 (30 min after VCR)
Calcium leucovorin   15 mg/m^2 i.v. every 3 hr for 8 doses (2 hr after MTX)

	Then
	15 mg/m^2 p.o. every 6 hr for 8 doses
HDMTX-Dox	
HDMTX as above plus	
Doxorubicin	75 mg/m^2 i.v. CI over 72 hr on day 6 (450 mg/m^2 max)

*HDMTX every week × 4; then HDMTX-Dox every 3 weeks × 6; then HDMTX every week × 4; then HDMTX-Dox every 3 weeks × 6; then HDMTX every week × 4

Source: Goorin AM, Perez-Atayde A, Gebhardt M, et al. Weekly high-dose methotrexate and doxorubicin for osteosarcoma: the Dana-Farber Cancer Institute/Children's Hospital: Study III. J Clin Oncol 1987;5:1178–1184.

RHABDOSARCOMA

Regimen 31

| Dactinomycin | 0.015 mg/kg/day, days 1–5 of weeks 0, 9, 18, 27, 36, 45 (max 0.5 mg/day) |
| Vincristine | 1.5 mg/m^2 i.v. day 1 of weeks 3–8, 12–17, 21–26, 30–35, 39–45, 48–53 (max 2 mg) |

Regimen 32

Same as Regimen 31 with XRT starting day 14

Regimen 33

| Same as Regimen 32 with Dox | |
| Doxorubicin | 30 mg/m^2 i.v. days 1, 2 of weeks 3, 6, 12, 15, 21, 24 |

Regimen 34

Dactinomycin (DAC)	0.015 mg/kg/day, days 1–5 of weeks 0–12, 16 (max 0.5 mg)
Vincristine (VCR)	1.5 mg/m^2 i.v. day 1 of weeks 0–12, 16 (max 2 mg)
Cyclophosphamide (CTX)	10 mg/kg/day, days 1–3 of weeks 0, 12, 16
	20 mg/kg day 1 of weeks 3, 6*, 9*

*Hold cyclophosphamide if bladder or extensive bone radiation

**Radiation starts week 6

***Repeat DAC, VCR, CTX every 4 weeks after XRT if in clinical or pathologic CR, through week 104

Regimen 38

Vincristine (VCR)	1.5 mg/m^2 i.v. weeks 0–11 (max 2 mg)
Cisplatin (CDDP)	90 mg/m^2 i.v. over 8 hr weeks 0, 3, 6, 9
Doxorubicin (Dox)	30 mg/m^2 i.v. day 1, 2 after cisplatin weeks 0, 3
Cyclophosphamide (CTX)	20 mg/kg day 1 of weeks 0, 6, 9

*Hold cyclophosphamide if bladder or extensive bone radiation

**Radiation starts week 6

***VCR, CDDP, Dox alternate with DAC as in regimen 31 every 4 weeks for weeks 12–52

Source: Strickland DK, Hakami N. Chemotherapy of pediatric solid tumors. In: Perry MC, ed. The chemotherapy source book. 2nd ed. Baltimore: Williams & Wilkins, 1997;1333–1344.

IRS-IV Pilot

Ifosfamide	1.8 g/m^2/day i.v. days 1–5 every 3 weeks × 3 with mesna; repeat weeks 9, 12, 16
Etoposide	100 mg/m^2/day i.v. days 1–5 every 3 weeks × 3
Vincristine	1.5 mg/m^2/week i.v. day 1 weekly × 9; then weeks 9, 10, 11, 12, 16 (max 2 mg)
XRT	Weeks 9–16

*Weeks 20–29, IFOS, ETOP, VCR repeated every 3 weeks × 2 (VCR is given weekly)

**Week 29 + repeat ETOP and VCR (3-week cycle) every 9 weeks for 4 cycles

Source: Arndt C, Tefft M, Gehan E, et al. A feasibility, toxicity, and early response study of etoposide, ifosfamide, and vincristine for the treatment of children with rhabdomyosarcoma: a report from the Intergroup Rhabdomyosarcoma Study (IRS) IV pilot study. J Pediatr Hematol Oncol 1997;19:124–129.

SOFT TISSUE SARCOMAS

ADIC

Doxorubicin	90 mg/m^2 i.v. CI over 96 hr
Dacarbazine	900 mg/m^2 i.v. CI over 96 hr

*Repeat every 21 days

Source: Zalupski M, Metch B, Balcerzak S, et al. Phase III comparison of doxorubicin and dacarbazine given by bolus versus infusion in patients with soft-tissue sarcomas: a Southwest Oncology Group Study. J Natl Cancer Inst 1991;83:920–926.

AI

Doxorubicin	50 mg/m^2 i.v. day 1
Ifosfamide	5 g/m^2 CI i.v. for 24 hr
Mesna	600 mg/m^2 i.v. prior to ifosfamide, then 2.5 g/m^2 in 3 L i.v. fluids to run with ifosfamide and 1.25 g/m^2 in 2L of i.v. fluids to run for 12 hr after the ifosfamide

*Repeat cycle every 3 weeks

Source: Santoro A, Tursz T, Mouridsen H, et al. Doxorubicin versus CY-VADIC versus doxorubicin plus ifosfamide in first-line treatment of advanced soft tissue sarcomas: a randomized study of the European Organization for Research and Treatment of Cancer Soft Tissue and Bone Sarcoma Group. J Clin Oncol 1995;13:1537–1545.

Or

Doxorubicin	30 mg/m^2 i.v. days 1, 2
Ifosfamide	3.75 g/m^2 i.v. over 4 hr days 1, 2
Mesna	750 mg/m^2 i.v. prior to each dose of ifosfamide, then 4 and 8 hr after the ifosfamide

*Repeat cycles every 3 weeks

Source: Edmonson JH, Ryan LM, Blum RH, et al. Randomized comparison of doxorubicin alone versus ifosfamide plus doxorubicin or mitomycin, doxorubicin, and cisplatin against advanced soft tissue sarcomas. J Clin Oncol 1993;11:1269–1275.

CYVADIC

Cyclophosphamide	500 mg/m^2 i.v. day 1
Vincristine	1.4 mg/m^2 i.v. day 1
Doxorubicin	50 mg/m^2 i.v. day 1
Dacarbazine	400 mg/m^2/day i.v. days 1–3

*Repeat every 21 days

Source: Bramwell V, Rouesse J, Steward W, et al. Adjuvant CYVADIC chemotherapy for adult soft tissue sarcoma: reduced local recurrence but no improvement in survival: a study of the European Organization for Research and Treatment of Cancer Soft Tissue and Bone Sarcoma Group. J Clin Oncol 1994;12:1137–1149.

Doxorubicin

Doxorubicin	75 mg/m^2 i.v. day 1

Repeat every 21 days

Source: Santoro A, Tursz T, Mouridsen H, et al. Doxorubicin versus CY-VADIC versus doxorubicin plus ifosfamide in first-line treatment of advanced soft tissue sarcomas: a randomized study of the European Organization for Research and Treatment of Cancer Soft Tissue and Bone Sarcoma Group. J Clin Oncol 1995;13:1537–1545.

Ifosfamide

Ifosfamide	60–80 mg/kg (2.5–3 g/m^2) i.v. over 4 hr days 1–5
Mesna	8–12 mg/kg i.v. at 0, 4, and 8 hr
Or	
Ifosfamide	5 g/m^2 CI i.v. over 24 hr
Mesna	600 mg/m^2 i.v. prior to ifosfamide, then 2.5 g/m^2 in 3 L i.v. fluids to run with ifosfamide and 1.25 g/m^2 in 2 L of i.v. fluids to run for 12 hr after the ifosfamide

*Repeat cycle every 3–4 weeks

Source: Schutte J, Kellner R, Seeber S. Ifosfamide in the treatment of soft tissue sarcomas: experience at the West German Tumor Center, Essen. Cancer Chemother Pharmacol 1993;31(suppl 2);194–198.

MAID

Mesna	2500 mg/m^2/day i.v. CI days 1–4
Doxorubicin	20 mg/m^2/day i.v. days 1–3
Ifosphamide	2500 mg/m^2/day i.v. days 1–3
DTIC	300 mg/m^2/day i.v. days 1–3

*Repeat every 21 days

Source: Elias AB, Ryan L, Aisner J, et al. Mesna, ifosfamide, dacarbazine (MAID) regimen for adults with advanced sarcoma. Semin Oncol 1990;17(2 Suppl 4):41–49.

Pulse VAC

Vincristine	2 mg/m^2 i.v. weekly for 12 (max 2 mg/week)
Actinomycin-D	0.075 mg/kg i.v. CI over 5 days every 3 months for 5 courses (max 0.5 mg/day)
Cyclophosphamide	10 mg/kg/day days 1–7 i.v. or p.o. every 6 weeks

Source: Wilbur JR, Suton WW, Sullivan MD, et al. Chemotherapy of sarcomas. Cancer 1975;36:765–769.

Standard VAC

Vincristine	2 mg/m^2 i.v. weekly for 12 (max 2 mg/week)
Actinomycin-D	0.075 mg/kg i.v. CI over 5 days every 3 months for 5 courses (max 0.5 mg/day)
Cyclophosphamide	2.5 mg/kg/day p.o. for 2 years

Source: Wilbur JR, Suton WW, Sullivan MD, et al. Chemotherapy of sarcomas. Cancer 1975;36:765–769.

PERFORMANCE SCALES

KARNOFSKY

100%	No evidence of disease
90	Normal activity; minor signs of disease
80	Normal activity with effort; signs of disease
70	Cannot do normal activity; cares for self
60	Requires occasional assistance
50	Requires considerable assistance; frequent medical care
40	Disabled; requires special care
30	Severely disabled; hospitalization may be indicated
20	Very sick; hospitalization necessary for supportive treatment
10	Moribund

ZUBROD

0	Asymptomatic; normal activity (Karnofsky 100%)
1	Symptomatic: fully ambulatory (Karnofsky 85%)
2	Symptomatic; in bed less than 50% of time (Karnofsky 65%)
3	Symptomatic; in bed more than 50% of time (Karnofsky 40%)
4	Bedridden 100% of time (Karnofsky 15%)

CALVERT FORMULA

Total dose in mg (not mg/m^2) = Target AUC $\times$ (GFR + 25)

CREATININE CLEARANCE

Males

$$\text{CrCl (mL/min)} = \frac{(140 - \text{age}) \text{ for weight (kg)}}{72 \text{ for creatinine (mg/dL)}}$$

Females

$$\text{CrCl (mL/min)} = \frac{(140 - \text{age}) \text{ for weight (kg)} \times 0.85}{72 \text{ for creatinine (mg/dL)}}$$

3
Toxicity Grading

John D. Wilkes

National Cancer Institute Common Toxicity Criteria

Toxicity	Grade 0	Grade 1	Grade 2	Grade 3	Grade 4
Hematologic					
WBC	≥4	3–3.9	2–2.9	1–1.9	<1.0
Plt (×10³)	WNL	75–normal	50–74.9	25–49.9	<25.0
Hgb g/100 mL	WNL	10–normal	8–10	6.5–7.9	<6.5
Hgb g/L	WNL	100–normal	80–100	65–79	<65.0
Hgb mmol/L	WNL	6.2–normal	4.95–6.2	4–4.9	<4.0
Granulocytes, bands	≥2	1.5–1.9	1–1.4	0.5–0.9	<0.5
Lymphocytes	≥2	1.5–1.9	1–1.4	0.5–0.9	<0.5
Other hematologic	None	Mild	Moderate	Severe	Life threatening
Clinical					
hemorrhage	None	Mild; no transfusion	Gross; 1–2 U transfusion per episode	Gross; 3–4 U transfusion per episode	Massive; >4 U transfusion per episode
Infection	None	Mild; no active treatment	Moderate; oral antibiotic	Severe; i.v. antibiotic, antifungal, or hospitalization	Life threatening
Gastrointestinal					
Nausea	None	Able to eat reasonable intake	Intake significantly decreased but able to eat	No significant intake	—

	None				
Vomiting	None	1 episode in 24 hr	2–5 episodes in 24 hr	6–10 episodes in 24 hr	>10 episodes in 24 hr or requires parenteral support
Diarrhea	None	Increase of 2–3 stools/day	Increase of 4–6 stools/day or nocturnal stools or moderate cramping	Increase of 7–9 stools/day or incontinence or severe cramping	Increase of ≥10 stools/day or grossly bloody diarrhea or need for parenteral support
Stomatitis	None	Painless ulcers, erythema, or mild soreness	Painful erythema, edema, or ulcers but can eat	Painful erythema, edema, or ulcers and cannot eat	Requires parenteral or enteral support
Esophagitis, dysphagia	None	Painless ulcers, erythema, mild soreness or dysphagia	Painful erythema, edema, or ulcers or moderate dysphagia but can eat without opioids	Painful erythema, edema, or ulcers and cannot eat solids or requires opioids to eat	Requires parenteral or enteral support; or complete obstruction or perforation
Anorexia	None	Mild	Moderate	Severe	Life threatening
Gastritis, ulcer	None	Antacid	Requires vigorous medical management or nonsurgical treatment	Uncontrolled by medical management; requires surgery	Perforation or bleeding
Small bowel obstruction	None	—	Intermittent; no intervention	Requires intervention	Requires operation
Intestinal Fistula	None	—	—	Yes	—

continued

National Cancer Institute Common Toxicity Criteria *continued*

Toxicity	Grade 0	Grade 1	Grade 2	Grade 3	Grade 4
Other GI	None	Mild	Moderate	Severe	Life threatening
Other mucosal	None	Erythema or mild pain not requiring treatment	Patchy and serosanguineous discharge or nonopioid for pain	Confluent fibrinous mucositis or ulceration or opioid for pain	Necrosis
Liver					
Bilirubin	WNL	—	<1.5 × normal	1.5–3 × normal	>3 × normal
Transaminases (SGOT/AST, SGPT/ALT)	WNL	≤2.5 × normal	2.6–5 × normal	5.1–20 × normal	>20 × normal
Alk phos or 5′ nucleotidase	WNL	≤2.5 × normal	2.6–5 × normal	5.1–20 × normal	>20 × normal
Liver, clinical	No change from baseline	—	—	Precoma	Hepatic coma
Other liver	None	Mild	Moderate	Severe	Life threatening
Renal and Bladder					
Creatinine	WNL	<1.5 × normal	1.5–3 × normal	3.1–6 × normal	>6 × normal
Proteinuria	No change	1+ or <0.3 g/100 mL or <3 g/L	2–3+ or 0.3–1 g/100 mL or 3–10 g/L	4+ or >1 g/100 mL or >10 g/L	Nephrotic syndrome
Hematuria	Negative	Micro only	Gross, no clots	Gross with clots	Requires transfusion
BUN (mg/100 mL)	WNL, <20	21–30	31–50	>50	—

	WNL, <7.5	7.6–10.9	11–18	>18	
Urea (mmol/L)					
Hemorrhagic cystitis	None	Blood on microscopic examination	Frank blood; no treatment required	Bladder irrigation required	Requires cystectomy or transfusion
Renal failure					Dialysis required
Incontinence	Normal	With coughing, sneezing, etc.	Spontaneous; some control	No control	—
Dysuria	None	Mild pain	Painful or burning urination controlled by pyridium	Not controlled by pyridium	—
Urinary retention	None	Residual >100 mL or occasional catheter or difficulty initiating stream	Self-catheterization required for voiding	Surgery required (TUR or dilation)	—
Increased frequency, urgency	No change	Frequency or nocturia up to twice normal	More than twice normal but less than hourly	With urgency and more than hourly frequency or requires catheter	—
Bladder cramps	None	—	Yes	—	—
Ureteral obstruction	None	Unilateral; no surgery required	Bilateral; no surgery required	Incomplete bilateral; nephrostomy tubes or surgery required	Complete bilateral obstruction
Genitourinary fistula	None	—	—	Yes	—
Other kidney, bladder	None	Mild	Moderate	Severe	Life threatening

continued

National Cancer Institute Common Toxicity Criteria *continued*

Toxicity	Grade 0	Grade 1	Grade 2	Grade 3	Grade 4
Alopecia	No loss	Mild hair loss	Pronounced or total hair loss	—	—
Pulmonary					
Dyspnea	None or no change	Asymptomatic, with abnormality in PFTs	Dyspnea on significant exertion	Dyspnea at normal levels of activity	Dyspnea at rest
PO_2, PCO_2	No change or PO_2 >85 and PCO_2 ≤40	PO_2 71–85 PCO_2 41–50	PO_2 61–70 PCO_2 51–60	PO_2 51–60 PCO_2 61–70	PO_2 ≤50 PCO_2 ≥70
DLCO	>90% of pretreatment	76–90% of pretreatment	51–75% of pretreatment	26–50% of pretreatment	≤25% of pretreatment
Pulmonary fibrosis	None	Radiographic changes; asymptomatic	—	Changes with symptoms	—
Pulmonary edema	None	—	—	Radiographic change; diuretics needed	Requires intubation
Pneumonia (noninfectious)	None	Radiographic changes; no steroids needed	Steroids required	Oxygen required	Assisted ventilation required
Pleural effusion	None	Present	—	—	—

	None	Mild	Moderate	Severe	Life threatening
ARDS	None	Mild	Moderate	Severe	Life threatening
Cough	No change	Mild; relieved by OTC medication	Requires opioid antitussive	Uncontrolled cough	—
Other pulmonary	None	Mild	Moderate	Severe	Life threatening
Cardiac					
Dysrhythmias	None	Asymptomatic, transient; no therapy required	Recurrent or persistent; no therapy required	Requires treatment	Requires monitoring; or hypotension, ventricular tachycardia, or fibrillation
Function	None	Asymptomatic; decline in resting ejection fraction by <20% of baseline value	Asymptomatic; decline in resting ejection fraction by >20% of baseline value	Mild CHF, responsive to therapy	Severe or refractory CHF
Ischemia	None	Nonspecific T-wave flattening	Asymptomatic; ST and T-wave changes suggest ischemia	Angina without evidence of infarction	Acute myocardial infarction
Pericardial	None	Asymptomatic effusion; no intervention required	Pericarditis (rub, chest pain, ECG changes)	Symptomatic effusion; requires drainage	Tamponade; drainage urgently required
Other cardiac	None	Mild	Moderate	Severe	Life threatening

continued

National Cancer Institute Common Toxicity Criteria *continued*

Toxicity	Grade 0	Grade 1	Grade 2	Grade 3	Grade 4
Blood Pressure					
Hypertension	None or no change	Asymptomatic transient increase by >20 mm Hg diastolic or >150/100 if previously WNL. No treatment required	Recurrent or persistent increase by >20 mm Hg diastolic or >150/100 if previously WNL. No treatment required	Requires therapy	Hypertensive crisis
Hypotension	None or no change	Changes requiring no therapy, including orthostatic hypotension	Requires fluid replacement or other therapy but not hospitalization	Requires therapy and hospitalization; resolves within 48 hr of stopping the agent	Requires therapy and hospitalization >48 hr after stopping the agent
Phlebitis, thrombosis, embolism	None	None	Superficial phlebitis (not local)	Deep vein thrombosis	Major event (cerebral, hepatic, pulmonary embolism)
Edema	None	1+ or dependent in evening only	2+ or dependent throughout the day	3+	4+; generalized anasarca
Neurologic					
Neurosensory	None or no change	Mild paresthesia; loss of deep tendon reflexes	Mild or moderate objective sensory loss; mild paresthesias	Severe objective sensory loss or paresthesias; interferes with function	—

Neuromotor	None	Subjective weakness; no objective findings	Mild objective weakness; no significant impairment of function	Objective weakness; impairment of function	Paralysis
Neurocortical	None	Mild somnolence or agitation	Moderate somnolence or agitation	Severe somnolence, agitation, or confusion; disorientation, or hallucinations	Coma, seizures, toxic psychosis
Neurocerebellar	None	Slight incoordination, dysdiadokinesis	Intention tremor, dysmetria, slurred speech, nystagmus	Locomotor ataxia	Cerebellar necrosis
Mood	No change	Mild anxiety or depression	Moderate anxiety or depression	Severe anxiety or depression	Suicidal ideation
Headache	None	Mild	Moderate or severe but transient	Unrelenting and severe	—
Constipation	None or no change	Mild	Moderate	Severe	Ileus >96 hr
Hearing	None or no change	Asymptomatic hearing loss on audiometry only	Tinnitus	Hearing loss interfering with function but correctable with hearing aid	Deafness not correctable
Vision	None or no change	—	—	Symptomatic subtotal loss of vision	Blindness
Pain	None	Mild	Moderate	Severe	Intolerable
Behavioral change	None	Change not disruptive to patient or family	Disruptive to patient or family	Harmful to others or self	Psychotic behavior

continued

National Cancer Institute Common Toxicity Criteria *continued*

Toxicity	Grade 0	Grade 1	Grade 2	Grade 3	Grade 4
Dizziness, vertigo	None	Not disabling	—	Disabling	—
Taste	Normal	Slightly altered taste	Markedly altered taste	—	—
Insomnia	Normal	Occasional difficulty sleeping; may need treatment	—	Difficulty sleeping despite medication	—
Other neurologic	None	Mild	Moderate	Severe	Life threatening
Dermatologic					
Skin	None or no change	Scattered macular or papular eruption or asymptomatic erythema	Scattered macular or papular eruption or erythema with pruritis or other associated symptoms	Generalized symptomatic macular, papular, or vesicular eruption	Exfoliative dermatitis or ulcerating dermatitis
Local	None	Pain	Pain and swelling with inflammation or phlebitis	Ulceration	Plastic surgery indicated
Allergy	None	Transient rash, drug fever <38°C, 100.4°F	Urticaria, drug fever >38°C, 100.4°F, mild bronchospasm	Serum sickness, bronchospasm; requires parenteral medications	Anaphylaxis
Flulike symptoms					
Fever in absence of infection	None	37.1–38°C 98.7–100.4°F	38.1–40°C 100.5–104°F	>40°C >104°F <24 hr	>40°C >104°F >24 hr or fever with hypotension

	None	Mild or brief	Pronounced or prolonged	—	—
Chills	None	Mild or brief	Pronounced or prolonged	—	—
Myalgias, arthralgia	Normal	Mild	Decrease in ability to move	Disabled	—
Sweats	Normal	Mild and occasional	Frequent or drenching	—	—
Malaise	None	Mild; able to continue normal activities	Impaired normal activity or bed rest <50% of waking time	In bed or chair >50% of waking time	Bedridden or unable to care for self
Other flulike symptoms	None	Mild	Moderate	Severe	Life threatening
Weight gain or loss	<5%	5–9.9%	10–19.9%	≥20%	—
Metabolic					
Hyperglycemia	<116 mg/dL	116–160	161–250	251–500	>500 or ketoacidosis
	<6.2 mmol/L	6.2–8.9	9–13.9	14–27.8	>27.8 or ketoacidosis
Hypoglycemia	>64 mg/dL	55–64	40–54	30–39	<30
	>3.6 mmol/L	3.1–3.6	2.2–3	1.7–2.1	<1.7
Amylase	WNL	<1.5 × normal	1.5–2 × normal	2.1–5 × normal	>5.1 × normal
Hypercalcemia	<10.6 mg/dL	10.6–11.5	11.6–12.5	12.6–13.5	>13.5
	<2.6 mmol/L	2.65–2.87	2.88–3.12	3.13–3.37	>3.37

continued

National Cancer Institute Common Toxicity Criteria continued

Toxicity	Grade 0	Grade 1	Grade 2	Grade 3	Grade 4
Hypocalcemia	>8.4 mg/dL	8.4–7.8	7.7–7.0	6.9–6.1	≤6.0
	>2.1 mmol/L	2.1–1.95	1.94–1.75	1.74–1.51	≤1.50
Hypomagnesemia	>1.4 mg/dL	1.4–1.2	1.1–0.9	0.8–0.6	≤0.5
Hyponatremia	WNL or >135 mmol/L	131–135	126–130	121–125	≤120
Hypokalemia	WNL or >3.5 mmol/L	3.1–3.5	2.6–3	2.1–2.5	≤2
Other metabolic	None	Mild	Moderate	Severe	Life threatening
Coagulation					
Fibrinogen	WNL	0.99–0.75 × normal	0.74–0.5 × normal	0.49–0.24 × normal	≤0.24 × normal
Prothrombin time	WNL	1.01–1.25 × normal	1.26–1.5 × normal	1.51–2 × normal	>2 × normal
Partial thromboplastin time	WNL	1.01–1.66 × normal	1.67–2.33 × normal	2.34–3 × normal	>3 × normal
Other coagulation	None	Mild	Moderate	Severe	Life threatening

Endocrine

Impotence, libido	Normal	Decrease in normal function	—	Absence of function	—
Sterility	No	Yes	—	—	—
Amenorrhea	No	Yes	—	—	—
Gynecomastia	None	Mild	Pronounced or painful	—	—
Hot flashes	None	Mild or <1/day	Moderate and ≥1/day	Frequent and interferes with normal function	—
Cushingoid	Normal	Mild	Pronounced	—	—
Other endocrine	None	Mild	Moderate	Severe	Life threatening

Eyes

Conjunctivitis, keratitis	None	Erythema or chemosis; no steroids or antibiotics	Steroids or antibiotics required	Corneal ulcerations or visible opacifications	—
Dry eye	Normal	—	Requires artificial tears	Requires enucleation	—
Glaucoma	No change	—	—	Yes	—
Other eyes	None	Mild	Moderate	Severe	Life threatening

WBC, white blood cell count; WNL, within normal limits; SGOT, serum glutamic-oxaloacetic transaminase; AST, aspartate amino transferase; SGPT, serum glutamate pyruvate transaminase; ALT, alanine aminotransferase; alk phos, alkaline phosphatase; BUN, blood urea nitrogen; DLCO, diffusing capacity for carbon dioxide; ARDS, acute respiratory distress syndrome; OTC, over the counter; CHF, congestive heart failure; ECG, electrocardiogram.

4
Chemotherapy Dose Modifications and Precautions

John D. Wilkes and Irfan Maghfoor

Chemotherapy doses must frequently be adjusted to the patient's age, performance status, hematologic parameters, hepatic function, renal function, or specific drug-induced toxicities. This chapter outlines recommended dose modifications and certain precautions for individual chemotherapeutic agents according to the manufacturer's official U.S. labeling. Further modifications may be required when agents are used in combinations or for off-label treatments. For dose modifications of combination regimens, referral to the original publication or protocol is strongly recommended.

Chemotherapeutic agents are highly toxic compounds with low therapeutic indices. These drugs must be used only under the direct supervision of physicians experienced in therapy with cytotoxic agents. In addition, many of these agents should be used only if adequate treatment facilities to manage these therapies and their complications are available. Dosage of chemotherapeutic drugs should be adjusted as needed according to the clinical response of the patient to achieve the optimum therapeutic result with the minimum adverse effects.

As a general guideline, any significant toxicity during the previous cycle of therapy should resolve before subsequent therapy is initiated. Specifically, hematologic parameters should be assessed prior to the administration of most agents. Similarly, an evaluation of the patient's hepatic and/or renal function is critical before patients receive agents that are metabolized or excreted by the liver or kidneys. Tables 4.1 through 4.3 give some general guidelines for dosing in patients with impaired organ function. More specific information is provided with each individual drug. Agents not listed in the following text and tables either have no reported dose modifications or precautions or are not yet commercially available. It is recommended that the clinician refer to published protocols for dosing and adjustments in these instances.

Table 4.1. General Guidelines for Percentage of Chemotherapy Dosage Based on Hematologic Parameters

Platelets	Granulocytes ($\times 10^6$ cells/L)			
	>2.0	1.5–1.99	1–1.49	<1
>100,000	100.0	75	50	0
50,000–99,000	50.0	50	50	0
<50,000	0.0	0	0	0

Table 4.2. General Guidelines for Percentage of Chemotherapy Dosage Based on Renal Function

Drug	Creatinine Clearance (mL/minute)			
	>60	30–60	10–30	<10
Asparaginases	NC	Omit	Omit	Omit
Bleomycin	NC	75	75	50
Carboplatin				Omit
Cisplatin	NC	50	Omit	Omit
Cyclophosphamide	NC	NC	NC	50
Dactinomycin	NC	WC	WC	WC
Daunorubicin	NC	75	50	WC
Estramustine	NC	WC	WC	WC
Etoposides	NC	75	75	WC
Fludarabine	NC	WC	WC	WC
Gallium	NC	WC	Omit	Omit
Gemcitabine	NC	WC	WC	WC
Hydroxyurea	NC	WC	WC	WC
Ifosfamide	NC	WC	WC	WC
Interleukin-2[a]				
Melphalan	NC	WC	WC	WC
6-Mercaptopurine	NC	WC	WC	WC
Methotrexate	NC	Omit	Omit	Omit
Mitomycin C	NC	Omit	Omit	Omit
Nitrosoureas	NC	Omit	Omit	Omit
Pentostatin	NC	WC	Omit	Omit
Streptozotocin	NC	75	75	50
Teniposide	WC	WC	WC	WC
6-Thioguanine	NC	WC	WC	WC
Topotecan	NC	50	50	Omit

NC, no change; WC, with caution.
[a]See Table 4.14.

Table 4.3. Percentage of Chemotherapy Dosage Based on Hepatic Function

Drug	Bilirubin 1.5–3 AST 60–180	Bilirubin 3.1–5 AST > 180	Bilirubin > 5
Anastrazole	WC	WC	WC
Androgens	Omit	Omit	Omit
Cyclophosphamide	100	75	Omit
Daunorubicin	75	50	Omit
Dactinomycin	WC	WC	WC
Docetaxel	Omit	Omit	Omit
Doxorubicins	50	25	Omit
Estramustine	NC	WC	WC
Estrogens	Omit	Omit	Omit
Etoposide	50	Omit	Omit
Fluorodeoxyuridine	WC	WC	Omit
5-Fluorouracil	100	100	Omit
Flutamide	WC	Omit	Omit
Gemcitabine	WC	WC	WC
Idarubicin	75	50	Omit
Interferon-α	NC	Omit	Omit
Ketoconazole	WC	Omit	Omit
Letrozole	WC	WC	WC
Medroxyprogesterone	Omit	Omit	Omit
Methotrexate	100	75	Omit
Mithramycin	WC	Omit	Omit
Mitoxantrone	WC	WC	WC
Paclitaxel	WC	WC	Omit
6-Thioguanine	WC	WC	Omit
Teniposide	WC	WC	WC
Tretinoin	NC	WC	Omit
Vinblastine	NC	50	Omit
Vincristine	NC	50	Omit
Vinorelbine	50	25	Omit

NC, *no change;* WC, *with caution.*

DNA-BINDING DRUGS: ALKYLATING AGENTS
BUSULFAN (MYLERAN)
Endocrine

Busulfan should be discontinued immediately if signs or symptoms suggest addisonian-like syndrome. These may include weakness, fatigue, anorexia, weight loss, nausea, vomiting, or melanoderma.

Hematologic

The use of busulfan in patients with marrow function compromised by prior irradiation or chemotherapy may lead to severe myelosuppression and should be undertaken with extreme caution. Doses of busulfan should be reduced in patients with impaired marrow or if busulfan is to be used with other myelosuppressive agents. However, there are no specific guidelines. In the treatment of chronic myelocytic leukemia, many investigators recommend discontinuation of the drug when the white blood cell count (WBC) falls to 10,000 to 15,000 cells/mm^3.

Hepatic

The risk of hepatic veno-occlusive disease increases with cumulative doses above 16 mg/kg of ideal body weight or when busulfan is combined with other alkylating agents. Serum aminotransferases and bilirubin should be periodically monitored.

Pulmonary

Busulfan should be discontinued immediately at the first sign or symptom of interstitial fibrosis, including dyspnea, cough, or congestion.

CARBOPLATIN (PARAPLATIN)

Hematologic

Pretreatment platelet count is an important prognostic factor for severity of myelosuppression. Table 4.4 reflects dose adjustments based on nadir blood counts following carboplatin dosing.

Renal

Renal excretion is the major route of elimination for carboplatin. Hence, patients with renal impairment may have significant hematologic toxicity following treatment with carboplatin. Dose adjustments may be based on creatinine clearance alone.

Table 4.4. Nadir Counts from Prior Cycle of Carboplatin (Cells/mm^3)

Platelets	Neutrophils	Adjusted Dose (% of prior dose)
>100,000	>2,000	125%
50–100,000	500–2,000	No adjustment
<50,000	<500	75%

This approach has largely been replaced by mathematical formulas that incorporate creatinine clearance with or without target platelet nadir. The use of these formulas allows compensation for variation from patient to patient in pretreatment renal function, which might lead to improper dosing. The Calvert formula for carboplatin dosing is as follows:

$$\text{Total dose in milligrams} = (\text{target AUC}) \times (\text{GFR} + 25)$$

Note: The total dose of carboplatin is in milligrams, *not* milligrams per square meter.

CARMUSTINE (BCNU, BiCNU, GLIADEL)

Hematologic

Carmustine dose must be reduced in patients with impaired marrow or when used with other myelosuppressive agents. Dose modifications should be based on nadir hematologic parameters as recommended in Table 4.5. There are no dose modifications for the carmustine wafers (Gliadel).

CHLORAMBUCIL (LEUKERAN)

Hematologic

The initial dose of chlorambucil should be reduced if radiation therapy or myelosuppressive chemotherapy has been administered within 4 weeks. Similarly, the initial daily dose should not exceed 0.1 mg/kg if pretreatment blood counts are depressed from bone marrow disease or prior therapy. Subsequent doses should be adjusted to hematologic parameters.

CISPLATIN (PLATINOL, DDP)

Ototoxicity

Cisplatin may produce cumulative ototoxicity, and many clinicians recommend routine audiometric testing prior to each course of therapy. Others have questioned the utility of this testing and

Table 4.5. Nadir Counts from Prior Cycle of Carmustine (cells/mm³)

Platelets	Leukocytes	Adjusted Dose (% of prior dose)
>100,000	>4000	100
75–99,999	3000–3999	100
25,000–74,999	2000–2999	50–70
<25,000	<2000	25–50

recommend audiometric testing at the first signs of clinical hearing loss. Clinically significant hearing changes may require dose reductions, delays, and/or discontinuation.

Renal

Renal toxicity becomes more prolonged and severe with repeat dosing of cisplatin. Renal function must return to normal (serum creatinine less than 1.5 mg/dL, blood urea nitrogen [BUN] less than 25 mg/dL) before retreatment with this drug. It is generally recommended that cisplatin not be administered to patients with a creatinine clearance less than 50 mL/minute. Concomitant use of aminoglycosides or other nephrotoxic agents may increase renal toxicity.

CYCLOPHOSPHAMIDE (CYTOXAN, NEOSAR)

Hematologic

For patients with compromised bone marrow function, an initial dose reduction of 33 to 50% is recommended. Subsequent doses may be adjusted to hematologic effects.

DACARBAZINE (DTIC)

Hematologic

A complete blood count should be performed prior to each dose of DTIC. If the WBC is less than 3,000 cells/mm^3 and/or the platelet count is less than 100,000 cells/mm^3, therapy should be suspended or discontinued.

IFOSFAMIDE (IFEX)

Hematologic

Significant myelosuppression is frequently observed with ifosfamide. WBC, hemoglobin, and platelets should be obtained before each dose and at appropriate intervals. Unless clinically essential, do not administer if WBC is less than 2,000 cells/mL and/or platelet count is less than 50,000 cells/μL.

Neurologic

Neurologic manifestations, including somnolence, confusion, hallucinations, and even coma, have been reported. While the central nervous system (CNS) effects are usually self-limited, drug must be withheld and supportive measures initiated immediately on manifestation of symptoms.

Renal and Urinary

Ifosfamide is toxic to the bladder mucosa. This drug should always be used with a uroprotective regimen, including aggressive hydration and mesna. A urine specimen should be obtained before each dose of ifosfamide. If microscopic hematuria (more than 10 red blood cells [RBC] per high-power field [HPF]) occurs, hold further doses until hematuria completely resolves. Administer further doses only with vigorous hydration. If more than 50 RBC per HPF are seen, the drug should be discontinued until hematuria resolves, then dose reduced by 50%. Ifosfamide should be used with caution in patients with renal impairment, although no specific dose modifications are provided.

LOMUSTINE (CCNU, CEENU)

Hematologic

Patients with impaired marrow function as a result of prior radiation or chemotherapy should receive a dose reduced 25% to 100 mg/m^2. Dose reductions based on hematologic nadirs are found in Table 4.6.

MECHLORETHAMINE (NITROGEN MUSTARD, MUSTARGEN)

Hematologic

Mechlorethamine, which most frequently used in combination regimens (i.e., MOPP), may cause significant marrow suppression. It is recommended that the drug be reduced by 50% if the leukocyte count is 3000 to 3999/mm^3. A dose reduction of 75% is recommended if the leukocyte count is 1000 to 2999/mm^3 and/or the platelet count is 50,000 to 100,000/mm^3. Mechlorethamine should be held if leukocyte counts are less than 1000/mm^3 or platelets less than 50,000/mm^3.

MELPHALAN (L-PHENYLALANINE MUSTARD [L-PAM], ALKERAN)

General

There are significant differences in the bioavailability between oral and intravenous melphalan. There is no conversion formula because of the variable absorption of oral melphalan. Clinicians should refer to published protocols for dosing guidelines.

Table 4.6. Nadir Counts from Prior Cycle of Lomustine (cells/mm^3)

Platelets	Leukocytes	Adjusted Dose (% of prior dose)
> 100,000	>4000	100
75–99,999	3000–3999	100
25,000–74,999	2000–2999	75
< 25,000	< 2000	50

Hematologic

Doses should be modified according to the nadir hematologic counts of the preceding cycle. The optimal therapeutic effect requires some degree of marrow suppression, which may lead to dose escalation or reduction based on hematologic toxicities.

Renal

Melphalan and its metabolites do appear in the urine after dosing. However, the inherent variable absorption of oral melphalan makes it difficult to recommend appropriate dose reductions in patients with renal impairment. Hence patients with azotemia must be closely observed for hematologic toxicity. For intravenous melphalan, doses should be reduced by 50% if the BUN is more than 30 mg/dL.

MITOMYCIN (MUTAMYCIN)

Hematologic

Mitomycin frequently produces significant bone marrow suppression. Hematologic parameters must be evaluated prior to each dose and at regular intervals for at least 8 weeks following therapy. The drug should be held if the platelet count is less than $100,000/mm^3$ or WBC is less than 4000 cells/mm^3 on the day of planned treatment. Doses of mitomycin should be adjusted according to the hematologic nadirs of the previous cycle of therapy as suggested in Table 4.7. See also next section for precautions related to hemolytic uremic syndrome.

Renal

The syndrome of microangiopathic hemolytic anemia, thrombocytopenia, and uremia (hemolytic uremic syndrome [HUS]) can occur at any time during treatment with mitomycin but is more common as cumulative doses approach 60 mg/m^2. Patients must be monitored carefully and the drug discontinued immediately if unexplained hemolysis, thrombocytopenia, or renal dysfunction occurs. Patients with a serum creatinine more than 1.7 should not be given mitomycin.

Table 4.7. Nadir Counts from Prior Cycle of Mitomycin

Platelets	Leukocytes	Adjusted Dose (% of prior dose)
>100,000	>4000	100
75–99,999	3000–3999	100
25,000–74,999	2000–2999	70
< 25,000	< 2000	50

PROCARBAZINE (MATULANE)

Hematologic

Procarbazine should be discontinued if the WBC is less than $4000/mm^3$ or if platelets less than $100,000/mm^3$, or bleeding or bleeding tendency occurs.

Gastrointestinal

Procarbazine should be discontinued if mucositis or diarrhea occurs.

Neurologic

Procarbazine should be discontinued if paresthesia, neuropathy, or confusion occurs.

STREPTOZOCIN (STREPTOZOTOCIN, ZANOSAR)

General

Repeat doses of streptozocin should not be administered until the patient's renal, hepatic, and hematologic parameters are within normal limits.

Renal

Renal parameters must be carefully monitored during therapy. Some clinicians recommend a 25% dose reduction for patients with creatinine clearance 10 to 50 mL/minute and a 50% dose reduction for patients with creatinine clearance less than 10 mL/minute.

THIOTEPA (THIO-TEPA, THIOPLEX)

General

Thiotepa should probably not be administered to patients with impaired renal or hepatic function. If necessary, the drug should be given in low doses and hepatic and renal function monitored carefully.

Hematologic

Therapy should be temporarily discontinued if the WBC falls to less than $3000/mm^3$ or the platelets fall to less than $150,000/mm^3$.

URACIL MUSTARD (URAMUSTINE)

Hematologic

As cumulative doses approach 1 mg/kg, irreversible bone marrow damage may occur. The drug must be temporarily discontinued if a sharp decline in WBC or platelets occurs.

ANTIMETABOLITES

CHLORODEOXYADENOSINE (CLADRIBINE, 2-CDA, LEUSTATIN)

Hepatic

The manufacturer recommends no specific dose modifications in the presence of hepatic impairment but suggests that hepatic function be monitored while patients are receiving therapy.

Immune

2-CdA can produce severe prolonged suppression of T cell–mediated immunity for as long as 12 months following therapy. Patients must be monitored carefully for opportunistic infections.

Renal

The manufacturer recommends no specific dose modifications in the presence of renal impairment but suggests that renal function be monitored while patients are receiving therapy.

CYTOSINE ARABINOSIDE (CYTARABINE, ARA-C)

Hepatic

Cytosine arabinoside should be used with caution and reduced doses in patients with hepatic disease. Specific dose reductions are not available.

Neurologic

Neurologic dysfunction has been associated with high-dose Ara-C regimens, especially in patients over 60 years of age. Patients should be monitored closely for signs of neurologic dysfunction with immediate interruption of therapy or significant reductions in dose as necessary to prevent irreversible neurotoxicity.

FLUDARABINE (FAMP, FLUDARA)

General

Doses of fludarabine should be delayed and/or reduced according to hematologic and nonhematologic toxicity with the prior cycle.

Renal

Though no specific dose modifications are provided, physicians should be aware that the clearance of 2-fluoro-ara-A (dephosphorylated fludarabine) correlates inversely with serum creatinine. Patients with impaired renal function may be at increased risk of toxicity and should be monitored carefully. Discontinuation or dose modification should be based on toxicities with prior cycles.

Neurologic

If there is any neurotoxicity, dose reductions, delays, or discontinuation should be strongly considered.

FLOXURIDINE (FLUORODEOXYURIDINE [FUDR])

General

Floxuridine is most frequently used as a continuous infusion for regional directed hepatic arterial therapy. Clinical parameters and hematologic and liver function tests must be monitored regularly. Therapy must be discontinued if WBC falls below $35,000/mm^3$ or platelet count falls below $100,000/mm^3$. Myocardial ischemia, abdominal pain, and mucositis are all indications to discontinue therapy immediately. The drug should also be used with extreme caution in patients who have received prior high-dose radiation therapy to the pelvis or alkylating therapy.

Hepatic

Rising liver function findings may be a sign of hepatic toxicity and necessitate dose reductions. Physicians should refer to specific protocols for dose reductions and delays for hepatic toxicity.

5-FLUOROURACIL (5-FU, ADRUCIL, EFUDEX, FLUOROPLEX)

General

Ideal body weight should be used for patients with obesity or significant fluid retention. Various doses, schedules, and combinations of 5-fluorouracil have appeared in the literature. The physician should refer to specific protocols of published materials for dose modifications. In general, dose modifications should be based on the level of toxicity caused by the previous cycle of therapy.

GEMCITABINE (GEMZAR)

General

The clearance of gemcitabine is low in women and older patients, so dose reductions may be necessary in these patients.

Hematologic

The dose of gemcitabine should be adjusted to hematologic parameters as recommended in Table 4.8. After completion of a full course of therapy with gemcitabine, patients may be considered for a 25% dose escalation if nadir absolute neutrophil count (ANC) was more than $1,500/mm^3$, platelets are more than

Table 4.8. Gemcitabine Dose Modifications Based on Hematologic Parameters on Date of Treatment

ANC	Platelets	Modification
>1,000	>100,000	None
500–999	50,000–99,999	75% of the full dose should be given weekly
<500	<50,000	Weekly dose should be withheld until counts exceed these levels

$100,000/mm^3$, no other nonhematologic toxicity greater than grade 1 was encountered. After another 3-week course, patients may undergo a second dose escalation to $1,500 \text{ mg}/m^2$ if the same criteria are met.

Hepatic

Data are insufficient to recommend specific dose adjustments for patients with hepatic dysfunction. It is recommended that caution be used when gemcitabine is administered to these patients.

Renal

Data are insufficient to recommend specific dose adjustments for patients with renal dysfunction. It is recommended that caution be used when gemcitabine is administered to these patients.

HYDROXYUREA (HYDREA)

General

For patients with significant fluid accumulation or obesity, ideal body weight should be used to calculate dosage. Elderly patients may be more sensitive to the effects of hydrea and may require a lower dose.

Hematologic

If bone marrow is suppressed, hydroxyurea doses should be held until hematologic parameters improve.

Renal

Hydroxyurea should be used with caution in patients with impaired renal function.

6-MERCAPTOPURINE (6-MP, PURINETHOL)

General

Allopurinol inhibits the oxidative metabolism of 6-MP. Thus, the initial dose of 6-MP should be reduced by 25 to 33% in patients who are taking allopurinol. Further reductions may be required according to the patient's response and toxicity. 6-MP may also interfere with the results of chemistry assays, giving falsely elevated levels of glucose and uric acid.

Renal

The dose of 6-MP should probably be reduced in patients with impaired renal function, although no specific guidelines exist.

METHOTREXATE (MTX, MEXATE)

General

Methotrexate should not be given if mucositis is present. Methotrexate accumulates in fluid collections, such as effusions. If possible, any significant effusion should be drained prior to treatments. Patients should be well hydrated before high-dose methotrexate is administered.

Hematologic

Administration of methotrexate should be delayed if the WBC is less than $1,500/\mu L$, ANC is less than $200/\mu L$, or platelet count is less than $75,000/\mu L$.

Hepatic

Administration of methotrexate should be delayed if the serum bilirubin is more than 1.2 mg/dL or alanine aminotransferase (ALT) is more than 450 U.

Renal

Patients must have a normal creatinine and creatinine clearance more than 60 mL/minute before therapy.

PENTOSTATIN (DEOXYCOFORMYCIN, NIPENT)

General

Pentostatin doses should be withheld from patients who develop a severe rash from the drug. Similarly, the drug should be withheld or discontinued in the event of nervous system toxicity.

Hematologic

Doses of pentostatin should be held if ANC drops from a baseline level more than $500/mm^3$ to less than $200/mm^3$. The drug may be resumed once the ANC returns to pretreatment levels.

Renal

There are insufficient data to recommend dose modifications for patients with renal insufficiency. The potential for significant toxicity does exist if pentostatin is administered to patients with creatinine clearance less than 60 mL/minute. Patients with renal insufficiency should receive pentostatin only if the potential benefits are thought to outweigh the possible risks.

6-THIOGUANINE (6-TG, THIOGUANINE)

Hematologic

Hematologic parameters must be monitored carefully in patients receiving thioguanine. Therapy should be withheld at the first signs of an abrupt drop in hemoglobin, platelets, or WBC. Therapy may be resumed once hematologic parameters return to acceptable levels.

Hepatic

Thioguanine should be discontinued immediately in the presence of signs or symptoms of hepatic dysfunction, including elevated liver enzymes, hepatomegaly, tenderness in the right upper quadrant, or jaundice. Patients with impaired liver function should receive reduced doses of thioguanine, although specific reductions are not clearly defined.

Renal

Patients with impaired renal function should receive reduced doses of thioguanine, although specific reductions are not clearly defined.

TRIMETREXATE (NEUTREXIN)

Trimetrexate is not yet approved in the United States for the treatment of malignancy, and dose and scheduling issues remain to be clarified. Thus, there are no specific dose modifications for this patient population. The drug is approved in combination with leucovorin for the treatment of *Pneumocystis carinii*, and dose modifications based on hematologic, hepatic, and renal parameters are available for this indication.

ANTITUMOR ANTIBIOTICS AND RELATED AGENTS

BLEOMYCIN (BLENOXANE)

Pulmonary

There are no guidelines for dose modification based on pulmonary impairment. The manufacturer recommends extreme caution when using bleomycin in patients with poor pulmonary status. If pulmonary symptoms arise, the drug should be discontinued immediately until it is clearly determined that these symptoms were unrelated to the drug. As the incidence of pulmonary toxicity depends on cumulative dose, extreme caution should be exercised when administering cumulative doses above 400 U. Patients who have received bleomycin are at increased risk for oxygen toxicity, and if oxygen is required, every attempt should be made to keep the FiO_2 as low as tolerated to maintain adequate oxygenation.

Renal

Clearance of bleomycin may be impaired in patients with renal dysfunction. There are no concrete guidelines for dose modifications, and the manufacturer recommends extreme caution when using bleomycin in patients with renal impairment.

DACTINOMYCIN (ACTINOMYCIN D, COSMEGEN)

Hepatic

The manufacturer recommends frequent evaluation of hepatic function, but no specific dose adjustments are reported.

Obesity

The dose of dactinomycin may have to be reduced in obese patients, although no specific modifications are reported. Dosage should be based on body surface area in obese or edematous patients.

Renal

The manufacturer recommends frequent evaluation of renal function, but no dose adjustments are reported.

DAUNORUBICIN (CERUBINE)

Cardiac

The manufacturer recommends obtaining an electrocardiogram (ECG) prior to each dose of daunorubicin. If the QRS voltage decreases by 30% or the left ventricular ejection drops below pretreatment levels, the clinician should carefully weigh the risk of cardiac damage against the potential benefits of additional therapy with this drug. In adults, the total dose of daunorubicin should not exceed 500 to 600 mg/m^2 because of risk of cumulative cardiac toxicity. In patients who have received radiation to the heart, the cumulative daunorubicin dosage should not exceed 400 to 450 mg/m^2. Higher doses may be administered if a cardioprotective agent such as dexrazoxane (Zinecard) is also given.

Hepatic

Patients with serum bilirubin of 1.2 to 3 mg/dL should receive only 75% of the planned dose of daunorubicin. If the bilirubin is more than 3 mg/dL, the dose should be reduced by 50%.

Renal

The dose of daunorubicin should be reduced by 50% in patients with a serum creatinine more than 3 mg/dL.

DOXORUBICIN (ADRIAMYCIN, RUBEX)

Cardiac

In adults, the total dose of doxorubicin should not exceed 550 mg/m^2 because of risk of irreversible cardiac toxicity. In patients who have received radiation to the heart or other cardiotoxic agents, the cumulative doxorubicin dosage should not exceed 400 mg/m^2. Higher doses may be administered if a cardioprotective agent such as dexrazoxane (Zinecard) is given concomitantly.

General

In patients with abnormal fluid retention, the ideal body weight should be used in dosing.

Hematologic

Doxorubicin doses may have to be reduced in patients with impaired marrow function, although there are no specific data on which to base recommendations.

Hepatic

Doxorubicin dose must be reduced for hepatic dysfunction. If the serum direct bilirubin is 1.2 to 3 mg/dL, 50% dose should be administered. If the bilirubin is more than 3 mg/dL, 25% of the scheduled dose should be administered.

DOXORUBICIN LIPOSOMAL (DOXIL)

Cutaneous

A common toxicity of liposomal doxorubicin is palmar-plantar erythrodysesthesia (hand-foot syndrome). Dose modifications for this cutaneous toxicity are listed in Table 4.9.

Hematologic

Dose modifications for hematologic toxicity are listed in Table 4.10.

Hepatic

In patients with impaired liver function, the manufacturer recommends the same dose reductions for encapsulated doxorubicin as for conventional doxorubicin. (See hepatic precautions listed under first discussion of doxorubicin).

Mucosal

Modifications based on mucosal toxicities are listed in Table 4.11.

Table 4.9. Dose Modifications for Cutaneous Toxicity Associated with Liposomal Doxorubicin

Toxicity Grade	Symptoms	Assessment 3 Weeks after Dose	Reassessment 4 Weeks after Dose
0	No symptoms	Redose at 3-week interval if grade 0	Redose at 3-week interval if toxicity improved to grade 0
1	Mild erythema, swelling, or desquamation not interfering with daily activities	Redose unless patient has had a grade 3 or 4 skin toxicity, in which case wait an additional week	Redose at 25% dose reduction if toxicity remained at grade 1; then return to 3 week interval if no worsening
2	Erythema, desquamation, or swelling with but not precluding normal physical activities; small blisters or ulcerations <2 cm in diameter	Wait an additional week	Redose at 50% dose reduction if toxicity remained at grade 2; then return to 3-week interval
3	Blistering, ulceration, or swelling interfering with walking or normal daily activities; cannot wear regular clothing	Wait an additional week	If no improvement, discontinue liposomal doxorubicin
4	Diffuse or local process causing infectious complications or a bedridden state or hospitalization	Wait an additional week	If no improvement to grade 2 or better, discontinue liposomal doxorubicin

IDARUBICIN (IDAMYCIN)

Cardiac

The use of idarubicin should be undertaken with extreme caution in patients with preexisting cardiac disease and in those

Table 4.10. Liposomal Doxorubicin Dose Modifications for Hematologic Toxicity

Toxicity Grade	ANC	Platelets	Modification
1	1500–1900	75,000–150,000	None
2	1000–1499	50,000–74,999	None
3	500–999	25,000–49,999	Wait until ANC >1,000 and/or platelets >50,000; then redose at 25% dose reduction
4	< 500	< 25,000	Wait until ANC >1,000 and/or platelets >50,000; then redose at 50% dose reduction

Table 4.11. Modifications in Liposomal Doxorubicin Based on Mucosal Toxicity

Toxicity Grade	Symptoms	Modification
1	Painless ulcers, erythema, or mild soreness	None
2	Painful erythema, edema, or ulcers but can eat	Wait 1 week; if symptoms improve, redose at full dose
3	Painful erythema, edema, or ulcers and cannot eat	Wait 1 week and if symptoms improve, redose at 25% dose reduction
4	Requires parenteral or enteral support	Wait 1 week and if symptoms improve, redose at 50% dose reduction

who have received cardiotoxic therapies in the past. The risk of irreversible cardiac damage must be weighed against any potential benefit of the drug in these patients.

Hematologic

If platelet count and/or neutrophil count markedly decreases or severe myelosuppression occurs, therapy should be discontinued to allow for marrow recovery. Idamycin should be used with extreme caution in patients with impaired marrow function or when used in conjunction with radiation of other myelosuppressive agents.

Hepatic

The majority of clinical trials evaluating idarubicin excluded patients with impaired liver function. A single phase III trial allowed for patients with bilirubin levels from 2.6 to 5 mg/dL with a 50% reduction in dose. Reductions in the dose of idarubicin are recommended for patients with evidence of hepatic impairment.

Mucosal

In patients with refractory acute myelogenous leukemia (AML) who develop severe mucositis with idarubicin, administration of a second course of the drug should be delayed until this toxicity has resolved. A 25% dose reduction is also recommended in this situation.

Renal

Dose reductions of idarubicin are recommended for patients with elevated serum creatinine levels, although no specific guidelines are available.

MITOXANTRONE (NOVANTRONE)

General

Decreased clearance of mitoxantrone may occur in patients with significant ascites or pleural effusions, and extra caution should be used when administering mitoxantrone to these patients.

Hepatic

Mitoxantrone is eliminated through the hepatobiliary system, and the safety of this drug in patients with severe hepatic impairment is not established. The available data are insufficient for recommendations of specific dose adjustments.

MICROTUBULE-TARGETING DRUGS

DOCETAXEL (TAXOTERE)

Hematologic

A 25% reduction in dose is recommended for patients who have severe or prolonged myelosuppression with the previous cycle of docetaxel (ANC less than 500 cells/mm^3 for 7 days or longer).

Hepatic

An increase in side effects has been reported in patients with mild to moderate liver impairment who receive docetaxel.

Therefore, this drug should not be administered to patients with elevated serum bilirubin levels or patients with aspartate amino transferase (AST) or alanine aminotransferase (ALT) levels more than 1.5 times normal or with alkaline phosphatase levels more than 2.5 times normal.

Other

A 25% reduction is dose is recommended for patients who experience severe cutaneous reactions or neurologic toxicity. If severe reactions persist, the drug should be discontinued.

PACLITAXEL (TAXOL, PAXENE)

Hematologic

Patients with severe neutropenia (neutrophils less than 500 cells/mm^3) with prior course of paclitaxel should receive a 20% reduction in dose. Repeat cycles of paclitaxel should be held until ANC is more than 1500/mm^3 and platelets more than 100,000/mm^3.

Hepatic

Paclitaxel should be used with extreme caution in patients with severe hepatic impairment, as this drug is metabolized in the liver. Specific dose modifications do not yet exist.

Neurologic

Patients who had severe peripheral neuropathy with prior doses of paclitaxel should have doses reduced by 20% with subsequent cycles.

VINBLASTINE (VELBAN)

General

Elderly patients and those with cachexia or ulcerated skin may be at increased risk for myelosuppression with vinblastine. Vinblastine should be used with extreme caution in these patients.

Hematologic

Doses of vinblastine should be withheld until WBC is more than 4000/mm^3. Doses may also have to be reduced in patients with recent exposure to radiation or myelosuppressive chemotherapy.

Hepatic

A 50% dose reduction is recommended for patients with a direct serum bilirubin more than 3 mg/dL or other evidence of significant hepatic dysfunction.

VINCRISTINE (ONCOVIN)

Hepatic

A 50% dose reduction is recommended for patients with a direct serum bilirubin more than 3 mg/dL or other evidence of significant hepatic impairment.

Neurologic

Elderly patients and those with underlying neurologic disorders may be particularly susceptible to the neurotoxic effects of vincristine. Most clinicians recommend reducing the dose or discontinuing the drug in the event of signs of nervous system toxicity, such as paresthesias, loss of deep tendon reflexes, and/or motor weakness.

VINORELBINE (NAVELBINE)

Hepatic

For patients with impaired hepatic function, the dose of vinorelbine should be adjusted as recommended in Table 4.12. For patients with both hepatic impairment and hematologic toxicity, the doses of vinorelbine should be reduced even further.

DNA TOPOISOMERASE INHIBITORS

ETOPOSIDE (VP-16, VEPESID)

Hepatic

Etoposide-induced hematologic toxicity appears to be worsened in patients with impaired hepatic function. Thus, etoposide should be used with caution, and patients with impaired hepatic function may need dose reductions. No specific guidelines are available.

Renal

The dose of etoposide should be reduced by 25% in patients with creatinine clearance of 15 to 50 mL/minute. Further reductions should be considered for patients with creatinine clearance less than 15 mL/minute.

Table 4.12. Dose Modifications for Vinorelbine in Patients with Hepatic Impairment

Serum Bilirubin (mg/dL)	Percent of Planned Dose
< 2.0	100
2.1–3.0	50
> 3.0	25

ETOPOSIDE PHOSPHATE (ETOPOPHOS)

Metabolic

Patients with low albumin may be at increased risk for toxicity. Although no dose modifications are recommended, clinicians should exercise added caution.

Renal

A 25% initial dose reduction is recommended for patients with a creatinine clearance between 15 and 50 mL/minute. Subsequent doses should be based on clinical effect and patient tolerance.

IRINOTECAN (CAMPTOSAR, CPT-11)

Gastrointestinal

Dose modifications based on diarrhea (National Cancer Institute common toxicity criteria listed in Chapter 3) are shown in Table 4.13. Subsequent doses of irinotecan should not be given until treatment-related diarrhea has resolved.

General

After an initial dose of irinotecan, subsequent doses should be modified according to the individual patient's tolerance and toxicity.

Hematologic

Dose modifications based on hematologic toxicities (National Cancer Institute common toxicity criteria listed in Chapter 3) are listed in Table 4.13. Subsequent doses of irinotecan should not be given until the ANC is more than $1500/mm^3$ and the platelets are more than $100,000/mm^3$.

TENIPOSIDE (VM-26, VUMON)

General

Patients with Down's syndrome are particularly sensitive to the myelotoxic effects of chemotherapy, and initial doses of teniposide should be reduced in these patients. Subsequent dose escalations may be possible depending on the degree of mucositis and myelosuppression seen with the previous cycles.

Hepatic

There are insufficient data to make recommendations regarding dose adjustments in patients with hepatic impairment. Dose reductions may be necessary in this population.

Renal

Adequate data on the use of teniposide in patients with renal impairment is lacking. Adjustments may be required.

Table 4.13. Dose Modifications for Irinotecan

Toxicity Grade[a]	During a Course of Therapy	At Start of Next Course of Therapy (dose compared with starting dose of previous course)
No toxicity	Maintain dose level	Increase dose by 25 mg/m² up to a max of 150 mg/m²
Hematologic toxicity grade		
1	Maintain dose level	Maintain dose level
2	Reduce by 25 mg/m²	Maintain dose level
3	Omit dose, then reduce by 25 mg/m² when toxicity < grade 2	Reduce dose by 25 mg/m²
4	Omit dose, then reduce by 50 mg/m² when toxicity < grade 2	Reduce dose by 50 mg/m²
Neutropenic fever	Omit dose, then reduce by 50 mg/m² when toxicity < grade 2	Reduce dose by 50 mg/m²
Diarrhea toxicity grade		
1	Maintain dose level	Maintain dose level
2	Reduce by 25 mg/m²	Maintain dose if only grade 2 toxicity
3	Omit dose; reduce by 25 mg/m² when toxicity < grade 2	Reduce dose by 25 mg/m² if only grade 3 toxicity
4	Omit dose, then reduce by 50 mg/m² when toxicity < grade 2	Reduce dose by 50 mg/m²
Nonhematologic toxicity grade		
1	Maintain dose level	Maintain dose level
2	Reduce by 25 mg/m²	Reduce dose by 25 mg/m²
3	Omit dose, then reduce by 25 mg/m² when toxicity < grade 2	Reduce dose by 50 mg/m²
4	Omit dose, then reduce by 50 mg/m² when toxicity < grade 2	Reduce dose by 50 mg/m²

[a]NCI common toxicity criteria, Chapter 3.

TOPOTECAN (HYCAMPTIN)

Renal

A 50% reduction in dose is recommended for patients with moderate renal impairment (creatinine clearance 20 to 39 mL/minute). There is insufficient data to recommend dose adjustments for patients with severe renal insufficiency.

ENZYMES

ASPARAGINASE (ELSPAR)

General

Prior to initiation of therapy and periodically during treatment, hematologic parameters, coagulation studies, and serum chemistries should be performed.

Hepatic

Asparaginase can significantly impair hepatic synthetic function. Coagulation studies should be performed regularly during therapy and doses held for hypofibrinogenemia.

Pancreatic

Asparaginase should be discontinued permanently at the first signs of pancreatitis. Serum amylase levels should be monitored frequently while on therapy.

Renal

Asparaginase should be discontinued at the first sign of renal failure.

PEGASPARGASE (PEG-ʟASPARAGINASE, ONCASPAR)

General

Prior to initiation of therapy and periodically during treatment, hematologic parameters, coagulation studies, and serum chemistries should be performed.

Hepatic

Pegaspargase should be used only with extreme caution in patients with impaired hepatic function or in combination with other hepatotoxic agents.

Pancreatic

Pegaspargase should be discontinued permanently at the first signs of pancreatitis. Serum amylase levels should be monitored frequently while on therapy.

Renal

Pegaspargase should be discontinued at the first sign of renal failure.

HORMONAL AGENTS

AMINOGLUTETHIMIDE (CYTADREN)

Endocrine

Aminoglutethimide produces adrenal insufficiency in a large percentage of patients, and monitoring for signs and symptoms, including electrolytes, is recommended. Replacement mineralo-corticoids and/or glucocorticoids may be required.

General

Dose reductions or discontinuations may be required for significant side effects, including drowsiness or severe skin rash. Mineralocorticoid replacement may be necessary for symptomatic orthostatic hypotension.

Hematologic

Periodic assessment of hematologic parameters is recommended, as patients taking aminoglutethimide may develop anemias or less commonly pancytopenia, which necessitates drug discontinuation.

ANASTROZOLE (ARIMIDEX)

Hepatic

Since 85% of anastrazole elimination occurs through hepatic metabolism, patients with moderate to severe liver dysfunction should be carefully monitored for toxicity. There are, however, no recommendations for dose reductions.

BICALUTAMIDE (CASODEX)

Hepatic

Bicalutamide should be used with caution in patients with moderate or severe hepatic impairment, as the drug is extensively metabolized in the liver. The manufacturer does not, however, provide dose modifications for patients with hepatic dysfunction.

DIETHYLSTILBESTROL (DES)

Hepatic

Estrogens should be discontinued at the first signs of hepatic impairment or jaundice. Estrogens are poorly metabolized in patients with liver impairment, and caution should be used when they are administered to this population.

Gynecologic

In women with an intact uterus, DES should be discontinued immediately if abnormal vaginal bleeding occurs, and a careful examination for endometrial carcinoma should be performed.

ESTRADIOL (ESTRACE, ESTRADERM)

Hepatic

Estrogens should be discontinued at the first signs of hepatic impairment or jaundice. Estrogens are poorly metabolized in patients with liver impairment, and caution should be used when they are administered to this population.

Gynecologic

In women with an intact uterus, estradiol should be discontinued immediately if abnormal vaginal bleeding occurs, and a careful examination for endometrial carcinoma should be performed.

FLUOXYMESTERONE (HALOTESTIN)

Hepatic

The use of androgens such as fluoxymesterone has been associated with potentially severe hepatic toxicity. Liver function tests should be monitored periodically, and the drug should be discontinued at the first sign of hepatitis or cholestasis.

Metabolic

Hypercalcemia may develop in immobilized patients or those with breast cancer, requiring discontinuation of the drug.

FLUTAMIDE (EULEXIN)

Hepatic

The use of flutamide has been associated with potentially severe hepatic toxicity. Liver function tests should be obtained at the first sign or symptom of liver dysfunction or unexplained flulike illness. If the patient develops jaundice or a twofold to threefold rise in transaminases, flutamide should be discontinued. If liver dysfunction reverses, flutamide may be cautiously reinitiated at a lower dose.

GOSERELIN (ZOLADEX)

Metabolic

Hypercalcemia and tumor flare reactions may occur in some patients with bone metastases during initial treatment with goserelin. The drug may have to be held until the serum calcium returns to safe levels. It is generally recommended that a testosterone antagonist such as flutamide be administered concurrently with luteinizing hormone–releasing hormone (LHRH) agonists to prevent such a reaction.

KETOCONAZOLE (NIZORAL)

Hepatic

Potentially fatal hepatic toxicity has been associated with the use of ketoconazole. Prompt recognition of liver injury and discontinuation of therapy are essential. Liver function tests should be monitored before initiation of therapy and at frequent intervals thereafter. Extreme caution should be used when prescribing ketoconazole to patients with preexisting liver disease or when the drug is used with other potentially hepatotoxic agents.

LETROZOLE (FEMARA)

Hepatic

Because letrozole is eliminated almost exclusively by the liver, patients with severe hepatic dysfunction should be dosed with extra caution.

LEUPROLIDE ACETATE (LEUPRON, LEUPRON DEPOT)

General

The pharmacokinetics of leupron have not been determined in patients with renal or hepatic dysfunction, and no dose modifications are available. Caution must be exerted when initiating leuprolide in patients with advanced prostate cancer, as an acute flare reaction may occur. It is generally recommended that a testosterone antagonist such as flutamide be administered concurrently with LHRH agonists to prevent such a reaction.

MEDROXYPROGESTERONE (DEPO-PROVERA, PROVERA)

Hepatic

Progestational agents should not be used in patients with hepatic impairment.

Ocular Disorders

Medroxyprogesterone should be immediately discontinued in the event of any ocular complaints, including loss of vision, proptosis, diplopia, or migraine. Similarly, if funduscopic examination reveals papilledema or vascular abnormalities, this drug should be discontinued.

Vascular and Thromboembolic

Progestational agents are associated with an increased risk of thromboembolic events, and clinicians should immediately discontinue this agent at the first clinical suspicion of such an event.

MEGESTEROL ACETATE (MEGACE)

Vascular and Thromboembolic

Progestational agents such as megestrol acetate have been associated with an increased risk of thromboembolic events, and clinicians should immediately discontinue this agent at the first clinical suspicion of such an event.

TAMOXIFEN (NOLVADEX)

Metabolic

Hypercalcemia may occur in some patients with bone metastases during initial treatment with tamoxifen. If hypercalcemia is severe, tamoxifen may have to be held until the serum calcium returns to safe levels. Tamoxifen may then be cautiously reinitiated at a reduced dosage or in conjunction with prednisone with careful monitoring of serum calcium.

TESTOLACTONE (TESLAC)

Metabolic

Hypercalcemia may occur in some patients with bone metastases during initial treatment with androgens such as testolactone. If hypercalcemia is severe, this drug may have to be held until the serum calcium returns to safe levels. Testolactone may then be cautiously reinitiated at a reduced dosage with careful monitoring of the serum calcium.

BIOLOGIC RESPONSE MODIFIERS

INTERFERON-α (IFN-α, INTRON A, ROFERON)

General

If serious adverse effects follow interferon administration, subsequent doses should be held, reduced, or delayed until adverse effects resolve. Therapy with interferon should be discontinued if serious adverse effects persist or recur despite modifications. Interferon should be used with great caution in patients with diabetes, congestive heart failure (CHF), or chronic lung disease.

Hematologic

Prior radiation or myelosuppressive chemotherapy may result in increased hematologic toxicity with interferon. If the ANC drops to less than $500/mm^3$, interferon should be held until hematologic recovery. The drug may be resumed at 50% dose.

Hepatic

For high-dose interferon regimens like those used in melanoma, a rise in transaminases (AST, ALT) by more than five times the upper limit of normal necessitates temporary discontinuation of drug until toxicity abates. The drug can be resumed at 50% dose. If hepatic toxicity recurs despite dose delays and reductions, interferon should be discontinued.

INTERLEUKIN-2 (PROLEUKIN)

General

The dosage of interleukin-2 must be adjusted carefully to patient tolerance and response. In high-dose regimens, doses should be withheld rather than reduced in the event of toxicity. Indications for withholding interleukin-2 are listed in Table 4.14.

MISCELLANEOUS AGENTS

ALTRETAMINE (HEXAMETHYLMELAMINE, HEXALEN)

Gastrointestinal

Dose reductions or discontinuation may be required if nausea and vomiting cannot be controlled with antiemetics.

Hematologic

Hexalen should be temporarily discontinued and resumed with a 25% dose reduction if WBC is less than $2000/mm^3$, ANC less than $1000/mm^3$, and/or platelet count less than $75,000/mm^3$.

Neurologic

Hexalen should be temporarily discontinued and resumed with a 25% dose reduction if the patient develops neurotoxicity (peripheral neuropathy, cerebellar symptoms, disorders of mood or consciousness). If neurologic symptoms do not resolve, the drug should be permanently discontinued.

AMIFOSTINE (ETHYOL)

Hemodynamics

Hypotension during infusion of amifostine may occur, requiring supportive measures and discontinuation of infusion. This reaction is most likely in patients who are volume depleted or taking antihypertensive agents. If the patient is asymptomatic and the blood pressure returns to baseline within 5 minutes, the infusion may be resumed. If therapy cannot be resumed because of hypotension, subsequent doses of amifostine should be reduced to 740 mg/m^2.

ESTRAMUSTINE (EMCYT)

Hepatic

Estramustine is poorly metabolized by patients with impaired liver function and should be used with caution in them.

Table 4.14. Criteria for Withholding and Resuming Interleukin-2 Based on Toxicity

Indications for Withholding Interleukin-2	Criteria for Resuming Therapy
ECG changes consistent with myocardial ischemia or infarction; chest pains suggestive of ischemia	ECG changes resolve and myocardial infarction is ruled out; chest pain resolves
Atrial fibrillation, supraventricular tachycardia, or bradycardia	Rhythm returns to normal sinus; symptoms resolve
Hypotension with systolic BP < 90 mm Hg or increasing vasopressor requirements	BP > 90 mm Hg or vasopressor requirements stabilize
Oxygen saturation < 94% on room air or 90% on 2 L oxygen	Oxygen saturation > 94% on room air or > 90% on 2 L nasal prongs
Mental status changes, including moderate confusion or agitation	Resolution of symptoms
Sepsis syndrome; patient clinically unstable	Sepsis resolves; patient is clinically stable; infection being treated
Serum creatinine > 4.5 mg/dL Or Serum creatinine > 4 mg/dL with acidosis, volume overload, or hyperkalemia	Serum creatinine < 4 mg/dL; fluid, electrolyte status stable
Oliguria with urine output < 10 mL/hr × 16–24 hr; increasing serum creatinine	Urine output > 10 mL/hr; decrease in serum creatinine ≥ 1.5 mg/dL or normal
Gastrointestinal bleeding with positive stool guaiac testing	Stool guaiac tests negative
Bullous dermatitis	Resolution
Signs of hepatic failure: encephalopathy, increasing ascites, liver pain, hypoglycemia	No further interleukin-2 on that course; subsequent courses may not begin until all signs and symptoms of hepatic failure resolved

Renal

Estramustine should be used with caution in patients with impaired renal function, although no specific dose modification guidelines are provided.

ETIDRONATE (DIDRONEL)

Renal

Etidronate has been associated with significant nephrotoxicity, especially when used in patients with underlying renal impairment or in conjunction with other nephrotoxins. A reduced dose of etidronate is advisable in patients with moderately impaired renal function (serum creatinine 2.5 to 4.9 mg/dL), although the effects of this agent in this population have not been systematically evaluated. Etidronate should be withheld from patients with severe renal impairment (serum creatinine more than 5 mg/dL).

GALLIUM NITRATE (GANITE)

Renal

Gallium nitrate is potentially nephrotoxic and should not be used in patients with serum creatinine more than 2.5 mg/dL. During therapy, hydration and monitoring of renal function are recommended. Gallium should be discontinued if signs of renal insufficiency arise.

LEVAMISOLE (ERGAMISOL)

Hematologic

The use of levamisole has been associated with severe cases of agranulocytosis. Frequent monitoring of hematologic parameters is recommended, and the drug should be discontinued if WBC is less than 3500 /mm^3 for more than 10 days despite holding 5-FU. Both 5-FU and levamisole should be held until platelet counts are more than 100,000 /mm^3.

Neurologic

The use of levamisole has been associated with multifocal leukoencephalopathy. Symptoms may be quite varied, ranging from lethargy, memory loss, speech disturbances, and weakness to coma. Levamisole and 5-FU must be discontinued immediately if acute neurologic symptoms develop.

MITHRAMYCIN (PLICAMYCIN)

Hematologic

Therapy should be interrupted if WBC is less than 4000/mm^3, the platelet count is less than 150,000/mm^3, or the prothrombin time is 4 seconds more than control. Mithramycin should be used with extreme caution in patients with impaired bone marrow function.

Hepatic

Mithramycin should be used with extreme caution in patients with hepatic insufficiency. The drug should be withheld if the AST is more than 600 U/mL or the LDH is more than 2000 U/mL. For the treatment of hypercalcemia, in patients with hepatic impairment, some clinicians recommend a single dose of mithramycin at 12.5 mg/m^2.

Renal

Renal function should be monitored carefully. Mithramycin should be used with extreme caution in patients with renal insufficiency. The drug should be withheld if the BUN is more than 25 mg/dL. For the treatment of hypercalcemia in patients with renal impairment some clinicians recommend a single dose of mithramycin at 12.5 mg/m^2.

MITOTANE (O,P'-DDD, LYSODREN)

General

The initial dose of mitotane is 1 to 6 g daily in divided doses. The dose should be gradually increased as tolerated to a dose of 9 to 10 g daily. If adverse effects occur, the drug should be titrated to a maximally tolerated dose for that patient.

PAMIDRONATE (AREDIA)

Renal

The clearance of pamidronate is delayed in patients with moderate renal impairment, although no dose modifications are required when standard doses and schedules are used. Pamidronate has not been evaluated in patients with severe renal insufficiency (serum creatinine more than 5 mg/dL), and clinical judgment should determine the risks and benefits of pamidronate in this population.

TRETINOIN (ALL *TRANS* RETINOIC ACID [ATRA] VESANOID)

Hepatic

Elevated liver function findings occur in 50 to 60% of patients receiving tretinoin but may resolve spontaneously without discontinuation of drug. If liver enzymes rise to more than 5 times normal levels, the clinician should consider temporarily discontinuing tretinoin.

Retinoic Acid Syndrome

Up to 25% of patients receiving tretinoin for acute promyelocytic leukemia develop a potentially fatal syndrome characterized by fever, dyspnea, weight gain, and pulmonary infiltrates. Prompt initiation of high-dose corticosteroids in addition to appropriate supportive measures is necessary. If severe, the retinoic acid syndrome may require temporary discontinuation of tretinoin.

BIBLIOGRAPHY

Anti-neoplastic agents. In: McKevoy GK, ed. American hospital formulary service drug information 1998. 39th ed. Bethesda: American Society of Health-System Pharmacists, 751–957.

Chemotherapeutic drugs. In: Perry MC, ed. The chemotherapy source book. 2nd ed. Baltimore: Williams & Wilkins, 1996;293–555.

PDR. Oncology prescribing guide. Montvale, NY: Medical Economics, 1997.

Physicians GenRx. The complete drug reference. St. Louis: Mosby–Year Book, 1997.

Section Two

Chemotherapeutic Agents

Section Two

Chemotherapeutic Agents

5
Drug Profiles

Clay M. Anderson

ALTRETAMINE
(Hexamethylmelamine [HMM], Hexalen)

Drug class, mechanism of action: Alkylating agent.

Form: 50-mg capsules.

Storage: Sealed bottles at room temperature; discard after expiration date.

Mixing instructions: None.

Drug interactions: Metabolism may be slowed by cimetidine or enhanced by phenobarbital.

Pharmacokinetics, metabolism: Well absorbed by mouth, metabolized extensively in the liver to inactive forms. Elimination half-life 4 to 13 hours.

Excretion: Metabolites largely excreted in urine.

Toxicity: Myelosuppression is dose-limiting. Leukopenia, thrombocytopenia, nausea, and vomiting are common. Neurologic toxicity, including confusion, lethargy, weakness, and sensory changes, is common.

Indications: Food & Drug Administration (FDA) approved for refractory ovarian carcinoma.

Dosing: 4 to 12 mg/kg per day in divided doses for 3 to 6 weeks, or 150 mg/m^2 per day for 14 days each cycle; higher doses have been used.

AMIFOSTINE
(Ethyol, WR-2721, Ethiofos)

Drug class, mechanism of action: Cytoprotectant; free radical scavenger.

Form: 500 mg powder in vial.

Storage: Powder form stable at −10°C to −20°C for 2 to 4 years; final solution stable at room temperature for 8 to 24 hours.

Mixing instructions: Reconstituted to 50 mg/mL in sterile water, then to 10 mg/mL in D$_5$W or normal saline for intravenous infusion.

Drug interactions: Not known to decrease the effectiveness of any cytotoxic drug but not yet adequately studied.

Pharmacokinetics, metabolism: Poorly absorbed in the gastrointestinal (GI) tract. After intravenous infusion, the drug is rapidly metabolized to inactive forms in the plasma compartment.

Excretion: Metabolites are cleared in the urine; less than 2% of unmetabolized drug found in the urine.

Toxicity: Transient hypotension is dose limiting. Nausea, vomiting, somnolence are common. Sneezing, hypocalcemia, flushing can be seen.

Indications: FDA-approved for pretreatment with cisplatin. Useful as a bone marrow, kidney, and nerve cytoprotectant. Useful with other alkylators as well.

Dosing: 740 mg/m^2 intravenous infusion over 15 minutes given 15 to 30 minutes before the cytotoxic agent.

AMINOGLUTETHIMIDE
(Cytadren)

Drug class, mechanism of action: Aromatase inhibitor; blocks adrenal conversion of cholesterol to δ-5-pregnenolone and peripheral conversion of androgens to estrogens.

Form: 250-mg tablets.

Storage: Sealed bottle at room temperature. Discard after expiration date.

Mixing instructions: None.

Drug interactions: Aminoglutethimide must be given with hydrocortisone. Induces metabolism of warfarin, theophylline, digoxin, medroxyprogesterone, and dexamethasone.

Pharmacokinetics, metabolism: Well-absorbed by mouth, 25% plasma protein-bound, metabolized in the liver, elimination half-life of 7 to 9 hours.

Excretion: Excreted as unchanged drug and metabolites in the urine.

Toxicity: Adrenal insufficiency is universal and must be treated with corticosteroids. Other common toxicities include fatigue, lethargy, rash, fever, virilization, and hypercholesterolemia.

Indications: FDA-approved for treatment of hormone-responsive breast cancer; may be useful in prostate cancer and adrenal carcinoma.

Dosing: 250 mg orally four times a day with 40 mg of hydrocortisone daily in divided doses. Usually started at 250 mg three times a day and increased after 2 weeks.

AMSACRINE
(AMSA, Acridinylanisidide)

Drug class, mechanism of action: Intercalating agent; topoisomerase II inhibitor.

Form: 75 mg/1.5 mL vials in N,N-dimethylacetamide with 13.5 mL lactic acid diluent.

Storage: Unopened vials stored at room temperature; dissolved drug stable for 48 to 96 hours at room temperature.

Mixing instructions: May precipitate in normal saline. Do not use plastic syringe for mixing. Dissolve AMSA solution in diluent; dilute with 500 mL D_5W plus 1 ampule $NaHCO_3$.

Drug interactions: None noted.

Pharmacokinetics, metabolism: Poorly available by oral route. Metabolized by the liver and excreted in bile and urine. Elimination half-life of 6 to 7 hours.

Excretion: Both biliary and urinary as metabolites and unchanged drug.

Toxicity: Myelosuppression is dose limiting. Leukopenia, thrombocytopenia, transient elevation of liver function tests, and local venous irritation are common; nausea, vomiting, and cardiac toxicity are seen; mucositis is rare.

Indications: Still investigational; used primarily for acute myeloid leukemia.

Dosing: 90 to 150 mg/m^2/day for 5 days; may be repeated after recovery of peripheral counts.

ANAGRELIDE
(Agrelin)

Drug class, mechanism of action: Inhibitor of platelet aggregation with an exploitable side effect of thrombocytopenia, for which the mechanism is unclear.

Form: 0.5 mg capsules.

Storage: Per package insert; discard after expiration date.

Mixing instructions: None.

Drug interactions: Sucralfate may decrease absorption.

Metabolism, pharmacokinetics: Good oral bioavailability. Maximum plasma concentration occurs after one hour. The plasma half life is 1.3 hours. The drug is metabolized extensively in the liver.

Excretion: Metabolites are excreted in the urine.

Toxicity: Other than thrombocytopenia, common toxicities include hypotension, headache, and palpitations. Rare toxicities include anemia, arrhythmias, angina pectoris, and congestive heart failure.

Indications: FDA-approved for treatment of essential thrombocytosis as an orphan drug.

Dosing: 0.5 mg four times daily or 1 mg twice daily.

ANASTRAZOLE
(Arimidex)

Drug class, mechanism of action: Nonsteroidal aromatase inhibitor; blocks estrogen production selectively.

Form: 1-mg tablets.

Storage: Sealed bottle at room temperature. Dispose after expiration date.

Mixing instructions: None.

Drug interactions: None noted.

Metabolism, pharmacokinetics: Well absorbed from the GI tract; maximum plasma levels within 2 hours. Terminal elimination half-life is 50 hours. The drug is extensively metabolized in the liver and eliminated in the urine as metabolites and 10% unchanged drug. Despite the importance of hepatic and renal clearance, no adjustments are needed for abnormal function of these organs because of the wide therapeutic index of this drug.

Excretion: Eliminated in the urine as metabolites and 10% unchanged drug.

Toxicity: The drug is very well tolerated. Asthenia, headache, and hot flashes occur in fewer than 15% of women. Diarrhea, abdominal pain, anorexia, nausea, and vomiting occur in 10% or fewer. Thrombophlebitis has been reported.

Indications: For treatment of postmenopausal women with breast carcinoma who have progressed on tamoxifen therapy.

Dosing: 1 mg orally daily. Higher doses are no more effective.

L-Asparaginase
(Elspar, Colaspase)

Drug class, mechanism of action: Naturally occurring enzyme derived from *Escherichia coli* or *Erwinia carotovora;* cleaves the essential amino acid asparagine, which is required by rapidly proliferating cells.

Form: 10,000-IU vial of lyophilized cake.

Storage: Intact vials are stored at 4°C; stable until expiration date. Diluted solutions are stable for 8 hours at room temperature and 14 days at 4°C. Cloudy solutions should be discarded.

Mixing instructions: Add 1 to 5 mL of sterile water or saline to the vial with gentle mixing; filter solution through a 0.5-μm filter and dilute in saline or D_5W to the desired concentration for intramuscular or intravenous injection.

Drug interactions: None noted.

Metabolism, pharmacokinetics: Not orally bioavailable. After intravenous or intramuscular injection, the drug is metabolized intravascularly by proteolysis. Elimination half-life is 8 to 30 hours.

Excretion: Not detected in urine.

Toxicity: Hypersensitivity can be life-threatening, requiring anaphylaxis precautions and a 2-U test dose. Coagulopathy is common and requires monitoring. Nausea, vomiting, abdominal cramps, anorexia, elevated liver function findings, and transient renal insufficiency are common. Lethargy, somnolence, fatigue, depression, and confusion are seen, as are pancreatitis and fever.

Indications: FDA-approved for acute lymphoblastic leukemia (ALL); also used in acute myeloid leukemia (AML), late-stage chronic myelocytic leukemia (CML), chronic lymphocytic leukemia (CLL), and non-Hodgkin's lymphomas.

Dosing: After a 2-U intradermal test dose, either an intramuscular dose of 6000 to 10,000 IU/m^2 every 3 days for nine doses or 1000 IU/kg per day intravenously over 30 minutes for 10 days has been used.

PEGASPARGASE
(Oncaspar, PEG-LAsparaginase)

Drug class, mechanism of action: Naturally occurring enzyme, covalently linked to polyethylene glycol to reduce immunogenicity, slow metabolism, and prolong half-life. The enzyme cleaves the essential amino acid asparagine, which is required by rapidly proliferating cells.

Form: 750 IU/mL in a 5-mL vial.

Storage: Follow package insert instructions and discard after expiration date.

Mixing instructions: No reconstitution or dilution necessary.

Drug interactions: None noted. Can reduce effectiveness of methotrexate if given beforehand due to inhibition of cell division.

Metabolism, pharmacokinetics: The drug is not absorbed by the GI tract. When given by intramuscular injection, it has an elimination half-life of approximately 5 days and is not detected in urine or bile.

Excretion: Metabolized completely; clearance does not depend on renal or hepatic function.

Toxicity: Although less immunogenic than the non-PEGylated form, hypersensitivity and anaphylaxis can still occur. Toxicities similar to those of the non-PEGylated forms include elevated liver enzymes, coagulopathy, hypercholesterolemia, pancreatitis, hyperglycemia, fever, chills, anorexia, lethargy, confusion, headache, seizures, and azotemia.

Indications: FDA-approved for treatment of ALL; like asparaginase, is also used for other leukemias and non-Hodgkin's lymphomas.

Dosing: 2500 IU/m^2 intramuscularly every 14 days with other chemotherapy agents for induction or maintenance.

AZACYTIDINE
(NSC-102816; Investigational)

Drug class, mechanism of action: Antimetabolite cytidine analogue; incorporated into nucleic acids, causing interruption of or errors in transcription and replication of DNA.

Form: 100-mg vial of lyophilized powder.

Storage: Unopened vials stable at 4°C for 2 to 4 years; must be diluted immediately after reconstitution. Diluted solution is stable for only 1 to 3 hours.

Mixing instructions: 100-mg vial diluted to 20 mL in sterile water, then rapidly diluted to a final concentration of 0.2 to 2 mg/mL in normal saline or D_5W.

Drug interactions: None noted.

Metabolism, pharmacokinetics: Not orally bioavailable. When administered by intravenous infusion, the drug is activated inside cells to the triphosphate form. It is deaminated in the liver. The elimination half-life is 3 to 6 hours.

Excretion: 90% of drug plus metabolites is excreted in the urine.

Toxicity: Myelosuppression is dose limiting. Leukopenia can be prolonged. Nausea and vomiting are common and can be severe. Diarrhea is common; stomatitis is rare. Hepatic enzyme elevation and liver functional compromise are common. Transient azotemia is seen. Lethargy, confusion, and coma have been reported.

Indications: Investigational agent for AML.

Dosing: 150 to 300 mg/m^2/d for 5 days every 3 weeks or 150 to 200 mg/m^2 twice a week for several weeks.

BACILLUS CALMETTE-GUÉRIN
(BCG, TICE, TheraCys)

Drug class, mechanism of action: Immunostimulant-vaccine; induces a cellular immune response at the site of instillation.

Form: Freeze-dried powder in vials, 27 mg per vial, supplied with diluent.

Storage: Sealed vials should be stored at 4°C, protected from light, and discarded after expiration date. Reconstituted drug should be used immediately.

Mixing instructions: Three reconstituted vials (81 mg total) should be diluted in 50 mL of sterile saline and administered into the bladder via an indwelling urethral catheter after complete bladder draining. After the catheter is removed, the patient should retain the instillation for 2 hours, with prone position changes during the first hour.

Drug interactions: Immunosuppressive drugs may block the reaction to BCG and may make the patient more prone to clinical infection from viable BCG organisms.

Metabolism, pharmacokinetics: BCG is a live attenuated bacteria culture, and as such it does not enter the body in viable form in any quantity. Therefore, it has no detectable pharmacokinetic fate. In rare cases, however, a clinical infection can result from treatment, indicating invasion of the body at the site of administration into the systemic circulation.

Excretion: None.

Toxicity: Urinary symptoms, including dysuria, hematuria, hesitancy, urgency, frequency, and secondary infection, predominate. Other toxicities include fever, chills, malaise, myalgias, arthralgias, anorexia, nausea, vomiting, and anemia. Clinical mycobacterial infection is rare, generally seen only in immunocompromised patients.

Indications: FDA-approved for noninvasive bladder cancer after removal of papillary tumors. Also used for some experimental vaccine programs as an adjuvant to the vaccine.

Dosing: 81 mg per treatment in 53 mL total volume as directed in paragraph on mixing instructions. Given once weekly for 6 doses, and then 3, 6, 12, 18, and 24 months after the induction.

BICALUTAMIDE
(Casodex)

Drug class, mechanism of action: Nonsteroidal antiandrogen.

Form: 50-mg tablets.

Storage: Store at room temperature; discard after expiration date.

Mixing instructions: None.

Drug interactions: Bicalutamide may enhance the anticoagulant effects of warfarin.

Metabolism, pharmacokinetics: Bicalutamide is well absorbed after oral administration. It is highly protein bound. It undergoes conversion to inactive metabolites in the liver via oxidation and glucuronidation. It has a terminal half-life of several days.

Excretion: Parent drug and metabolites are excreted in the urine and feces.

Toxicity: Constitutional symptoms, including hot flashes, decreased libido, depression, weight gain, edema, gynecomastia, early pain at the disease site (flare reaction), and constipation, predominate. Nausea, vomiting, anorexia, diarrhea, and dizziness are uncommon. Dyspnea, anemia, fever, and rash are rare.

Indications: FDA-approved for stage D2 prostate cancer in combination with a luteinizing hormone–releasing hormone (LHRH) agonist agent.

Dosing: 50 mg by mouth daily in combination with an LHRH agonist agent.

BLEOMYCIN
(Blenoxane, Bleo)

Drug class, mechanism of action: Antitumor antibiotic; causes DNA strand breaks directly in normal and neoplastic cells.

Form: Available as 15-U (15 mg) vials of lyophilized powder.

Storage: Unopened vials at 4°C; discard after expiration date. Reconstituted drug stable for 14 to 28 days.

Mixing instructions: 3 mL of normal saline injected into the 15-U vial, mixed, and then further diluted in normal saline or D_5W.

Drug interactions: None noted.

Metabolism, pharmacokinetics: Bleomycin is not orally bioavailable. After an intravenous infusion, it has an elimination half-life of 3 to 5 hours. Bleomycin is incompletely metabolized by intracellular aminopeptidase.

Excretion: Bleomycin in excreted in the kidney, half as unchanged drug and half as metabolites.

Toxicity: Pulmonary toxicity, including reversible and irreversible fibrosis, is dose limiting. Other common toxicities include fever, chills, rash, exfoliation, and anorexia. Nausea, vomiting, myelosuppression, anaphylaxis, and mucositis are rare.

Indications: FDA-approved for germ cell tumors, Hodgkin's disease, and squamous cell cancers. Used off-label for melanoma, ovarian cancer, and Kaposi's sarcoma. Also used as a sclerosing agent for malignant pleural or pericardial effusions.

Dosing: After 1 to 6 hours of observation following a 2-U intravenous test dose given over 15 minutes, the full dose can be given. The usual dose is 10 to 20 U/m^2 intravenous, intramuscular, or subcutaneously one to two times per week or 15 to 20 units/m^2 per day as a continuous infusion over 3 to 7 days. As a sclerosing agent 60 U is generally used.

BUSERELIN
(Suprefact, HOE 766)

Drug class, mechanism of action: Peptide anti–sex hormone agent, LHRH agonist, shuts off secretion of luteinizing hormone (LH) and follicle-stimulating hormone (FSH), producing chemical castration.

Form: Available as vials for injection at 1 mg/mL and as an intranasal spray in a 10-mL canister.

Storage: Follow package insert instructions.

Mixing instructions: None.

Drug interactions: May cause pain flares in bone metastases if not given with a direct hormonal antagonist.

Metabolism: Intravascular and extravascular proteolysis.

Excretion: None.

Toxicity: Flare reactions as noted under paragraph on drug interactions, which can be prevented. Castration symptoms such as hot flashes and decreased libido are common. Other nonspecific symptoms include headache, nausea, vomiting, diarrhea, constipation, weakness.

Indications: Prostate cancer, breast cancer.

Dosing: 500 μg subcutaneously three times a day for the first week; then 200 μg per day or 800 μg three times a day followed by 400 μg daily intranasally.

BUSULFAN
(BSF, Myleran)

Drug class, mechanism of action: Alkylating agent.

Form: 2-mg scored tablets; an intravenous form is not yet widely available.

Storage: Store tablets at room temperature and discard after expiration date.

Mixing instructions: None.

Drug interactions: None.

Metabolism, pharmacokinetics: Excellent oral bioavailability; peak levels in serum occurring at about 1 hour; elimination half-life of 2.5 hours. Metabolized partially in liver.

Excretion: Parent drug and metabolites excreted in the urine.

Toxicity: Myelosuppression, partly chronic and cumulative, is dose limiting. Other common toxicities include nausea, vomiting, anorexia, mucositis, hyperpigmentation, and elevated liver function findings (veno-occlusive disease of the liver at transplant doses). Neurologic toxicity, including blurred vision, dizziness, and confusion, and interstitial lung disease are less common.

Indications: Regular dose therapy in CML (FDA-approved) and polycythemia vera. High-dose therapy in bone marrow transplant.

Dosing: Regular dose is 4 to 8 mg /day. High dose is 8 to 16 mg/kg total dose.

CARBOPLATIN
(Paraplatin, Carbo, CBDCA)

Drug class, mechanism of action: Atypical alkylator, produces intrastrand and interstrand crosslinks in DNA via covalent bonds with the platinum molecule, leading to DNA strand breakage during replication.

Form: Available as powder in glass vials of 50, 150, and 450 mg.

Storage: Store vials at room temperature and discard after expiration date. Reconstituted solution is stable for 8 to 24 hours at room temperature, longer when refrigerated.

Mixing instructions: Dilute to 10 mg/mL in water, saline, or D_5W, then further dilute as needed in D_5W for intravenous infusion.

Drug interactions: None noted.

Metabolism, pharmacokinetics: Carboplatin is not orally bioavailable. It is rapidly cleared from the bloodstream after intravenous infusion, with a terminal half-life of 2.5 hours. It is cleared largely as unchanged drug.

Excretion: Carboplatin is cleared by the kidneys exclusively.

Toxicity: Myelosuppression, especially thrombocytopenia, is dose limiting. Nausea and vomiting are mild. Renal and neuronal toxicity are rare.

Indications: FDA-approved for ovarian cancer and used extensively in testicular cancer, squamous cell cancers of the head and neck and cervix, and lung cancer.

Dosing: Dosing can be per meter squared or through any of several formulas, such as Calvert's formula, that take into account renal function and desired level of thrombocytopenia. Typical doses with normal renal function are in the 300- to 500-mg/m^2 range as an intravenous infusion.

CARMUSTINE
(BiCNU, BCNU, bis-Chloronitrosourea)

Drug class, mechanism of action: Alkylator agent in the nitrosourea class. Cell cycle–independent mechanism.

Form: 100 mg vial of carmustine powder and a 3-mL vial of ethanol.

Storage: Store vials in the refrigerator; do not expose to heat. Discard after expiration date. The reconstituted drug is stable for 8 hours at room temperature and for more than 40 hours at 4°C. Protect drug from light.

Mixing instructions: Reconstitute 100 mg of drug in 3 mL of ethanol. Then add 27 mL of sterile water. Dilute this stock to desired concentration with D_5W or normal saline.

Incompatibilities: Polyvinyl chloride intravenous bags, sodium bicarbonate solutions.

Drug interactions: None noted.

Metabolism, pharmacokinetics: Poorly available by the oral route. After an intravenous infusion, the drug is rapidly taken up by tissues, including the central nervous system. Extensively metabolized in the liver. The serum half-life is only 15 to 20 minutes.

Excretion: The parent drug and metabolites are cleared by the kidney.

Toxicity: Myelosuppression, which is slow in onset and cumulative, is dose limiting. Nausea and vomiting are common and can be severe. Hyperpigmentation and renal toxicity can be seen. Interstitial lung disease, including fibrosis, is rare but can occur with any dose. Transplant doses can cause severe liver toxicity and more frequently, lung toxicity.

Indications: FDA-approved for brain tumors, multiple myeloma, Hodgkin's disease, lymphoma. Also used for breast cancer, melanoma, stomach cancer, colon cancer, and liver cancer.

Dosing: Single-agent dose is 150 to 200 mg/m^2 every 6 weeks. For transplant, the dose is as high as 600 mg/m^2, along with other drugs.

CHLORAMBUCIL
(Leukeran)

Drug class, mechanism of action: Alkylating agent, cell cycle independent.

Form: 2-mg tablets.

Storage: Stored in bottles, initially sealed, at room temperature. Discard after expiration date.

Mixing instructions: None.

Drug interactions: None noted.

Metabolism: Excellent oral bioavailability. Maximum plasma level at 1 hour and an elimination half-life of 1 to 2 hours. Extensively metabolized in the liver to active and inactive metabolites.

Excretion: Metabolites excreted via the kidneys.

Toxicity: Myelosuppression, which is dose limiting and universal, can be cumulative. Nausea, vomiting, and diarrhea are mild and uncommon. Sterility and alopecia occurs in a minority of patients. Pulmonary fibrosis and neurologic side effects are quite rare.

Indications: FDA-approved for chronic lymphocytic leukemia and low-grade lymphomas. Also used for Waldenstrom's macroglobulinemia, multiple myeloma, hairy cell leukemia, and rarely for some solid tumors.

Dosing: 16 mg/m^2 per day for 5 days every 4 weeks, or 0.4 mg/kg every 2 to 4 weeks, or 0.1 to 0.2 mg/kg/d for 3 to 6 weeks.

CISPLATIN
(DDP, Platinol, Cisplatinum, cis-Diamminedichloroplatinum II [cDDP])

Drug class, mechanism of action: Atypical alkylator, produces intrastrand and interstrand crosslinks in DNA via covalent bonds with the platinum molecule, leading to DNA strand breakage during replication.

Form: Lyophilized powder in sealed vials of 10 mg and 50 mg and as a 1-mg/mL solution in bottles of 50 and 100 mg/bottle.

Storage: Vials and solutions are stored at room temperature. Diluted drug is stable at room temperature for 96 hours.

Mixing instructions: Dilute powder to 1 mg/mL in normal saline, then dilute in half-normal or normal saline to desired total volume.

Incompatibilities: Unstable in D_5W; may precipitate with aluminum; should not be mixed with metoclopramide, sodium bicarbonate solutions, sodium thiosulfate, 5-fluorouracil, or mesna.

Drug interactions: None noted.

Metabolism, pharmacokinetics: Poor oral bioavailability. After intravenous infusion, rapid distribution to tissues takes place, and the drug is more than 90% protein bound. While the distribution half-life is less than 1 hour, the terminal half-life is 60 to 90 hours because of tissue retention. Not extensively metabolized.

Excretion: Elimination is via the kidneys.

Toxicity: Nephrotoxicity is dose limiting for an individual dose; neurotoxicity, especially painful peripheral neuropathy, is dose limiting for cumulative doses. Myelosuppression is mild. Nausea and vomiting are common but manageable, and anorexia and diarrhea are common. Cumulative ototoxicity is also common. Chronic renal magnesium and potassium wasting is common and sometimes not reversible. Elevated liver transaminases can be seen; alopecia and cardiac conduction abnormalities are rare.

Indications: Used for almost every class of solid tumor and lymphoma. FDA-approved for testicular and ovarian cancer and transitional cell carcinoma.

Dosing: Cisplatin can be given all in one intravenous infusion or daily as an intravenous infusion for several days for each cycle. Daily divided doses are tolerated somewhat better. The total dose per cycle ranges from 80 to 160 mg/m^2. Continuous infusion can also be used. Dose should be reduced for a creatinine clearance below 60 mL/minute. Adequate renal perfusion and urine output are critical for minimizing renal toxicity, and therefore prehydration and adequate posttreatment hydration are used, usually with normal saline with or without mannitol, potassium, and magnesium, along with the cisplatin. Cisplatin 100 to 200 mg/m^2 is also used intraperitoneally for ovarian cancer.

CLADRIBINE
(Leustatin, chlorodeoxyadenosine, 2-CdA)

Drug class, mechanism of action: Anti-metabolite, purine analogue, cytotoxic to dividing and nondividing cells via disruption of DNA function through inhibition of DNA polymerase, DNA ligase, and ribonucleotide reductase; also incorporation into DNA. Strand breaks in DNA accumulate and cause cell death within 48 hours.

Form: 1 mg/mL solution in 20 mL vials.

Storage: Store unopened vials at 4°C. Discard after expiration date. When diluted, stable for up to 7 days at room temperature.

Mixing instructions: Contents of original vial are filtered and then diluted in normal saline to desired concentration (up to 100 mL total for outpatient infusion or 1 L for inpatient infusion).

Drug interactions: None noted.

Metabolism, pharmacokinetics: Not orally bioavailable. After intravenous administration, it has a distribution half-life of 36 minutes and an elimination half-life of 7 hours. Resistant to adenosine deaminase. Chemical conversion to the active form takes place intracellularly in all cells that have deoxycytidine kinase activity. Further information on metabolism and excretion is not available.

Excretion: Poorly characterized in humans.

Toxicity: Renal toxicity is dose limiting, but at the typical doses used, myelosuppression, including universal lymphopenia, and common neutropenia and thrombocytopenia are most prominent. Fever is common; nausea and vomiting are rare and mild, and neurologic reactions are rare.

Indications: FDA-approved for hairy cell leukemia. Also used in chronic and acute leukemias, lymphoma, and mycosis fungoides.

Dosing: For hairy cell leukemia, the dose is 0.1 mg/kg per day for 7 days as a continuous intravenous infusion, as a single treatment or repeated once. Other doses have ranged from 0.1 to 0.3 mg/kg per day for 5 to 7 days. Can also be given subcutaneously.

CYCLOPHOSPHAMIDE
(CPM, Cytoxan, Neosar, CTX, Cy)

Drug class, mechanism of action: Prototypical alkylator drug. Cell cycle independent.

Form: 25-mg and 50-mg tablets for oral use; vials of powder of 100, 200, 500, 1000, and 2000 mg for intravenous administration.

Storage: Tablets and vials are stored at room temperature and should be discarded after the expiration date. Reconstituted drug is stable for 7 days at room temperature, for at least 14 days at 4°C, and for more than 15 weeks if frozen.

Mixing instructions: Vials of powder should be dissolved in sterile water or normal saline to a concentration of 20 mg/mL and then further diluted in saline or D_5W as needed for administration.

Drug interactions: None noted.

Metabolism, pharmacokinetics: 75% oral bioavailability. Peak serum levels occur approximately 1 hour after administration. Activated by hepatic enzymes and metabolized to inactive forms in the liver as well. Elimination half-life is 3 to 10 hours.

Excretion: Parent drug and metabolites are excreted in the urine.

Toxicity: Myelosuppression is dose limiting, with leukopenia being most significant. Nausea and vomiting are common and can be chronic with oral administration. Hemorrhagic cystitis is uncommon with standard dose but is common with doses over 2 g/m². Other toxicities of high-dose therapy include syndrome of inappropriate antidiuretic hormone secretion (SIADH), pulmonary fibrosis, and hemorrhagic myocarditis. Secondary malignancies are well documented but rare.

Indications: FDA-approved for many malignancies and used for even more. Most commonly used for breast carcinoma, non-Hodgkin's lymphoma, ovarian carcinoma, and testicular cancer.

Dosing: Doses range from 50 mg/m² for 14 days every 28 days to standard intravenous doses of 600 to 2,000 mg/ m² once every 21 to 28 days to transplant doses of 60 mg/kg intravenously for 2 days.

CYTARABINE
(Cytosar-U, Ara-C, Cytosine Arabinoside)

Drug class, mechanism of action: Antimetabolite. Incorporated into DNA during replication, leading to strand termination. This drug is S-phase specific.

Form: Comes in 100 mg through 2000 mg vials of powder.

Storage: Store unopened vials at room temperature and discard after expiration date. Concentrated solution is stable for 8 days at room temperature and longer if refrigerated; a dilute solution at 50 mg/mL is stable for 28 days at room temperature.

Mixing instructions: Add sterile water to the vials to a final concentration of 50 to 100 mg/mL, and then dilute this solution in D_5W or normal saline to arrive at the total dose.

Incompatibilities: incompatible in solution with most penicillins, 5-FU, and heparin.

Drug interactions: None noted.

Metabolism: Parenteral bioavailability only. After an intravenous dose, it is rapidly distributed into tissues, where it is converted to AraCTP and rapidly deaminated in the blood. It has an elimination half-life of 2 to 3 hours.

Excretion: Eliminated through the kidneys.

Toxicity: Myelosuppression, often severe and prolonged, is dose limiting. It affects all lineages. Nausea, vomiting, anorexia, mucositis, and diarrhea are common. Skin erythema with exfoliation is common. Keratitis and conjunctivitis are common. Hepatic inflammation and elevation of liver function tests are common. Flulike syndrome with fever is common. Neurologic toxicity, mostly central with ataxia being predominant, is common and usually mild, but it is dose dependent and may leave permanent dysfunction. It is more common with intrathecal administration. Pulmonary infiltrates after administration are uncommon but can be fatal. Cardiac complications are rare.

Indications: Acute myeloid leukemia, acute lymphoblastic leukemia, non-Hodgkin's lymphoma. Intrathecal use in acute leukemia.

Dosing: Doses range from 100 mg/m^2 per day for 7 days as bolus or continuous infusion to 3 g/m^2 every 12 hours for 3 days. Doses less than 500 mg/m^2 are considered standard; doses of 1 g/m^2 or more are considered high dose. The intrathecal dose is generally 12 mg total dose to 30 mg/m^2, given intermittently during systemic treatment.

DACARBAZINE
(DTIC-Dome, DTIC, DIC, Imidazole Carboxamide)

Drug class, mechanism of action: Atypical alkylator, methylates guanine base preferentially, non–cell cycle dependent.

Form: Vials of lyophilized drug containing 100 mg, 200 mg, or 1,000 mg.

Storage: Vials are stored at 4°C protected from light. Reconstituted drug is stable for 96 hours if refrigerated and protected from light, and diluted solutions are stable for 8 hours at room temperature.

Mixing instructions: Mix the contents of a vial with sterile water to a final concentration of 10 mg/mL, and protect this solution from light. Discard if the solution turns pink or red. Dilute the final solution in normal saline or D$_5$W to give the total dose in a volume of 100 to 500 mL.

Incompatibilities: Hydrocortisone, heparin.

Metabolism, pharmacokinetics: Not orally bioavailable. After intravenous administration, the drug is activated by demethylation by microsomal enzymes in the liver and further metabolized to inactive forms. The elimination half-life is 3 to 5 hours.

Excretion: Active and inactive metabolites are largely excreted in the urine.

Toxicity: Myelosuppression is dose limiting. Nausea and vomiting are severe without aggressive antiemetic therapy. Fever is common and flulike syndrome is uncommon, as are diarrhea, stomatitis, alopecia, rash, or significant liver or renal toxicity.

Indications: FDA-approved for the treatment of malignant melanoma and Hodgkin's disease; also used for adult sarcomas and neuroblastoma.

Dosing: Given by intravenous piggyback in doses of 375 to 1,450 mg/m^2 every 2 to 3 weeks or 50 to 250 mg/m^2 per day for 5 to 10 days every 3 to 4 weeks.

DACTINOMYCIN
(ACT-D, Cosmegen, Actinomycin D)

Drug class, mechanism of action: Antitumor antibiotic; inhibits transcription by complexing with DNA.

Form: Vials of 0.5 mg lyophilized.

Storage: Unopened vials are stored at room temperature. Discard after expiration date. Stock solutions of the drug are stable at room temperature for 2 months.

Mixing instructions: Dissolve the contents of a single vial in 1.1 mL sterile water for a final concentration of 0.5 mg/mL. This solution can be used for slow intravenous push through a running intravenous line or further diluted in 50 mL of D$_5$W or normal saline and given as an intravenous rapid infusion.

Drug interactions: None noted.

Metabolism, pharmacokinetics: Poor oral bioavailability. After an intravenous dose, the drug is widely distributed except to the cerebrospinal fluid. It is metabolized in the liver. It has an elimination half-life of 30 to 40 hours.

Excretion: Dactinomycin and its metabolites are excreted in both bile and urine.

Toxicity: This drug is a moderate vesicant. Myelosuppression is dose limiting. Nausea, vomiting, skin erythema, acneiform lesions, and hyperpigmentation are common; mucositis, diarrhea, and anorexia are uncommon. Hepatitis, ascites, fever, and hypocalcemia are rare.

Indications: FDA-approved for Wilms' tumor, Ewing's sarcoma, rhabdomyosarcoma, uterine carcinoma, germ cell tumors, and sarcoma botryoides; also used for other sarcomas, melanoma, acute myeloid leukemia, ovarian cancer, and trophoblastic neoplasms.

Dosing: 1 to 2 mg/m^2 every 3 weeks or continuous infusions of 0.25 to 0.6 mg/m^2 per day for 5 days every 3 to 4 weeks.

DAUNORUBICIN
(Daunomycin, Cerubidine, Rubidomycin)

Drug class, mechanism of action: Anthracycline antitumor antibiotic, intercalating agent.

Form: 20-mg vials of powdered drug for reconstitution.

Storage: Store vials at room temperature and discard after expiration date. Reconstituted drug is stable for 48 hours at room temperature, longer if refrigerated.

Mixing instructions: Dissolve one vial in 4 mL of normal saline; draw this solution into a syringe containing 15 mL of normal saline.

Incompatibilities: Heparin, 5-FU, and dexamethasone.

Drug interactions: None noted.

Metabolism, pharmacokinetics: Not orally bioavailable. After intravenous bolus, the drug is widely distributed and metabolized in the liver to active and inactive metabolites. The elimination of the parent drug is 18 hours, and that of the active metabolite daunorubicinol is about 25 hours.

Excretion: Elimination of parent drug and metabolites is via the biliary and renal routes.

Toxicity: Daunorubicin is a vesicant. Precautions are necessary. Myelosuppression is dose limiting. Alopecia, nausea, vomiting, and stomatitis are common. Diarrhea, rash, elevated liver function tests, and transient arrhythmias are uncommon. Dose-related cardiomyopathy is uncommon below cumulative doses of 500 to 550 mg/m^2.

Indications: FDA-approved for acute myeloid leukemia and acute lymphoblastic leukemia.

Dosing: Given as a single intravenous injection daily for 1 to 5 days. Total dose per course up to 150 mg/m^2. A typical dose is 45 mg/m^2 per day for 3 days.

DEXAMETHASONE
(DXM, Decadron, Dex)

Drug class, mechanism of action: Corticosteroid; pleomorphic properties in various body tissues. Directly toxic to benign and malignant lymphocytes. Potent anti-inflammatory action.

Form: Tablets ranging from 0.25 to 6 mg; oral solution at 0.1 mg/mL and solution for injection at 4 to 24 mg/mL.

Storage: Store at room temperature; discard after expiration date. Diluted drug is stable for 24 hours at room temperature.

Mixing instructions: Vials of solution for intravenous dosage are diluted in D_5W or normal saline with the total dose to be given in 50 to 100 mL.

Drug interactions: Drugs that induce hepatic microsomal enzymes can enhance the metabolism of dexamethasone and decrease its effectiveness. This includes phenytoin (Dilantin) and carbamazepine (Tegretol).

Metabolism, pharmacokinetics: Well absorbed by the GI tract. Metabolized in the liver. Elimination half-life is 3 to 4 hours.

Excretion: Elimination of metabolites is primarily renal, with some biliary component.

Toxicity: Toxicities, which are shared with other corticosteroids, include leukocytosis, hyperglycemia, mood changes, euphoria, insomnia, increased appetite, weight gain, dyspepsia, exacerbation of peptic ulcer disease, cataracts, adrenal suppression, edema, and osteoporosis.

Indications: Used for many purposes in oncology and hematology patients, including treatment of multiple myeloma, chronic and acute lymphoid leukemia, non-Hodgkin's lymphoma, immune thrombocytopenic purpura, and hemolytic anemia. Also used to alleviate symptoms from brain or spinal cord metastases and other metastatic sites where there is edema and inflammation. Used as an adjunctive antiemetic medication as well.

Dosing: Oral and parenteral dosing are equivalent. Dosage for acute indications or active treatment entails total daily doses of 16 to 40 mg, sometimes with an initial bolus dose of up to 100 mg. Tapering treatments decrease to 1 to 2 mg/day. As an antiemetic, 10 to 20 mg is the standard dose.

DEXRAZOXANE
(Zinecard, ADR-529, ICRF-187)

Drug class, mechanism of action: Iron chelating-agent that serves as a free radical scavenger and cytoprotectant.

Form: Lyophilized powder, 500 mg per vial, with diluent.

Storage: Vials are stored at room temperature. Solutions of dexrazoxane are stable for 6 hours at room temperature.

Mixing instructions: Add 50 mL of diluent to vial of drug for a final concentration of 10 mg/mL.

Drug interactions: None noted.

Metabolism, pharmacokinetics: The drug is not bioavailable by the oral route. After an intravenous dose, distribution in the body is widespread and rapid. Metabolism is predominantly hepatic. The terminal half-life is 3 to 4 hours.

Excretion: Parent drug and metabolites are excreted by the kidneys.

Toxicity: Dexrazoxane appears to worsen slightly the leukopenia induced by doxorubicin. Mild nausea and vomiting are common; fever, stomatitis, fatigue, anorexia, and hypotension are uncommon. Seizure, respiratory arrest, deep venous thrombosis, and significant liver toxicity are rare.

Indications: FDA-approved as an orphan drug to prevent doxorubicin-induced cardiomyopathy.

Dosing: Administered just prior to a dose of doxorubicin as a 15- to 30-minute infusion at 500 to 1,000 mg/m^2.

DIETHYLSTILBESTEROL
(DES, Stilphostrol, stilbestrol)

Drug class, mechanism of action: Synthetic steroidal pro-estrogen hormone.

Form: 1-, 2.5-, and 5-mg tablets. An intravenous formulation is rarely used and not available.

Storage: Sealed bottles are stored at room temperature. Discard after expiration date.

Mixing instructions: None.

Drug interactions: None noted.

Metabolism, pharmacokinetics: Good oral bioavailability. Metabolized to inactive forms in the liver. The terminal half-life is about 24 hours.

Excretion: The majority of metabolites are excreted in the urine.

Toxicity: Toxicity profile is typical for an estrogenic compound. Common side effects include nausea and vomiting, bloating, cramps, headache, vaginal spotting weight gain, rash, hirsutism, pruritus, and hyperpigmentation. Less common toxicities include hyperlipidemia, hyperbilirubinemia, venous thromboembolism, hypertension, and cardiac dysfunction. DES is a carcinogen and a mutagen.

Indications: FDA-approved for prostate carcinoma and breast carcinoma.

Dosing: For prostate cancer, the usual dose is 1 to 5 mg per day. For breast cancer, the dose is higher, typically 15 mg/day but it is rarely used today.

DOCETAXEL
(Taxotere, RP-56976)

Drug class, mechanism of action: Docetaxel is a semisynthetic taxane, a class of compounds that inhibit the mitotic spindle apparatus by stabilizing tubulin polymers, leading to death of mitotic cells.

Form: 20- and 80-mg vials at a concentration of 40 mg/mL in polysorbate 80 solvent.

Storage: Vials are stable at 4°C for 6 months. The concentrated solution in diluent is stable at room temperature for 8 hours.

Mixing instructions: Dilute the total contents of a vial in the provided diluent to a concentration of 10 mg/mL; dilute the administered dose of this stock solution in 250 mL of D_5W or normal saline.

Incompatibilities: Not to be infused through polyvinyl chloride (PVC) equipment or tubing, as the drug and diluent leach dibutyl phthalate from PVC materials.

Drug interactions: Docetaxel given concurrently with cisplatin has been reported to increase the incidence and severity of peripheral neuropathy.

Metabolism, pharmacokinetics: Docetaxel has poor oral bioavailability. After a 1- hour infusion, it is widely distributed. It has a triphasic elimination course, with a distribution half-life of 4 minutes, an elimination half-life of 1 hour, and a terminal half-life of 18 hours. Extent and byproducts of metabolism are not well-known.

Excretion: Biliary excretion of drug into the feces is the main route.

Toxicity: Myelosuppression is universal and dose limiting. Alopecia is also universal. Edema and fluid accumulation, including pleural effusions and ascites, are common and can be dose limiting. Fluid accumulation is partially preventable with corticosteroid treatment before and after each cycle of docetaxel. Mild sensory or sensorimotor neuropathy is common. Mucositis and diarrhea are common and usually mild. Hypersensitivity reactions are uncommon and can largely be prevented through premedication with corticosteroids and antihistamines. Rash and elevated liver function findings are uncommon.

Indications: FDA-approved for metastatic breast cancer. Clinical experience increasing in non-small cell lung cancer, ovarian cancer, and other epithelial neoplasms.

Dosing: The standard dose is 100 mg/m^2 intravenously over 1 hour every 3 weeks. Higher doses and other schedules have been used.

DOXORUBICIN
(Adriamycin, Rubex, Adria, Hydroxydaunorubicin)

Drug class, mechanism of action: Anthracycline antitumor antibiotic; intercalating agent.

Form: Available in vials of lyophilized powder containing 10 to 150 mg of drug and as vials of 2 mg/mL solution in 10 to 200 mg vials.

Storage: Powder vials are to be stored at room temperature; vials of solution should be refrigerated; discard after expiration date. Stock solutions of the drug are stable for 35 days at room temperature and 6 months at 4°C or when frozen. Diluted solutions in saline are stable for 14 days at room temperature.

Mixing instructions: Vials in solution are ready to use or dilute further in saline. The powder should be dissolved in preservative-free normal saline to a concentration of 2 mg/mL.

Drug interactions: None noted.

Metabolism, pharmacokinetics: Doxorubicin has poor oral bioavailability. After an intravenous dose, it is widely distributed in tissues and is 70% protein-bound. It is metabolized in the liver to active and inactive forms. It has an elimination half-life of 18 hours or more.

Excretion: Most of the drug and metabolites are excreted through the biliary route.

Toxicity: Doxorubicin is a potent vesicant, and extravasation precautions are a must. Myelosuppression is universal and usually dose limiting with each cycle. Cardiotoxicity is common and can be dose limiting, though usually subclinical. Chronic, cumulative cardiomyopathy is expected when total dose exceeds 400 to 500 mg/m^2. This toxicity can be lessened by addition of dexrazoxane or by longer infusions. Acute cardiac effects, including arrhythmias, are less often seen and are unpredictable. Nausea and vomiting are common but manageable. Diarrhea and stomatitis are common but usually mild. Alopecia, rash, and hyperpigmentation are common.

Indications: FDA-approved for a variety of cancers and used for many more. Most commonly used for breast carcinoma, adult sarcomas, pediatric solid tumors, Hodgkin's disease, non-Hodgkin's lymphomas, and ovarian cancer.

Dosing: Standard doses range from 60 to 90 mg/m^2 intravenously as a bolus or continuous infusion over 48 to 72 hours every 3 to 4 weeks. Weekly and biweekly schedules are also used with lower doses. Doses are usually reduced for elevated bilirubin levels.

EDATREXATE
(10-EDAM)

Drug class, mechanism of action: Antifolate antimetabolite, cell cycle–dependent.

Form: Lyophilized powder at 50 mg per vial.

Storage: Vials stored at room temperature, to be discarded after expiration date.

Mixing instructions: Dilute contents of the vial to 12.5 mg/mL with normal saline.

Drug interactions: Folinic acid reverses toxic and antitumor effects of this drug, similar to methotrexate.

Metabolism, pharmacokinetics: Edatrexate has poor oral bioavailability. When given intravenously, it is metabolized in the liver. It has an elimination half-life of about 12 hours.

Excretion: Parent drug and metabolites are excreted via the kidney.

Toxicity: Stomatitis is expected and is dose limiting. Leucovorin rescue may diminish this toxicity. Nausea, vomiting, and diarrhea are uncommon. Myelosuppression is common but mild. Elevated coagulation times may also occur. Skin rash and elevated transaminases are common. Renal insufficiency, pulmonary toxicity, and alopecia are uncommon.

Indications: Investigational agent used in non-small cell lung cancer and head and neck squamous cell carcinoma.

Dosing: The usual dose is 80 mg/m^2 intravenous bolus per week.

ERYTHROPOIETIN
(EPO, Epogen, Procrit, Epoetin-α)

Drug class, mechanism of action: Hematopoietic growth factor. Stimulates erythrocytic precursors.

Form: Vials of 2,000, 4,000, and 10,000 U in solution.

Storage: Vials should be refrigerated and discarded after expiration date. Single-use vials should not be reused even if refrigerated after opening.

Mixing instructions: None.

Drug interactions: Erythropoietin may temporarily decrease the effectiveness of heparin when the two drugs are given simultaneously. Oral aluminum-containing antacids may decrease the effectiveness of erythropoietin.

Metabolism, pharmacokinetics: This peptide must be given parenterally. After intravenous or subcutaneous dosing, it is detectable in plasma for 24 hours. It is distributed to a volume approximating the total blood volume. It is degraded by proteolysis within the blood compartment. The half-life ranges from 4 to 27 hours. Onset of therapeutic effect takes at least 7 days.

Excretion: Excretion of intact peptide is negligible.

Toxicity: Hypertension is common but usually mild and not dose limiting. Injection site pain is common but mild. Flulike syndrome and diaphoresis are uncommon. Nausea and vomiting are rare. Seizures have been reported in dialysis patients receiving the drug. Iron deficiency anemia can occur after prolonged therapy, and concomitant iron administration may increase the effectiveness of erythropoietin. Hematocrit should be monitored closely to prevent polycythemia and hyperviscosity.

Indications: The oncology indication is symptomatic chemotherapy-induced anemia. Also used for anemia of chronic renal failure and human immunodeficiency virus (HIV)–associated anemia.

Dosing: Starting doses of 150 U/kg subcutaneously three times a week are recommended, with increases up to 300 U/kg if there is suboptimal effect after 6 to 8 weeks.

ESTRAMUSTINE
(Emcyt)

Drug class, mechanism of action: A conjugate of estrogen and an alkylating moiety, estramustine appears to work through estrogen-binding proteins to kill malignant cells through a non-alkylator mechanism, perhaps by inhibition of microtubules.

Form: 140-mg capsules.

Storage: Capsules should be refrigerated in the original container. Discard after expiration date. Capsules stable at room temperature for 30 days.

Mixing instructions: None.

Drug interactions: None noted.

Metabolism, pharmacokinetics: Well absorbed by mouth; subject to hepatic metabolism; terminal half-life is about 20 hours.

Excretion: Not clearly delineated.

Toxicity: Nausea and vomiting are common and dose limiting but diminish over time. Headache, edema, decreased libido, and impotence are common. Gynecomastia and breast tenderness can be seen. Rash, alopecia, myelosuppression, hepatic toxicity, and thromboembolic events are rare.

Indications: FDA-approved for the treatment of prostate cancer. Not used commonly for any other types of cancer.

Dosing: The usual dose for prostate cancer is 15/mg/kg per day, which is typically given as 420 mg orally three times a day.

ETOPOSIDE
(Vespid, VP-16, epipodophyllotoxin; also available as etoposide phosphate, or Etopophos)

Drug class, mechanism of action: Plant alkaloid, topoisomerase II inhibitor, partially cell cycle dependent.

Form: Etoposide comes in oral form as 50-mg capsules and in parenteral form as 100-mg multidose vials in solution at 20 mg/mL. Etoposide phosphate is available in 100-mg single dose vials as lyophilized powder.

Storage: Capsules should be refrigerated and discarded after expiration date. Vials of parenteral etoposide can be stored at room temperature. After dilution to 0.2 to 0.4 mg/mL in D_5W or normal saline, solutions are stable for 72 to 96 hours at room temperature. Etoposide phosphate vials should be refrigerated and discarded after expiration date. In solution, etoposide phosphate is stable for 24 hours at room temperature.

Mixing instructions: Etoposide solution 20 mg/mL should be diluted in D_5W or normal saline to 0.2 to 0.4 mg/mL for a total volume of 250 to 500 mL per daily dose. Etoposide phosphate can be diluted to 5 to 10 mg/mL in normal saline for rapid infusion in a total volume of 20 to 50 mL.

Incompatibilities: Etoposide and idarubicin are not compatible in solution.

Drug interactions: None noted.

Metabolism, pharmacokinetics: Etoposide phosphate is rapidly converted to etoposide after intravenous infusion. Etoposide itself is extensively protein-bound and metabolized in the liver; it has an elimination half-life of about 10 hours. About 50% of oral etoposide is absorbed via the GI tract, requiring oral doses to be twice as high as parenteral doses.

Excretion: Excreted both unchanged in the urine and as metabolites in the bile.

Toxicity: Myelosuppression, primarily leukopenia, is universal and dose limiting. Nausea and vomiting are common with oral administration but rare when the drug is given intravenously. Stomatitis and diarrhea are rare with normal doses but common with high doses. Alopecia is mild or absent. Hepatic toxicity and neurologic (peripheral neuropathy and central nervous system changes) effects are rare. Hypotension can occur with rapid administration of etoposide but does not occur commonly when etoposide phosphate is infused over 5 minutes. Secondary AML has been reported after etoposide.

Indications: FDA-approved for germ cell tumors and small cell lung cancer. Also used for lymphomas, acute myelogenous leukemia, brain tumors, non-small cell lung cancer, and as high-dose therapy in the transplant setting for breast cancer, ovarian cancer, and lymphomas.

Dosing: Etoposide can be given either over several days or at lower doses over many days. Typical doses are 50 to 120 mg/m^2 per day for 3 to 5 days intravenously. Oral doses are generally double the intravenous dose. A typical protracted oral course is 50 mg/m^2 per day for 21 days given every 28 days. Transplant doses up to 1,200 mg/m^2 over 1 to 3 days have been used.

FILGRASTIM
(Neupogen, G-CSF)

Drug class, mechanism of action: Hematopoietic growth factor, relatively specific for the granulocyte lineage.

Form: Available in single-use vials of 300 and 480 μg in solution.

Storage: Store single-use vials in the refrigerator and discard after the expiration date. Once a vial is drawn into a syringe, it should be refrigerated until use and used within 24 hours.

Mixing instructions: Vials are ready to use for subcutaneous administration but can be diluted in D$_5$W to a concentration of 5 to 15 μg/mL with human albumin added for intravenous administration.

Drug interactions: None noted.

Metabolism, pharmacokinetics: After a bolus subcutaneous

injection, peak plasma levels of filgrastim occur in 2 to 6 hours; the elimination half-life is generally 7 hours or less. Metabolism is proteolytic in the blood compartment.

Excretion: Intact molecule largely absent from bile or urine.

Toxicity: Mild bone pain is common. Low-grade fever, myalgias, arthralgias, and transient hypotension are uncommon, as is hyperuricemia and elevation of lactate dehydrogenase and alkaline phosphatase. Leukocytosis leading to hypoxia or capillary leak syndrome has been reported. Anaphylaxis or allergic reaction is rare.

Indications: FDA-approved for minimization of granulocytopenia after myelosuppressive chemotherapy. Also used to speed recovery of granulocytes in the setting of neutropenic fever after chemotherapy, for myelodysplastic syndromes, for congenital agranulocytosis, for cyclic neutropenia, and for mobilization of peripheral blood stem cells from patients or donors for transplant.

Dosing: Starting dose is 5 μg/kg/day until neutrophil recovery (discontinue the drug at an absolute neutrophil count of 10,000 or more), although generally either the whole 300 μg or the 480 μg vial is used. For posttransplant or high-dose chemotherapy applications, 10 μg/kg per day is the typical dose. There is no known maximum dose.

FLOXURIDINE
(FUDR, FUdR, Fluorodeoxyuridine)

Drug class, mechanism of action: Pyrimidine nucleotide analogue, antimetabolite, cell cycle dependent.

Form: 500-mg vials of lyophilized powder.

Storage: Vials should be stored at room temperature. Reconstituted drug is stable in solution for at least 2 weeks at room temperature.

Mixing instructions: Dissolve the vial contents in 5 mL of sterile water for a stock solution at 100 mg/mL, which can in turn be diluted in 100 to 500 mL of D_5W or normal saline for rapid or slow infusion.

Drug interactions: Leucovorin enhances the toxicity of floxuridine.

Metabolism: After infusion into the hepatic artery, the drug is phosphorylated to the active monophosphate form and incorporated into cells. Further hepatic metabolism to inactive forms is rapid. The elimination half-life is 30 minutes.

Excretion: Metabolites are cleared by the kidneys.

Toxicity: When given as a bolus, myelosuppression is dose limiting; diarrhea and stomatitis are the dose limiting toxicities of the more common protracted infusions. Other gastrointestinal toxicities, all rare, include nausea, vomiting, anorexia, gastritis, cramping, enteritis, and duodenal ulcers. Liver toxicity, usually a cholestatic picture, is dose limiting with intrahepatic arterial infusions. Serious neurologic side effects, including ataxia and visual changes, are rare, as is fever.

Indications: FDA-approved for regional (intra-arterial) treatment of GI adenocarcinomas metastatic to the liver. Sometimes used intravenously for the same tumors.

Dosing: Protracted intra-arterial infusions are generally given at 0.1 to 0.6 mg/kg per day until grade III toxicity, sometimes according to a circadian schedule. Intravenous doses range up to 60 mg/kg per week by various infusion schedules.

FLUDARABINE
(Fludara, FAMP)

Drug class, mechanism of action: Purine nucleotide analogue antimetabolite, only partially cell cycle dependent.

Form: Vials containing 50 mg of lyophilized drug.

Storage: Vials should be refrigerated. Reconstituted drug at concentrations as low as 1 mg/mL are stable for 16 days at room temperature and at 0.04 mg/mL, for 48 hours at room temperature.

Mixing instructions: Add 2ml of sterile water to the vial to make a 25-mg/mL solution, and then dilute the desired dose further to a concentration of 0.04 to 1 mg/mL depending on the infusion schedule.

Drug interactions: None noted.

Metabolism, pharmacokinetics: Fludarabine is available only by the parenteral route. After intravenous administration, the drug is metabolized to 2-fluoro-araA and widely distributed in tissues. It has an elimination half-life of 9 to 10 hours.

Excretion: The drug and metabolite are excreted primarily by the kidneys.

Toxicity: Neurotoxicity, including cortical blindness, confusion, somnolence, coma, and demyelinating lesions, is dose limiting, but the lower doses conventionally used rarely produce these side effects. At these doses, mild myelosuppression is the most common toxicity, with cumulative lymphopenia being the most clinically important. Nausea, vomiting, and other GI toxicities are rare. Alopecia and rash are also rare.

Indications: FDA-approved for the treatment of chronic lymphocytic leukemia. Also used for low-grade lymphomas and for acute myeloid leukemia.

Dosing: The standard regimen is 25 mg/m^2 per day for 5 days by short intravenous infusion. Prolonged infusions have also been used.

5-FLUOROURACIL
(5-FU, Adrucil, Efudex)

Drug class, mechanism of action: Pyrimidine antimetabolite, partially cell cycle dependent, inhibitor of thymidylate synthase.

Form: Available in solution in 0.5- to 5-g ampules or vials at a concentration of 50 mg/mL.

Storage: Store stock vials at room temperature protected from light and discard after expiration date. Diluted solutions in D_5W are stable for up to 16 weeks if refrigerated.

Mixing instructions: The stock solution can be diluted in D_5W or saline to the desired concentration, depending on the infusion schedule.

Incompatibilities: Incompatible with doxorubicin, cisplatin, cytarabine, and diazepam.

Drug interactions: None noted.

Metabolism: Parenteral bioavailability only. After an intravenous dose, 80% of the drug is metabolized to the inactive dihydro-5-FU by dihydropyrimidine dehydrogenase in the liver. The rest of the drug is activated to fluorodeoxyuridine monophosphate in the target cells. The elimination half-life is about 20 minutes.

Excretion: Parent drug and active and inactive metabolites are excreted by the kidneys.

Toxicity: GI toxicities, primarily mucositis for bolus injection and diarrhea for prolonged infusions, are dose limiting. Rare patients with dihydropyrimidine dehydrogenase deficiency have excessive GI toxicity. Myelosuppression is generally less mild with continuous infusion schedules. Nausea and vomiting are uncommon and mild. Dermatitis and other cutaneous toxicities, including hand–foot syndrome, are common. Cerebellar ataxia and myocardial ischemia are rare.

Indications: FDA-approved for colon, rectum, gastric, pancreas, and breast carcinomas and used for a wide range of other neoplasms in combination regimens. Used for intrahepatic arterial infusion for liver metastases from GI tumors; also used topically for various cutaneous neoplasms and disorders.

Dosing: Intravenous dosing schemes include weekly bolus, five days of bolus every 28 days, 4- to 5-day continuous infusion, and prolonged continuous infusions. Doses range from 300 to 3,000 mg/m^2 per day depending on the dosing scheme and schedule.

FLUOXYMESTERONE
(Halotestin , Oro-Testryl)

Drug class, mechanism of action: Synthetic steroidal androgen. Antagonizes estrogenic effects in estrogen-dependent target cells.

Form: 2-, 5-, and 10-mg tablets.

Storage: Store bottles at room temperature and discard after expiration date.

Mixing instructions: None.

Drug interactions: None noted.

Metabolism, pharmacokinetics: The drug is available by the oral route, is metabolized in the liver, and has an elimination half-life of about 10 hours.

Excretion: The routes of excretion are unknown.

Toxicity: Androgenic effects predominate. Hirsutism, amenorrhea, hoarseness, acne, and increased libido occur in women; men may have gynecomastia. Mild edema is common. Liver abnormalities, which are fairly common, include transaminitis, fatty change, cholestatic jaundice, and rarely carcinoma. Polycythemia may occur.

Indications: FDA-approved for the treatment of hormone-sensitive breast cancer and for hypogonadism in males.

Dosing: The total daily dose for breast cancer is usually 10 to 40 mg, divided into 2 or 3 doses per day.

FLUTAMIDE
(Eulexin)

Drug class, mechanism of action: Nonsteroidal antiandrogen.

Form: 125-mg capsules.

Storage: Store capsules at room temperature and discard after expiration date.

Mixing instructions: None.

Drug interactions: None noted.

Metabolism, pharmacokinetics: Good oral bioavailability, with peak plasma levels after an oral dose at 1 to 2 hours. The drug is metabolized to active and inactive forms in the liver. The elimination half-life is 8 to 10 hours.

Excretion: Parent drug and metabolites are excreted in the urine.

Toxicity: Generally well tolerated. Gynecomastia, galactorrhea, and impotence are common. Nausea, vomiting, diarrhea, mild myelosuppression, myalgias, and elevated liver function findings are rare.

Indications: FDA-approved for prostate carcinoma.

Dosing: Standard is 250 mg orally three times daily. Often given in conjunction with an LHRH agonist, such as leuprolide, to create complete androgen blockade.

GALLIUM NITRATE
(Ganite)

Drug class, mechanism of action: Heavy metal that is cytotoxic to cancer cells because of its ability to antagonize iron metabolism in tumor cells preferentially. Causes hypocalcemia by a similar mechanism.

Form: 500-mg vials (20-mL vials of a 25-mg/mL solution).

Storage: Vials should be stored at room temperature. Diluted solutions are stable at room temperature for at least 24 hours.

Mixing instructions: Contents of the vials corresponding to the total dose are diluted in 500 to 1,000 mL of normal saline or D_5W for infusion.

Drug interactions: None noted.

Metabolism, pharmacokinetics: This drug is not metabolized; it has an elimination half-life of about 5 hours.

Excretion: Cleared as unchanged drug in the urine.

Toxicity: Renal toxicity, including glomerular and tubular defects, is dose limiting but partly preventable with adequate hydration during therapy. Hypocalcemia is expected and common and can be dose limiting. Nausea, vomiting, diarrhea, and anorexia are not uncommon. Mild myelosuppression, rashes, hearing loss or tinnitus, visual disturbances, and transient neurologic symptoms are rare.

Indications: FDA-approved for the treatment of malignancy-related hypercalcemia. Also used for advanced bladder carcinoma.

Dosing: The standard dose and schedule are 300 mg/m² per day for 7 days by continuous intravenous infusion in a volume of 1 L per day of normal saline.

GEMCITABINE
(Gemzar)

Drug class, mechanism of action: Antimetabolite. Gemcitabine is a nucleoside analogue that exhibits cell cycle dependent and S-phase specific cytotoxicity, likely due to inhibition of DNA synthesis.

Form: Supplied as lyophilized powder in vials containing 200 and 1,000 mg of drug.

Storage: Vials of powdered drug should be discarded after expiration date. Reconstituted drug is stable at room temperature for at least 24 hours.

Mixing instructions: Add 5 mL or 25 mL of normal saline to 200 mg or 1,000-mg vial, respectively, and shake to dissolve. This 40-mg/mL solution can be further diluted in normal saline to give the total drug amount in 100 mL to 250 mL.

Drug interactions: None noted.

Metabolism, pharmacokinetics: Gemcitabine has poor oral bioavailability. After intravenous infusion, it is rapidly distributed and has a half-life of less than 2 hours. It is metabolized throughout the body to inactive forms.

Excretion: Parent drug and metabolite are excreted principally by the kidneys.

Toxicity: Myelosuppression, including anemia, is mild but dose limiting. Nausea and vomiting are mild but common. Diarrhea and edema are sometimes seen. Elevated transaminases are common, as is fever during drug administration. Hematuria and proteinuria are uncommon. Acute dyspnea and rash are uncommon. Paresthesias and central nervous system depression are rare.

Indications: FDA-approved for advanced pancreatic adenocarcinoma. Also used in non-small cell lung cancer, breast cancer, and bladder cancer.

Dosing: The usual dose in pancreatic cancer is 1,000 mg/m^2 as an intravenous bolus weekly for up to 7 weeks, followed by a week of rest before another cycle is begun.

GOSERELIN ACETATE
(Zoladex)

Drug class, mechanism of action: LHRH agonist; inhibits pituitary–gonadal axis function. This drug causes steroid hormone withdrawal from dependent tissues, including prostate cancer and breast cancer cells.

Form: 3.6-mg prefilled syringes.

Storage: Store syringes at room temperature and discard after expiration date.

Mixing instructions: None.

Drug interactions: None noted.

Metabolism, pharmacokinetics: After the contents of the syringe are injected subcutaneously into adipose tissue, the depot of drug is slowly released over 28 days and peaks at 12 to 15 days. The elimination half-life is 4 hours, and the drug is not appreciably metabolized.

Excretion: Excretion in almost entirely urinary.

Toxicity: Mild. Endocrine side effects, which are most prominent, include hot flashes, diminished libido, impotence, gynecomastia, amenorrhea, and breakthrough vaginal bleeding. Other toxicities include flares of pain early during treatment in sites of disease, local tenderness at injection sites, headache, nausea, depression, and elevated cholesterol levels.

Indications: FDA-approved for advanced prostate cancer; used also in metastatic breast cancer.

Dosing: 3.6 mg subcutaneously, usually in the abdomen, every 28 days.

HYDROXYUREA
(Hydrea, Hydrocarbamide)

Drug class, mechanism of action: Antimetabolite, inhibitor of ribonucleotide reductase, which converts nucleotides to the deoxyribose forms for DNA synthesis. Cell cycle dependent.

Form: 500 mg-capsules.

Storage: Store bottles at room temperature and discard after expiration date.

Mixing instructions: None.

Drug interactions: None noted.

Metabolism: After oral administration the drug is well absorbed, and drug levels peak in the blood 2 hours after a dose. The elimination half-life is 2 to 5 hours. Metabolism to inactive forms occurs in the liver.

Excretion: Renal excretion is the route of elimination for parent compound and inactive metabolites.

Toxicity: Myelosuppression is common and dose limiting. Other toxicities include rash, headache, fever, and hyperuricemia. Nausea and vomiting are uncommon. Liver toxicity and serious neurologic toxicity are rare.

Indications: FDA-approved for chronic myelogenous leukemia (CML), used commonly for other myeloproliferative disorders and occasionally for metastatic melanoma and refractory ovarian carcinoma.

Dosing: For CML the dose is 1,000 to 3,000 mg per day; for solid tumors the dose is either 80 mg/kg every third day or 1.25 g/m^2 every 8 hours for five doses once a week.

IDARUBICIN
(Idamycin, 4-Demethoxydaunorubicin)

Drug class, mechanism of action: Anthracycline intercalating agent; non-cell cycle dependent.

Form: Lyophilized powder in vials of 5 mg and 10 mg.

Storage: Vials are stored at room temperature. Drug in solution is stable for 7 days when refrigerated and 3 days at room temperature.

Mixing instructions: Dilute the contents of a vial to 1 mg/mL with saline or sterile water for intravenous injection.

Incompatibilities: Idarubicin is known to be incompatible in solution with 5-FU, etoposide, dexamethasone, heparin, hydrocortisone, methotrexate, and vincristine.

Drug interactions: None noted.

Metabolism, pharmacokinetics: Idarubicin has poor oral bioavailability. After an intravenous dose it is metabolized in the liver to active and inactive forms. The elimination half-life of the parent compound is 13 to 26 hours.

Excretion: Metabolites and some of the unchanged drug are almost exclusively excreted in bile.

Toxicity: Myelosuppression is common and generally dose

limiting for each dose. The cumulative dose-limiting toxicity is cardiomyopathy, but idarubicin is less cardiotoxic than daunorubicin or doxorubicin. Nausea and vomiting are common but usually mild. Diarrhea and stomatitis are sometimes seen. Idarubicin is a weak vesicant or irritant in the setting of extravasation.

Indications: FDA-approved for the treatment of acute myeloid leukemia.

Dosing: The standard dose as part of a 7 plus 3 regimen with cytarabine is 12 mg/m^2 per day for 3 days for induction, reinduction, or intensification. Other doses have been used.

IFOSFAMIDE
(Ifex)

Drug class, mechanism of action: Classic alkylating agent, non–cell cycle dependent.

Form: Available in 1- and 3-g vials of powdered drug.

Storage: Undissolved vials of drug are stored at room temperature. Diluted solutions of drug in D_5W, normal saline, or Ringer's solution are stable at room temperature for 1 week and at 4°C for 6 weeks. The drug is also stable at 10 to 80 mg/mL in PVC pump infusion cassettes for 8 days.

Mixing instructions: Dissolve the contents of a vial in sterile water to a concentration of 50 mg/mL, and then dilute the total dose in an appropriate buffer at a concentration appropriate for the method of administration.

Drug interactions: None noted.

Metabolism, pharmacokinetics: After an intravenous dose, ifosfamide is activated by hepatic microsomal enzymes. It is then converted to inactive metabolites in the liver. The active form of the drug is the same as that for cyclophosphamide. The elimination half-life of the drug is 7 to 15 hours.

Excretion: The metabolites and some unchanged drug are excreted in the urine.

Toxicity: Myelosuppression, hemorrhagic cystitis, and central nervous system toxicity are all fairly common and can be dose limiting. Hemorrhagic cystitis can largely be prevented by coadminstration of the uroprotective agent mesna, and nausea and vomiting are minimized with modern antiemetic regimens. The central nervous system toxicity, including lethargy, stupor, coma, myoclonus, and seizures, is usually mild and completely reversible. It is worse with impaired renal function. Reversible renal dysfunction is also seen with ifosfamide. Hepatic toxicity, diarrhea, and rash are rare.

Indications: FDA-approved for the treatment of recurrent germ cell tumors. Used for many other tumor types, including adult sarcomas, lymphoma, Hodgkin's disease, breast cancer, and ovarian cancer.

Dosing: Ifosfamide is generally given intravenously over 3 to 5 days with a total dose of 8 to 12 g/m^2 per cycle, repeated every 3 to 4 weeks. It can be given as a short infusion each day or as a continuous infusion. Mesna is given intravenously concurrently, also by short or continuous infusion. Hydration of more than 3 L per day total, with saline or alkali solutions, is also recommended.

INTERFERON-α
(IFN-α, Intron A, Roferon, α-interferon)

Drug class, mechanism of action: Biologic response modifier, antiviral, immunostimulant.

Form: Available in vials of lyophilized powder or aqueous solution in quantities of 3 million to 50 million IU per vial.

Storage: Unreconstituted drug and drug in solution should be stored at 4°C. Reconstituted drug should be used within 30 days after reconstitution. Vials of powdered drug should be discarded after the expiration date.

Mixing instructions: Lyophilized drug should be resuspended in the provided diluent to reach a final concentration depending on the dose required but generally such that the total dose is diluted in 1 to 2 mL for injection into the skin or muscle. For intravenous administration, the drug is further diluted in saline to a concentration of 100,000 IU/mL or weaker.

Drug interactions: None noted.

Metabolism, pharmacokinetics: After parenteral administration, peak levels of interferon-α in the blood occur in 30 minutes to 8 hours depending on the route. The elimination half-life is 2 to 9 hours. Interferon-α is catabolized through proteolysis, throughout the body but primarily in the renal tubules.

Excretion: Excretion of intact drug is minimal and not significantly affected by organ function.

Toxicity: Constitutional symptoms are predominant side effects and are dose limiting both in the short term and long term in low dose schedules. Acute side effects include fever, chills, nasal congestion, diarrhea, and malaise. Chronic side effects include fatigue, anorexia, weight loss, and depression. Neutropenia and thrombocytopenia, both of which are transient, are dose limiting at higher doses. Anemia may also occur, albeit with more chronic administration. Cardiac toxicity, including congestive heart failure and arrhythmias, is rare and almost always reversible. Serious central nervous system toxicity, including delirium and psychosis, and peripheral neuropathies are also rare and reversible. Hypocalcemia and hyperglycemia can also occur.

Indications: FDA-approved for nonmalignant conditions and

malignancies including melanoma, chronic myelogenous leukemia, hairy cell leukemia, Kaposi's sarcoma, cutaneous T-cell lymphoma. Also used in multiple myeloma and low-grade lymphomas.

Dosing: Dose depends on both the diagnosis and the brand or type of interferon-α. The doses for malignant conditions range from 2 million to 30 million U/m^2 by the subcutaneous, intramuscular, or intravenous route and from three times a week to every day. Adjustments are based on tolerance and laboratory parameters.

INTERFERON-γ
(Actimmune)

Drug class, mechanism of action: Biologic response modifier, antiviral, immunostimulant.

Form: Vials of sterile aqueous solution containing 100 μm (3 million U) of drug.

Storage: Unopened vials are stored at 4°C. Drug withdrawn into a syringe should be used within 12 hours. Unused reconstituted drug should be discarded.

Mixing instructions: None.

Drug interactions: None noted.

Metabolism, pharmacokinetics: The peak serum level after a subcutaneous injection occurs at about 7 hours, and the drug is eliminated with a half-life of 40 minutes. It is metabolized via proteolysis.

Excretion: There is little excretion of intact drug.

Toxicity: Dose-limiting side effects are constitutional symptoms, including headache, lethargy, fatigue, fever, chills, night sweats, and diarrhea. Transient decrease in peripheral platelet and leukocyte counts also can be dose limiting. Other toxicities, which are rare, include central nervous system changes (Parkinsonism, delirium), pneumonitis, arrhythmias, acute renal failure, coagulopathy, transaminase elevation, and hyponatremia.

Indications: Not FDA-approved for any malignances but has shown modest activity in renal cell carcinoma.

Dosing: A typical dose in renal cell carcinoma trials has been 50 μg/m² subcutaneous injection once a week.

INTERLEUKIN-2
(IL-2, Proleukin, Aldesleukin)

Drug class, mechanism of action: Interleukin-2 is a glycoprotein cytokine, previously known at T-cell growth factor, which stimulates antigen-specific and nonspecific T-cell and other lymphocyte subsets and triggers an inflammatory cytokine cascade. Its antineoplastic effects depend on an intact immune system.

Form: Vials of lyophilized drug containing 18 million IU.

Storage: Store intact vials at 4°C. Reconstituted drug is stable at room temperature for at least 48 hours.

Mixing instructions: Add sterile water (1.2 mL) to each vial carefully so as to avoid foaming. Swirl gently to dissolve. Further dilute this stock solution in 50 mL D_5W for intravenous infusion.

Incompatibilities: Do not dissolve IL-2 in normal saline or piggyback it into normal saline, as much of the drug will be lost to precipitation in normal saline.

Drug interactions: None noted.

Metabolism, pharmacokinetics: IL-2 is available by the parenteral route only. It has an elimination half-life of 30 to 60 minutes. It is catabolized by proteolysis throughout the body.

Excretion: Negligible amounts of intact drug are found in urine or bile.

Toxicity: IL-2 has a wide range of moderate to severe toxicities that depend on both dose and schedule. Toxicities tend to follow immediately after a bolus dose but gradually accumulate during a continuous infusion. Toxicities are higher for a given dose with continuous infusion than with bolus dosing. Capillary leak syndrome, which is dose limiting for most IL-2 administration schedules, results in hypotension, edema, pulmonary congestion, renal insufficiency, arrhythmias, diarrhea, and possibly some of the central nervous system and hepatic toxicity seen. Transient myelosuppression or more prolonged anemia occur commonly, as does transient hyperbilirubinemia, elevation of transaminases, and electrolyte imbalances. Other constitutional symptoms include fever, chills, malaise, arthralgia, myalgias, erythroderma, nasal congestion, rhinorrhea, nausea, and vomiting. Other serious and less common toxicities include lethargy or delirium, angina pectoris, congestive heart failure, frank respiratory failure, and infections, particularly gram-positive bacteremia.

Indications: FDA-approved for high-dose bolus treatment of metastatic renal cell cancer. Also used at low to high doses for metastatic melanoma and at lower doses for maintenance treatment of acute myeloid leukemia.

Dosing: The FDA-approved dose for renal cell carcinoma is 600,000 IU/kg intravenous bolus every 8 hours for a maximum of 15 doses on days 1 to 5 and 11 to 15 every 6 weeks. Lower doses are more commonly used, especially continuous infusions of 3 million to 18 million IU/m^2 per day for 96 hours. Subcutaneous administration at similar daily doses has also been attempted with reasonable tolerance.

IRINOTECAN
(Camptosar, CPT-11)

Drug class, mechanism of action: Semisynthetic camptothecin; functions as a topoisomerase I inhibitor; partly cell cycle dependent.

Form: Available in 100-mg vials as a 20-mg/mL aqueous solution.

Storage: Unopened vials should be stored at room temperature protected from light. Reconstituted drug is stable in ambient light at room temperature for at least 24 hours.

Mixing instructions: The appropriate dose should be diluted from unopened vials of drug in normal saline or D_5W in a total volume up to 500 mL.

Drug interactions: None noted.

Metabolism, pharmacokinetics: Irinotecan is available only by the parenteral route. After intravenous administration, the drug is converted partially from the active lactone form to the inactive carboxylate form through hydrolysis. The parent drug is metabolized in the intestine, liver, and plasma. The active metabolite of irinotecan, SN-38, also exists in the lactone and inactive carboxylate form in equilibrium in plasma. SN-38 is inactivated by glucuronidation in the liver. SN-38 is responsible for most antitumor activity attributed to the parent drug. The elimination half-life of irinotecan is 8 hours; the elimination half-life of SN-38 is about 12 hours.

Excretion: Excretion of parent drug and metabolites is largely via the bile.

Toxicity: Myelosuppression, primarily neutropenia, is common and dose limiting. Diarrhea is also common and can be dose limiting. Diarrhea can occur as part of a cholinergic syndrome, along with cramping, nausea, and vomiting, during or immediately after drug administration, or for several days after drug administration. Anticholinergics and antidiarrheals curtail the immediate diarrhea and other GI symptoms partially but are less effective in treating the delayed diarrhea. Flushing, rash, and alopecia are common. Significant hepatic, renal, neurologic, or pulmonary toxicities are rare.

Indications: Irinotecan is FDA-approved for refractory or recurrent metastatic colon cancer, and it has been used in other malignancies, including lung cancer, ovarian cancer, and lymphoma.

Dosing: The recommended dosage for recurrent colon cancer is 125 mg/m^2 as a 90-minute intravenous infusion every week for 4 weeks, with this cycle repeated every 6 weeks. Other rates and schedules have been used.

ISOTRETINOIN
(Accutane, 13-cis-Retinoic acid, 13-CRA)

Drug class, mechanism of action: Isotretinoin is a retinoid derivative of vitamin A, which binds to specific nuclear receptors and leads to changes in gene expression. This results in apoptosis or differentiation of many malignant or premalignant cell lines.

Form: 10-, 20-, and 40-mg capsules.

Storage: Bottles of drug should be stored at room temperature protected from light and discarded after the expiration date.

Mixing instructions: None.

Drug interactions: None noted.

Metabolism, pharmacokinetics: Oral bioavailability is about 25%, and the drug is highly protein bound in plasma. It is metabolized in the liver and has an elimination half-life of 10 to 20 hours.

Excretion: Parent compound and metabolite are excreted in both the urine and feces.

Toxicity: Isotretinoin is teratogenic and should not be given to women of child-bearing age without adequate contraception. Mucocutaneous side effects that are common and dose limiting include xerostomia, stomatitis, conjunctivitis, dry skin, pruritus, cheilitis, rash, patchy alopecia, fragility of nails and skin, photosensitivity, and epistaxis. Other less common side effects include elevations in transaminases and bilirubin or frank hepatitis, hyperlipidemia, nausea, vomiting, anorexia, diarrhea, headache, fatigue, depression, myalgias, and arthralgias. Anemia and pseudotumor cerebri are rare.

Indications: FDA-approved for acne vulgaris. Has been used and has shown some effectiveness in chemoprevention of aerodigestive malignancies. Ongoing studies are testing its chemopreventive potential in other malignancies.

Dosing: Daily oral doses of 0.5 to 4 mg/kg per day for 2 to 6 months have been used in the chemoprevention trials.

LEUCOVORIN CALCIUM
(Wellcovorin, Citrovorum Factor, Folinic Acid [FA], LV)

Drug class, mechanism of action: Tetrahydrofolate derivative and enzyme cofactor for thymidylate synthase and other purine and pyrimidine synthesis steps. Leucovorin bypasses the dihydrofolate reductase step, which is inhibited by methotrexate and therefore can be used to rescue normal cells from the toxicity of methotrexate after high doses are administered. In addition, leucovorin potentiates the toxicity of fluoropyrimidines such as fluorouracil by strengthening the association of the drug with its target enzyme, thymidylate synthase.

Form: Tablets in 5- to 25-mg sizes, powder for oral solution, and vials of powder 50 to 350 mg.

Storage: All unreconstituted forms should be stored at room temperature. The oral solution is stable for 14 days after reconstitution at 4°C or 7 days at room temperature. Reconstituted parenteral drug is stable for 7 days at room temperature at 10 mg/mL or for 24 hours at less than 1 mg/mL in normal saline or D_5W. The tablets should be discarded after the expiration date.

Mixing instructions: Add sterile water to the vials to reach a concentration of 10 mg/mL. This solution can be further diluted in normal saline or D_5W for intravenous infusion.

Incompatibilities: Incompatible in intravenous solution with sodium bicarbonate, foscarnet, and droperidol.

Drug interactions: Reduces the effectiveness and toxicity of dihydrofolate reductase inhibitors such as methotrexate.

Metabolism, pharmacokinetics: Leucovorin has excellent bioavailability by the oral or parenteral route. It is oxidized in cofactor reactions throughout the body and is partly metabolized. It has an elimination half-life of 2 to 4 hours.

Excretion: Parent drug and metabolites are excreted in the urine.

Toxicity: Leucovorin is generally very well tolerated. It occasionally causes stomach upset or nausea, rash, diarrhea, and headache. Allergic reactions have been reported.

Indications: Used for rescue of high-dose methotrexate therapy for a variety of neoplasms and as a potentiator of fluoropyrimidine therapy in GI malignancies, particularly colorectal cancer.

Dosing: For rescue from methotrexate the usual dose is 10 to 25 mg/m^2 orally or intravenously every 6 hours starting up to 24 hours after the methotrexate, until methotrexate levels are less than 1×10^{-8} molar. To potentiate 5-FU, doses ranging from 20 to 500 mg/m^2, depending on the 5-FU dose and usually given intravenously, have been used.

LEUPROLIDE ACETATE
(Leupron, Leuprorelin Acetate)

Drug class, mechanism of action: Gonadotropin-releasing hormone agonist; paradoxically shuts down the pituitary release of gonadotropins with chronic exposure. This results in a dramatic decrease in gonadal estrogens and androgens and growth inhibition of hormone-dependent neoplasms.

Form: Available in vials for weekly administration (depot) containing 3.75 and 7.5 mg of powder, along with diluent and syringe. A multidose vial containing 2.8 mL of a 5-mg/mL solution along with syringes is also available for daily administration.

Storage: Powdered drug is stored at room temperature and is stable for 24 hours after reconstitution. Vials of drug for injection (already dissolved) should be stored at 4°C in the dark; an opened vial is stable for at least a month at room temperature.

Mixing instructions: 1 mL of diluent is used to dissolve each vial of drug; this 1 mL solution is drawn up completely into the provided syringe for injection.

Drug interactions: None noted.

Metabolism, pharmacokinetics: Leuprolide is bioavailable only by the parenteral route. After a subcutaneous injection, about 90% of the drug is eventually absorbed. The depot form of the drug is absorbed slowly over days; the injectable solution is absorbed over several hours. The elimination half-life of the drug once in the serum is 3 hours. Metabolism is not well delineated but is clinically unimportant.

Excretion: Not well delineated but clinically unimportant.

Toxicity: Usually well tolerated, but side effects can affect many systems, including endocrine (hot flashes, impotence, gynecomastia, breast tenderness, diminished libido, amenorrhea, atrophic vaginitis, increased cholesterol), GI (nausea, constipation, anorexia, diarrhea), hepatic (elevation of transaminases), dermatologic (rash, changes in body hair composition, pruritus), or neuropsychiatric (insomnia, depression, emotional lability, lethargy, memory loss). Significant cardiac toxicity is rare.

Indications: FDA-approved for the treatment of hormone-dependent advanced prostate cancer. Also used for breast cancer and endometriosis.

Dosing: The usual dose for prostate cancer is 7.5 mg of the depot form by subcutaneous injection once every month or 1 mg of the injectable solution subcutaneously daily.

LEVAMISOLE
(Ergamisol, L-tetramisole, ICI-59623)

Drug class, mechanism of action: This drug is an anti-helminthic agent that seems to have immune-potentiating effects in humans.

Form: 59-mg tablets (50 mg of drug).

Storage: Store unopened tablets at room temperature. Discard after expiration date.

Mixing instructions: None.

Drug interactions: Levamisole may prolong the prothrombin time in patients receiving warfarin and predispose to bleeding complications. Close monitoring and dose adjustment are warranted.

Metabolism: Levamisole is rapidly and completely absorbed from the GI tract following oral administration. It is extensively metabolized in the liver to the parahydroxyl form and conjugated to glucuronic acid. It has an elimination half-life of 3 to 6 hours.

Excretion: Levamisole and its metabolites are excreted in the urine.

Toxicity: Common adverse reactions to levamisole include reversible leukopenia (agranulocytosis and thrombocytopenia are rare), altered taste and smell, nausea, vomiting, diarrhea, skin rash (usually mild), and arthralgias. Less common toxicities include vasculitis and central nervous system symptoms (anxiety, insomnia, dizziness, confusion, depression). Seizures and encephalopathy are rare.

Indications: FDA-approved for adjuvant therapy of completely resected Duke's C colon cancer.

Dosing: 50 mg orally every 8 hours for 3 days, repeated every 14 days for 1 year, along with 5-FU 5-day intravenous bolus followed 28 days later by weekly intravenous bolus.

LOMUSTINE
(CeeNU, CCNU)

Drug class, mechanism of action: Nitrosourea alkylating agent, cell cycle independent.

Form: Available as 10-, 20-, and 100-mg capsules.

Storage: Capsules should be stored at 4°C and discarded after expiration date.

Mixing instructions: None.

Drug interactions: None noted.

Metabolism, pharmacokinetics: Well-absorbed after oral administration. Widely distributed in the body, including the cerebrospinal fluid. Metabolized extensively in the liver to active metabolites. Elimination half-life is 72 hours.

Excretion: Metabolites are excreted in the urine.

Toxicity: Myelosuppression is dose limiting and tends to be cumulative. Nausea and vomiting are common but usually mild. Anorexia is also common but short-lived. Pulmonary fibrosis can occur with long-term administration. Other toxicities, including central nervous system effects, hepatic and renal dysfunction, and secondary leukemia, are rare.

Indications: FDA-approved for primary brain tumors and Hodgkin's disease. Also used in melanoma, multiple myeloma, other lymphomas, and breast cancer.

Dosing: The recommended dose for brain tumors is 100 to 130 mg/m^2 orally every 6 weeks. Other doses and schedules have been used.

MECHLORETHAMINE
(HN$_2$, Mustargen Nitrogen Mustard)

Drug class, mechanism of action: Classic alkylating agent, cell cycle independent.

Form: 10-mg vials of lyophilized powder.

Storage: Store intact vials at room temperature. Reconstituted drug is unstable and should be used within 1 hour of mixing.

Mixing instructions: Add 10 mL of sterile water to each vial to make a 1-mg/mL solution for intravenous administration. May be prepared in alcohol and diluted in Aquaphor for topical administration.

Incompatibilities: Incompatible with other drugs of any kind because of its instability.

Drug interactions: None noted.

Metabolism, pharmacokinetics: Mechlorethamine is not orally bioavailable. After an intravenous dose, the drug is rapidly deactivated in the blood by reaction with biomolecules. It has an elimination half-life of 15 minutes and has no significant organ metabolism.

Excretion: Virtually no excretion of the drug is detected in urine or stool.

Toxicity: This drug is a powerful vesicant, so optimal extravasation precautions are a must, as is rapid infusion. Tissue necrosis occurs if the drug extravasates, although sodium thiosulfate is a somewhat effective antidote. Vein discoloration and scarring are common. Nausea and vomiting are common, potentially severe, and often dose limiting. Myelosuppression is expected and also often dose limiting. Alopecia and infertility are often seen. Less common toxicities include anorexia, diarrhea, jaundice, tinnitus, and skin rash (common with topical treatment). Secondary leukemia and permanent hearing loss are rare.

Indications: FDA-approved for a variety of hematologic malignancies and solid tumors but generally used less in the past decade. Still used for Hodgkin's disease and topically for cutaneous T-cell lymphoma.

Dosing: The standard dose for Hodgkin's disease as part of the MOPP regimen is 6 mg/m^2 intravenously over 1 to 5 minutes on day 1 and day 8 of a 28-day cycle. The topical form is usually a 10-mg/60-mL solution or 10 mg/dL ointment.

MEDROXYPROGESTERONE ACETATE
(Provera, Depo-Provera)

Drug class, mechanism of action: Steroidal progestational agent.

Form: Tablets 2.5, 5, and 10 mg and suspension for depot injection as 100 or 400 mg/mL.

Storage: Both forms should be stored at room temperature and discarded after the expiration date.

Mixing instructions: The suspension should be shaken well before withdrawal into the syringe.

Drug interactions: The metabolism of medroxyprogesterone acetate may be enhanced by aminoglutethimide, leading to decreased effect for a given dose.

Metabolism, pharmacokinetics: This drug has good oral bioavailability. It is metabolized in the liver to inactive metabolites and has an elimination half-life of up to 60 hours.

Excretion: Parent drug and metabolites are excreted in the urine and bile.

Toxicity: Mostly constitutional and not dose limiting. It includes menstrual changes, amenorrhea, gynecomastia, hot flashes, edema, weight gain, fatigue, acne, hirsutism, anxiety, depression, sleep disturbance, and headache. Nausea, significant skin reactions or allergy, jaundice, and thrombophlebitis are uncommon.

Indications: FDA-approved for treatment of advanced endometrial or renal cell carcinoma. Also used occasionally for breast or prostate cancer.

Dosing: Loading doses of up to 1,000 mg intramuscularly weekly and 400 mg intramuscularly every month have been used; oral doses range from 100 to 300 mg per day. Much lower doses are used for gynecologic indications.

MEGESTROL ACETATE
(Megace, Megestrol)

Drug class, mechanism of action: Steroidal progestational agent.

Form: 20- and 40-mg tablets; oral solution 40 mg/mL.

Storage: Tablets and oral solution are stored at room temperature and should be discarded after the label expiration date.

Mixing instructions: None.

Drug interactions: None noted.

Metabolism, pharmacokinetics: The drug is well absorbed by mouth, is metabolized in the liver to inactive compounds, and has an elimination half-life of 15 to 20 hours.

Excretion: Parent drug and metabolites are excreted in the urine.

Toxicity: Similar to those of other progestins, as noted earlier. They include menstrual changes, hot flashes, edema, weight gain, fatigue, acne, hirsutism, anxiety, depression, sleep disturbance, and headache. Urinary frequency can also occur. Nausea, vomiting, diarrhea, skin rash or allergy, jaundice, and thrombophlebitis are uncommon.

Indications: FDA-approved for treatment of breast and endometrial carcinoma. Also used for renal cell carcinoma and for appetite stimulation in HIV disease and cancer patients.

Dosing: The standard dose for cancer treatment is 160 mg per day in divided doses or a single dose. The dose for appetite stimulation may be as high as 800 mg per day, which is why the concentrated oral solution is useful.

MELPHALAN
(Alkeran, L-PAM, L-Phenylalanine Mustard, L-Sarcolysin)

Drug class, mechanism of action: Classical alkylating agent, cell cycle independent.

Form: 2 mg tablets, and vials for injection at 50 mg/vial.

Storage: Tablets and vials should be stored at room temperature and discarded after expiration date. Reconstituted drug in solution is unstable and should be used within 1 hour.

Mixing instructions: Contents of a vial should be dissolved in 10 mL of the provided diluent. This 5 mg/mL solution should be filtered and then diluted to no more than a 2-mg/mL solution in normal saline.

Drug interactions: None noted.

Metabolism, pharmacokinetics: Melphalan has unpredictable GI absorption, is highly protein bound, and is rapidly autometabolized by hydrolysis in the plasma. It has an elimination half-life of about 2 hours.

Excretion: 10 to 15% as unchanged drug in the urine.

Toxicity: Myelosuppression is expected and is dose limiting. Recovery may be prolonged, and effects can be cumulative. Large doses may cause significant nausea and vomiting. Diarrhea and stomatitis are uncommon. Vein reactions including scarring may occur, but this agent is not known as a vesicant. Other skin reactions are uncommon, as are pulmonary fibrosis, vasculitis, infertility, alopecia, and secondary leukemia.

Indications: Used primarily for multiple myeloma, but also FDA-approved for ovarian carcinoma. May also be useful in high-dose chemotherapy and transplant settings and in regional perfusion of extremities for melanoma and sarcoma.

Dosing: Doses for myeloma are typically in the range of 0.1 mg/kg per day for 2 to 3 weeks up to 6 mg/m^2 per day for 5 days every 6 weeks. Transplant doses (intravenous or oral) range up to 140 mg/m^2 total. Doses for perfusion are either 0.45 to 0.9 mg/kg or a certain concentration in the perfusate.

MERCAPTOPURINE
(Purinethol, 6-Mercaptopurine, 6-MP)

Drug class, mechanism of action: Purine analogue antimetabolite, predominantly S-phase specific.

Form: 50-mg tablets. An intravenous formulation is investigational.

Storage: Tablets are stored at room temperature and should be discarded after the label expiration date.

Mixing instructions: None.

Drug interactions: Allopurinol inhibits first-pass metabolism of mercaptopurine in the liver by xanthine oxidase, and therefore dose reduction is required if allopurinol is also being given.

Metabolism, pharmacokinetics: 6-MP has good oral bioavailability, undergoes extensive first-pass metabolism in the liver, and has an elimination half-life of about 7 hours.

Excretion: Intact drug and metabolites are excreted by the kidneys.

Toxicity: Myelosuppression is common and dose limiting. Nausea and vomiting occur occasionally but are usually mild. Diarrhea, anorexia, and stomatitis are less common. Headache and rash are uncommon. Fulminant hepatic toxicity is very rare, but lesser degrees of cholestasis and hepatitis are sometimes seen.

Indications: Mercaptopurine is FDA-approved for treatment of acute lymphoblastic leukemia. It is occasionally used for other hematologic malignancies. There is an investigational intravenous formulation that does not yet have clinical indications.

Dosing: The usual dose is 70 to 100 mg/m^2 per day for a defined period of days during induction or maintenance.

MESNA
(Mesnex, Mercaptoethanesulfonate Sodium, Uromitexan)

Drug class, mechanism of action: Thiol uroprotectant binds to and inactivates the highly reactive metabolite of cyclophosphamide and ifosfamide, acrolein, helping to prevent hemorrhagic cystitis.

Form: Aqueous solution at 100 mg/mL.

Storage: Ampules should be stored at room temperature and discarded after listed expiration date. Diluted mesna solutions are stable for at least 24 hours at 4°C. Diluted solutions are stable at room temperature for up to 72 hours depending on the concentration and fluid composition used. The most stable solution is 1 mg/mL in D5/0.45% saline.

Mixing instructions: The 100-mg/mL solution can be used undiluted; more typically it is diluted in any of a number of fluids to concentrations of 1 to 20 mg/mL for rapid or prolonged infusions.

Incompatibilities: Mesna is not compatible in solution with cisplatin.

Drug interactions: Mesna does not decrease the effectiveness of cytotoxic drugs or radiation.

Metabolism: Mesna has an oral bioavailability of about 50% and is usually given by vein. After an intravenous dose, mesna is converted in the plasma to dimesna, is filtered by the kidneys, and is reconverted into mesna in the urine. It has an elimination half-life of 1 hour.

Excretion: As in the preceding paragraph.

Toxicity: Mesna is usually very well tolerated. It has occasionally caused nausea, vomiting, diarrhea, rash, fatigue, headache, hypotension, or arthralgias.

Indications: FDA-approved for use as a uroprotectant when administering ifosfamide. Also effective for high-dose cyclophosphamide.

Dosing: The usual dose of mesna is 60% of the daily milligram amount of the ifosfamide, given three times daily by intravenous bolus before, 4 hours after, and 8 hours after the chemotherapy or as a continuous infusion with a loading dose before the chemotherapy. Mesna may be continued for up to 24 hours after the chemotherapy has been completed.

METHOTREXATE
(MTX, Mexate, Folex, Amethopterin)

Drug class, mechanism of action: Antifolate antimetabolite; interferes with nucleotide synthesis by inhibiting dihydrofolate reductase. Cell cycle dependent.

Form: 2.5-mg tablets, 20- to 1,000-mg vials of powder for injection; 2.5- and 25-mg/mL aqueous solution for injection.

Storage: Unopened drug should be stored at room temperature protected from light. Tablets should be discarded after expiration date. Reconstituted stock solutions are stable for 14 days at room temperature. Diluted solutions at 2 to 25 mg/mL are stable for 90 days at room temperature.

Mixing instructions: Vials of powder can be reconstituted in a number of fluids to a concentration up to 25 mg/mL. This stock solution and the vials of solution for injection can be diluted further in D_5W or 0.45% to 0.9% saline.

Incompatibilities: not compatible in solution with bleomycin, doxorubicin, droperidol, idarubicin, metaclopramide, prednisolone, or ranitidine.

Drug interactions: None noted.

Metabolism, pharmacokinetics: Methotrexate has good oral

bioavailability at low doses. After oral or intravenous dosing, it is distributed throughout the body water compartment. It will accumulate in third-space fluid compartments and exhibit prolonged toxicity and therefore should be used with caution if at all in patients with significant pleural or peritoneal fluid. The drug is minimally metabolized in the liver and has an elimination half-life of about 3 hours, and even low concentrations of drug after most of the drug is eliminated can contribute to significant toxicity. Therefore, dosing based on renal function is critical.

Excretion: Excretion of this drug is entirely renal.

Toxicity: Myelosuppression is expected and is usually dose limiting. Stomatitis and diarrhea are common. Nausea and vomiting are uncommon. Renal toxicity is uncommon and usually reversible but can be severe. Many types of skin reactions can occur but are uncommon. Pulmonary fibrosis and hepatic fibrosis are rare. Encephalopathy is rare with moderate-to-low–dose therapy, but is more common with high doses, intrathecal administration, or concomitant central nervous system radiation. It can be severe and permanent.

Indications: FDA-approved for a wide spectrum of malignant and nonmalignant diseases. Most often used for acute leukemias, lymphomas, breast cancer, bladder cancer, squamous cell cancers, and sarcomas.

Dosing: For malignant conditions, doses up to 100 mg/m^2 are considered low; 100 to 1,000 mg/m^2, moderate; and over 1,000 mg/m^2, high. Moderate and high doses require leucovorin rescue. Doses can be given weekly or at longer intervals. Intravenous infusions can be 30 minutes or longer, including 24-hour continuous infusions. Methotrexate is also commonly given intrathecally, usually as a 12-mg dose in 10 mL of preservative-free saline.

MITOMYCIN C
(Mutamycin)

Drug class, mechanism of action: Antitumor antibiotic, which inhibits DNA and RNA synthesis.

Form: Vials of powder, 5, 20, and 40 mg.

Storage: Vials should be stored at room temperature and discarded after the listed expiration date. Reconstituted drug is stable for 7 days at room temperature at 0.5 mg/mL. More dilute solutions are less stable and should be used within 3 hours.

Mixing instructions: Add sterile water to the vials to reach a concentration of 0.5 mg/mL. This solution can be further diluted in D_5W or normal saline.

Incompatibilities: Bleomycin loses activity when combined in solution with mitomycin C.

Drug interactions: None noted.

Metabolism, pharmacokinetics: Poor oral bioavailability. After an intravenous dose, mitomycin C is rapidly metabolized to inactive forms in the liver, spleen, and kidneys, with an elimination half-life of about 1 hour.

Excretion: Parent drug and inactive metabolites are excreted in the urine.

Toxicity: Mitomycin C is a vesicant; extravasation precautions are a must. Myelosuppression is expected and is dose limiting, with a WBC nadir at 4 weeks and full recovery at 6 to 7 weeks. Mild nausea, vomiting, anorexia, and fatigue are common. Uncommon toxicities include diarrhea, stomatitis, rash, fever, and renal insufficiency. Rare toxicities include veno-occlusive disease of the liver, hemolytic-uremic syndrome, and interstitial pneumonitis.

Indications: FDA-approved for adenocarcinomas of the stomach and pancreas. Also used commonly in breast cancer and lung cancer.

Dosing: The usual dose is 10 to 20 mg/m^2 intravenously over 2 to 5 minutes every 6 to 8 weeks.

MITOTANE
(Lysodren, o,p'-DDD)

Drug class, mechanism of action: Adrenal cortical cytotoxin.

Form: 500-mg tablets.

Storage: Store at room temperature and discard after expiration date.

Mixing instructions: None.

Drug interactions: None noted.

Metabolism, pharmacokinetics: This drug has moderate oral bioavailability, with a peak plasma level about 4 hours after an oral dose. Significant therapeutic effect is not seen until up to 4 weeks of continuous usage. Mitotane is metabolized in the liver and has a variable elimination half-life (due to storage of the drug in adipose tissue) of up to 160 hours.

Excretion: Mitotane is eliminated in the urine and bile.

Toxicity: Adrenal insufficiency is expected and must be abrogated with concomitant oral glucocorticoids (and sometimes mineralocorticoids as well). Anorexia, nausea, vomiting, sedation, and lethargy are common. Hypercholesterolemia and elevation of liver function findings are also common. Rash is common but is usually mild. Myelosuppression, diarrhea, fever, wheezing, changes in blood pressure, and flushing are uncommon. Permanent central nervous system changes, retinopathy, nephrotoxicity, and hemorrhagic cystitis are rare.

Indications: FDA-approved for adrenal cortical carcinoma.

Dosing: The initial dose is usually 1 g per day in four divided doses, and this is increased up to 10 g per day as tolerated.

MITOXANTRONE
(DHAD, Novantrone, Dihydroxyanthracenedione)

Drug class, mechanism of action: Anthracycline antitumor antibiotic.

Form: Vials of 2 mg/mL solution.

Storage: Unopened vials should be stored at room temperature. Diluted drug (0.02 to 0.5 mg/mL) is stable for at least 7 days at room temperature.

Mixing instructions: Dilute the desired dose in at least 50 mL of D_5W or normal saline for intravenous infusion.

Incompatibilities: Incompatible in solution with heparin and hydrocortisone.

Drug interactions: None noted.

Metabolism, pharmacokinetics: Mitoxantrone has poor oral bioavailability. After an intravenous dose, it exhibits a large volume of distribution, undergoes metabolism in the liver, and has an elimination half-life of 24 to 37 hours.

Excretion: Mitoxantrone is eliminated through the bile.

Toxicity: Mitoxantrone is not a tissue vesicant. Myelosuppression, mostly limited to leukopenia, is expected and dose limiting. Nausea and vomiting are common but mild, stomatitis is common, and diarrhea and anorexia are less common. Elevated liver function findings are common, but significant hepatic toxicity is rare. Cardiotoxicity is uncommon and dose dependent. Lung or neurologic toxicity are rare.

Indications: FDA-approved for acute myelogenous leukemia and prostate carcinoma. Also used for breast cancer, lymphoma, and hepatocellular carcinoma.

Dosing: For acute myeloid leukemia (AML), the typical dose is 10 to 12 mg/m^2 per day for 3 days by 30-minute infusion, along with Ara-C. For solid tumors, 12 mg/m^2 is given over 30 minutes every 3 to 4 weeks.

OCTREOTIDE
(Sandostatin, L-Cysteinamide)

Drug class, mechanism of action: Synthetic peptide analogue of somatostatin; inhibits other GI peptides, such as serotonin, insulin, glucagon, gastrin.

Form: Ampules of 0.05, 0.1, and 0.5 mg in 1 mL aqueous solution.

Storage: Unopened ampules should be stored at 4°C and used within 12 hours of opening. Discard after expiration date. Drug diluted in saline to 5 to 100 μg/mL is stable at room temperature for 4 days.

Mixing instructions: Drug can be injected after withdrawal from the ampule or further diluted in normal saline for intravenous infusion.

Incompatibilities: Is not compatible with lipid infusions but is compatible with total parenteral nutrition solutions.

Drug interactions: May interfere with insulin action, requiring increase in insulin dosage.

Metabolism, pharmacokinetics: Not orally bioavailable but rapidly absorbed after subcutaneous administration. Metabolized by hydrolysis throughout the body. No active metabolites. The half-life of elimination is about 1.5 hours.

Excretion: Intact drug is cleared via the kidneys.

Toxicity: GI side effects, which are dose limiting, include abdominal pain, vomiting, loose stool, occasional fat malabsorption, bloating, and cholelithiasis. Elevations of liver function findings can also occur, but frank hepatitis is rare. Skin reactions, such as pain at the injection site or flushing, rash, or skin thinning, are sometimes seen. Constitutional symptoms, including rhinorrhea, xerostomia, sweating, throat discomfort, and vertigo can be bothersome. Either hyperglycemia or hypoglycemia can occur. Cardiac side effects, including angina, congestive heart failure, and hypotension or hypertension, are uncommon. Anxiety, depression, fatigue, and anorexia are uncommon; seizures are rare.

Indications: FDA-approved for carcinoid tumors causing carcinoid syndrome and for vasoactive peptide-secreting tumors. Also used for refractory diarrhea, either cancer related or treatment related, in cancer patients.

Dosing: Doses from 50 μg twice a day to 1,000 μg four times a day injected subcutaneously have been used. Continuous intravenous infusions or administration of drug in total parental nutrition solutions have also been used.

OPRELVEKIN
(Neumega, Interleukin-11 [IL-11])

Drug class, mechanism of action: Recombinant polypeptide cytokine molecule with multiple cellular actions, including stimulation of megakaryocyte proliferation and platelet production from megakaryocytes.

Form: Vials, 5 mg lyophilized powder.

Storage: Unopened vials should be stored at 4°C and discarded after expiration date. Reconstituted drug is stable at room temperature for 3 hours.

Mixing instructions: Add 1 mL of sterile water to each vial, mix with gentle swirling until clear, and then draw up the desired dose into a syringe for subcutaneous administration.

Drug interactions: None noted.

Metabolism, pharmacokinetics: Oprelvekin is available only by parenteral routes. With subcutaneous administration, it is absorbed into the circulation with a peak plasma concentration of 3 hours and has an elimination half-life of about 7 hours. This polypeptide agent is metabolized throughout the body by proteolysis.

Excretion: Because of degradation, excretion of drug is not substantial.

Toxicity: Headache, fever, malaise, dyspnea, rash, conjunctival irritation, fluid retention, and edema are common during administration but not usually severe. Oral thrush, dizziness, diarrhea, pleural effusions, and transient anemia are uncommon. Paresthesias, ocular hemorrhage, atrial arrhythmias, and exfoliative dermatitis are rare.

Indications: FDA-approved for prevention of severe chemotherapy-related thrombocytopenia.

Dosing: 50 μg/kg per day subcutaneous injection until the post-nadir platelet count is above 50,000/mm^3, starting 1-day after the completion of chemotherapy.

PACLITAXEL
(Taxol)

Drug class, mechanism of action: Naturally occurring taxane molecule inhibits depolymerization of tubulin in the spindle apparatus, inducing apoptosis in dividing cells.

Form: Vials containing 30 and 100 mg of drug in nonaqueous solution.

Storage: Unopened vials should be stored at room temperature and discarded after expiration date. Reconstituted drug is stable at room temperature for 27 hours.

Mixing instructions: The desired dose should be dissolved in normal saline or D$_5$W to a final concentration of 0.3 to 1.2 mg/mL, and this solution should be stored in a glass or polypropylene container or bag and administered through polyethylene-lined tubing to prevent leaching of plasticizer chemicals from polyvinyl chloride materials.

Drug interactions: Cisplatin administered before paclitaxel may enhance the myelosuppressive effect of paclitaxel. Coadministration of paclitaxel and doxorubicin may enhance the cardiotoxicity of doxorubicin.

Metabolism, pharmacokinetics: Paclitaxel has poor oral bioavailability. After intravenous administration, the drug exhibits a large volume of distribution and undergoes metabolism in the liver. The elimination half-life is 15 to 50 hours.

Excretion: Excretion of drug and metabolites is predominantly via the bile.

Toxicity: Paclitaxel is an irritant or mild vesicant when extravasated into subcutaneous tissue. Myelosuppression, predominantly neutropenia, is expected and is dose limiting. Shorter infusions of the same dose produce less neutropenia. Mucositis is also very common, particularly with longer infusions. Peripheral neuropathy, which is common and usually mild, increases with cumulative dose. Acute neuromyopathy is also common; it occurs for several days after each dose. This syndrome may require opioid analgesics to control pain. Cardiovascular side effects, including hypertension, hypotension, premature contractions, and bradyarrhythmias, are common but rarely require intervention. Hypersensitivity reactions to paclitaxel, including urticaria, wheezing, chest pain, dyspnea, and hypotension, are common but are reduced in frequency and severity by premedication with corticosteroids, H_1-antihistamines, and H_2-antihistamines (the recommended regimen is dexamethasone 20 mg orally 12 and 6 hours prior to paclitaxel and diphenhydramine 50 mg and cimetidine 300 mg intravenously 30 minutes prior to paclitaxel). Alopecia, usually complete, is expected. Other toxicities are uncommon; they include nausea, vomiting, diarrhea, liver toxicity, and interstitial pneumonitis.

Indications: FDA-approved for salvage therapy in ovarian cancer and breast cancer. Used also in lung, head and neck, and bladder cancer.

Dosing: 135 mg/m² to 225 mg/m² intravenously over 3 hours or 24 hours every 3 weeks. Weekly schedules and longer infusions have also been used.

PAMIDRONATE
(Aredia, Aminohydroxypropylidene Diphosphonate, APD)

Drug class, mechanism of action: Organic bisphosphonate; inhibitor of bone resorption by osteoclasts.

Form: 30-mg vials of lyophilized powder.

Storage: Vials should be stored at room temperature and discarded after listed expiration date. Reconstituted drug at 3 mg/mL is stable for at least 24 hours at 4°C; drug diluted in D_5W or normal saline to 0.03 to 0.09 mg/mL is stable for at least 24 hours at room temperature.

Mixing instructions: Dissolve each 30-mg vial in 10 mL of

sterile water to yield a 3-mg/mL stock solution, which can then be dissolved in 1 L of normal saline or D_5W.

Incompatibilities: incompatible with lactated Ringer's solution.

Drug interactions: None noted.

Metabolism, pharmacokinetics: Pamidronate is available only by the parenteral route. After intravenous administration, the drug concentrates in the bone, spleen, and liver. Its metabolism is not well characterized. It has a terminal half-life is about 27 hours.

Excretion: 50% of the parent drug is eliminated in the urine.

Toxicity: Pamidronate is usually quite well tolerated. Hypotension, syncope, tachycardia, and even atrial fibrillation have been reported uncommonly during the infusion. Hypocalcemia, hypophosphatemia, hypokalemia, and hypomagnesemia occur commonly but only rarely require intervention. Nausea, vomiting, and somnolence are rare.

Indications: FDA-approved for malignancy-induced hypercalcemia. May lead to pain relief and even tumor shrinkage of bone metastases in multiple myeloma, breast cancer, and prostate cancer.

Dosing: 60 mg/m² to 90 mg/m² intravenously over 24 hours, although the clinical experience with infusions of 1 to 3 hours is extensive. Treatment may be repeated every 1 to 3 weeks. Peak effect occurs 3 to 7 days after a dose.

PENTOSTATIN
(Nipent, Covidarabine, 2'-Deoxycoformycin [dCF])

Drug class, mechanism of action: Purine analogue antimetabolite; inhibits adenosine deaminase. Partly cell cycle dependent.

Form: 10-mg vials of lyophilized powder.

Storage: Store unopened vials at 4°C and discard after expiration date. Solutions of drug at 2 mg/mL are stable for 72 hours at room temperature. Dilute solutions (0.02 mg/mL) are stable at room temperature for 24 hours in D_5W and 48 hours in normal saline.

Mixing instructions: Dissolve contents of 10-mg vials in 5 mL sterile water; further dilute the desired dose to 1 mg/mL or less concentration in normal saline or D_5W.

Drug interactions: None noted.

Metabolism, pharmacokinetics: Available only as an intravenous preparation, pentostatin has an elimination half-life of about 5 hours and undergoes very little metabolism.

Excretion: Most of a dose is eliminated in the urine as unchanged drug.

Toxicity: Myelosuppression is expected and dose limiting. Lymphopenia is severe and can lead to opportunistic infections. Anemia and thrombocytopenia are also common. Nausea and vomiting are common but mild. Fever and fatigue are also common. Anorexia, diarrhea, stomatitis, rash, elevated liver function findings, significant nephrotoxicity, and headache are uncommon. Hepatitis, acute tubular necrosis, and central nervous system alterations, including coma and seizures, are rare.

Indications: FDA-approved for the treatment of hairy cell leukemia. Also used occasionally for non-Hodgkin's lymphoma and chronic lymphocytic leukemia.

Dosing: The usual dose is 4 mg/m^2 intravenous bolus (with 1 to 2 L intravenous hydration) every 2 weeks.

PLICAMYCIN
(Mithracin, Mithramycin)

Drug class, mechanism of action: Antitumor antibiotic, partly cell cycle dependent.

Form: Supplied as lyophilized powder in vials containing 2.5 mg of drug.

Storage: Vials of drug should be stored at 4°C and discarded after the expiration date. Reconstituted drug is stable for at least 24 hours at room temperature.

Mixing instructions: Add 4.9 mL sterile water to a vial to yield a 0.5-mg/mL solution; dilute the desired dose in 100 to 500 mL of normal saline or D_5W.

Incompatibilities: Do not combine plicamycin with iron or other trace element solutions, and do not use a cellulose ester filter with this drug.

Drug interactions: None noted.

Metabolism, pharmacokinetics: Available only by the intravenous route. After an intravenous dose, the drug is metabolized by the liver and has an elimination half-life of about 2 hours.

Excretion: Parent drug and metabolites are eliminated via the kidneys.

Toxicity: Plicamycin is a vesicant if extravasated into soft tissues. Hemorrhage, due to both thrombocytopenia and/or coagulopathy, is dose limiting. Other hematologic toxicities are uncommon. Nausea and vomiting are common but not severe. Stomatitis, diarrhea, and anorexia are less common. Rash is common, but severe cutaneous reactions such as toxic epidermal necrolysis are rare. Depletion of calcium, potassium, phosphate, and magnesium are expected but rarely require intervention. Renal toxicity, including proteinuria and azotemia, is uncommon.

Elevated liver function findings and neurologic toxicity, including lethargy, weakness, anxiety, somnolence, and headache, are uncommon.

Indications: FDA-approved for treatment of malignancy-induced hypercalcemia and for treatment of germ cell tumors. Also has been used for chronic myelogenous leukemia in blast crisis.

Dosing: The typical dose for germ cell tumors is 25 to 30 $\mu g/kg$ per day intravenous infusion over 60 minutes for 8 to 10 days. For hypercalcemia, the same dose is given one to three times per week.

PREDNIMUSTINE
(Sterecyt)

Drug class, mechanism of action: Corticosteroid–alkylator conjugate with a poorly understood mechanism of action.

Form: 20-mg tablets.

Storage: Store tablets at room temperature and discard after expiration date.

Mixing instructions: None.

Drug interactions: None noted.

Metabolism, pharmacokinetics: Oral bioavailability is adequate. The drug is metabolized in the liver.

Excretion: Parent drug and metabolites are excreted in the feces.

Toxicity: Myelosuppression is common and dose limiting. Nausea, vomiting, and anorexia are common and mild. Diarrhea is less common. Confusion, euphoria, hypertension, and edema are uncommon.

Indications: No FDA-approved indications, but available as an orphan drug for use against chronic lymphocytic leukemia, lymphoma, breast cancer, prostate cancer, and ovarian carcinoma.

Dosing: Common dosing schemes are either chronic daily administration at 20 to 30 mg per day or 100 to 160 mg/m^2 per day for 5 days every 10 to 14 days.

PREDNISONE
(Deltasone)

Drug class, mechanism of action: Corticosteroid.

Form: Tablets from 1 mg to 50 mg and oral solution.

Storage: Tablets and liquid are stored at room temperature and should be discarded after the label expiration date.

Mixing instructions: None.

Drug interactions: None noted.

Metabolism, pharmacokinetics: Prednisone has good oral bioavailability and is extensively metabolized in the liver, primarily to the active form of the drug, prednisolone. It has an elimination half-life of approximately 4 hours. Liver disease may decrease conversion to the active form, requiring use of prednisolone instead of prednisone.

Excretion: Routes of excretion of the parent drug and metabolites are not well delineated.

Toxicity: Mostly constitutional symptoms, including mood changes (depressive, anxious, or euphoric), insomnia, indigestion, enhanced appetite, weight gain, acne, and cushingoid features. Other side effects may be more serious but are less common. Hyperglycemia and increased stomach acid, predisposing to acute ulceration; osteopenia, cataracts, skin atrophy, and adrenal insufficiency occur with prolonged use.

Indications: FDA-approved for a wide variety of malignant and nonmalignant conditions. Used in oncology for lymphoid malignancies, for palliative care, and for management of side effects and toxicities.

Dosing: Lympholytic doses are generally in the range of 50 to 100 mg/m^2 per day for 5 to 14 days. Higher or lower doses, depending on the indication, are also used.

PROCARBAZINE
(Matulane, Natulanar, N-Methylhydrazine)

Drug class, mechanism of action: Alkylating agent; cell cycle independent.

Form: 50-mg capsules.

Storage: Store at room temperature and discard after listed expiration date.

Mixing instructions: None.

Drug interactions: This drug has monoamine oxidase inhibitory activity and therefore should not be taken with certain types of food, including beer, wines, fermented cheese, chocolate and fava beans, or with certain medications, including ethanol, decongestants, tricyclic antidepressants, antihypertensives, antihistamines, opioids, barbiturates, phenothiazines, or other monoamine oxidase inhibitors.

Metabolism, pharmacokinetics: Well absorbed by the oral route, reaching peak plasma levels in 1 hour, with good distrubution to the cerebrospinal fluid. Procarbazine is metabolized by the liver and has an elimination half-life of about 1 hour.

Excretion: Parent drug and metabolites are largely excreted in the urine.

Toxicity: Myelosuppression is expected and dose limiting,

but anemia is uncommon. Nausea and vomiting are common and can be dose limiting as well. Rash, hives, and photosensitivity sometimes occur. Other side effects are uncommon; they include anorexia, diarrhea, stomatitis, hypotension, tachycardia, syncope, flulike syndrome, interstitial pneumonitis, central nervous system excitation including seizures, and secondary malignancies.

Indications: FDA-approved for Hodgkin's disease; may also be useful in non-Hodgkin's lymphoma, multiple myeloma, brain tumors, melanoma, and lung cancer.

Dosing: In Hodgkin's disease regimens such as MOPP, the dose is 100 mg/m^2 per day for 14 days during each cycle.

RITUXIMAB
(Rituxan)

Drug class, mechanism of action: Monoclonal antibody directed against the B-cell surface antigen CD20.

Form: Sterile vials containing 100 mg and 500 mg of antibody in aqueous solution (10 mg/mL).

Storage: This agent should be stored at 4°C, and vials should be discarded after the listed expiration date. Diluted drug should be used within 12 hours.

Mixing instructions: Dilute the desired dose to 1 to 4 mg/mL in normal saline or D$_5$W.

Drug interactions: None noted.

Metabolism, pharmacokinetics: Not available by the oral route, but when given intravenously, it is taken up by B lymphocytes and degraded throughout the body by proteolysis, with a wide-ranging serum half-life of 11 to 105 hours (mean 60 hours) with the first dose.

Excretion: No appreciable excretion of this polypeptide agent occurs.

Toxicity: Fever, chills, and malaise are common during administration, even with premedication with acetaminophen and diphenhydramine. Other infusion-related symptoms include nausea, vomiting, flushing, urticaria, angioedema, hypotension, dyspnea, bronchospasm, fatigue, headache, rhinitis, and pain at disease sites. These symptoms are generally self-limited, improve with slowing of the infusion, and resolve after infusion. Short-lived myelosuppression, abdominal pain, and myalgia are uncommon. Arrhythmias and angina pectoris are rare.

Indications: FDA-approved for relapsed or refractory low-grade or follicular CD20-positive B-cell lymphomas.

Dosing: The recommended dose is 375 mg/m^2 by intravenous infusion starting at 50 mg/hour and increasing to 400 mg/hr maximum weekly for 4 weeks.

SARGRAMOSTIM
(Leukine, Leukomax, Granulocyte-Macrophage Colony–Stimulating Factor [GM-CSF])

Drug class, mechanism of action: Cytokine; exhibits pleiotropic stimulatory effects on bone marrow progenitor cells.

Form: 250-, 400- and 500-μg vials of lyophilized GM-CSF.

Storage: Vials should be stored at 4°C and discarded after the label expiration date. Reconstituted drug for subcutaneous injection in stable for 24 hours (Leukomax) or 30 days (Leukine); drug diluted 10 μg/mL or higher) is stable for 72 hours at room temperature.

Mixing instructions: Add sterile water to the vials and mix gently before withdrawing for dilution in normal saline or D_5W or into the syringe for injection.

Drug interactions: None noted.

Metabolism, pharmacokinetics: Not available by the oral route but similar bioavailability when given intravenous or subcutaneously. Degraded throughout the body, predominantly in the liver and kidneys, with an elimination half-life of 2 hours.

Excretion: No appreciable excretion of this peptide occurs.

Toxicity: Constitutional symptoms, which tend to decrease over time, predominate at standard doses. Higher doses may cause capillary leak syndrome. Side effects include flushing, hypotension or hypertension, dyspnea, fever, nausea, vomiting, fatigue, myalgias, bone pain, headache, and skin rash. Thrombocytopenia may also occur. Fluid retention and edema are rare at standard doses. Progression of myelodysplastic syndrome has been documented in patients on GM-CSF.

Indications: FDA-approved for the treatment of myelosuppression after autologous bone marrow transplantation. May be useful to minimize myelosuppression after standard-dose chemotherapy or to shorten the course of neutropenic fever. Immunostimulatory properties of GM-CSF are still being investigated.

Dosing: 250 μg/m^2 per day for 21 days or 5 μg/kg per day for 10 to 14 days.

STREPTOZOCIN

Drug class, mechanism of action: Alkylating agent; cell cycle independent.

Form: 1-g vials of lyophilized streptozocin.

Storage: Streptozocin vials should be stored at 4°C protected from light. Reconstituted solutions are stable for 48 hours at room temperature and 96 hours at 4°C.

Mixing instructions: Dissolve the contents of the 1-g vial in

9.5 mL of D_5W or normal saline (100 mg/mL), and then dilute the desired dose in D_5W or normal saline.

Drug interactions: None noted.

Metabolism, pharmacokinetics: Streptozocin is bioavailable only by the intravenous route. It is metabolized primarily in the liver and has an elimination half-life of less than an hour.

Excretion: Parent drug and metabolites are excreted in the urine.

Toxicity: GI side effects (nausea, vomiting, and cramping) and nephrotoxicity (glomerular and tubular damage) are common and potentially dose limiting. Myelosuppression is less often dose limiting. Elevated liver function findings occasionally occur but are rarely clinically significant. Fever, delirium, and depression occur rarely. Streptozocin is an irritant if extravasated into perivenous soft tissue.

Indications: FDA-approved for metastatic islet cell carcinoma and may also be useful for advanced carcinoid tumor, pancreatic carcinoma, and Hodgkin's disease.

Dosing: The usual dose is 500 to 1,000 mg/m^{2}per day by intravenous bolus for 5 days every 4 weeks.

SURAMIN
(Germanin, Moranyl, Bayer 205)

Drug class, mechanism of action: Novel polyanionic antiparasitic agent; antagonizes cellular effects of various basic growth factors.

Form: 1-g vials of lyophilized powder.

Storage: Vials should be stored at room temperature and discarded after the expiration date. Reconstituted drug at 2 to 10 mg/mL in D_5W or normal saline is stable for 24 hours at room temperature.

Mixing instructions: Add 10 mL of sterile water to the 1-g vial; further dilute the desired dose to 2 to 10 mg/mL with D_5W or normal saline.

Drug interactions: None noted.

Metabolism, pharmacokinetics: No oral bioavailability. After intravenous administration, the drug is tightly bound to plasma proteins and is not appreciably metabolized. The elimination half-life is more than 40 days.

Excretion: Drug is cleared via the kidneys.

Toxicity: Severe toxicity can occur at high plasma concentrations, necessitating pharmacokinetic monitoring. Fever, malaise, nausea, vomiting, erythematous rash, and proteinuria are common, as is mild coagulopathy. Constipation is often seen. Adrenal insufficiency is also common and frequently requires steroid replacement transiently or sometimes permanently.

Leukopenia, anemia, and thrombocytopenia are uncommon. Significant neurologic toxicity, including paresthesias and neuropathy, is uncommon with monitoring of serum levels. Renal insufficiency, significant liver dysfunction, and vortex keratopathy are also uncommon.

Indications: Not FDA-approved, it has orphan drug status for oncology and may be useful in many malignancies. It has been studied most extensively in metastatic prostate cancer.

Dosing: 350 mg/m^2 per day by continuous intravenous infusion to reach a serum level of 250 to 300 μg/mL, repeated every 2 months. Other doses and schedules have been used.

TAMOXIFEN
(Nolvedex)

Drug class, mechanism of action: Nonsteroidal antiestrogen with cytostatic effects on both estrogen-dependent and estrogen-independent malignant cells.

Form: 10-mg tablets.

Storage: Store at room temperature and discard after the listed expiration date.

Mixing instructions: None.

Drug interactions: None noted.

Metabolism, pharmacokinetics: Tamoxifen has good oral bioavailability, is metabolized in the liver, and has an elimination half-life of about 7 days.

Excretion: Neither tamoxifen nor its major metabolite is found in the bile or urine.

Toxicity: Tamoxifen is usually very well tolerated. Constitutional symptoms are most prevalent and usually dose limiting. Hot flashes, sweating, mood changes, weight gain or loss, and stomach upset are most common. Nausea, vomiting, diarrhea, and constipation are less common. Menstrual changes, including significant vaginal bleeding, are uncommon. Venous thromboembolism, myelosuppression, and retinopathy are rare.

Indications: FDA-approved for the treatment of breast cancer, generally in postmenopausal patients or those with estrogen receptor–positive tumors. Also used for melanoma and pancreatic cancer.

Dosing: The standard dose for breast cancer is 10 mg orally three times a day or 20 mg once a day.

TENIPOSIDE
(Vumon, VM-26, PTG)

Drug class, mechanism of action: Inhibitor of topoisomerase II; similar in action to etoposide.

Form: Vials of 10 mg/mL solution containing 50 mg of drug.

Storage: Store vials at 4°C and discard after expiration date. After dilution of the drug to 0.1 to 0.4 mg/mL in normal saline or D_5W, it is stable for 24 hours in a glass container. Teniposide in D_5W precipitates in plastic containers.

Mixing instructions: The desired dose should be diluted in a glass container to 0.1 to 0.4 mg/mL in normal saline or D_5W for slow intravenous infusion.

Drug interactions: Metabolism of teniposide is increased by inducers of liver microsomal enzymes, such as phenobarbital and carbamazepine.

Metabolism, pharmacokinetics: Teniposide is available only by the intravenous route. It is extensively protein-bound in the plasma and undergoes nearly complete metabolism in the liver. It has an elimination half-life of 5 hours.

Excretion: Metabolites are excreted in the bile and urine.

Toxicity: Myelosuppression, predominantly leukopenia, is universal and dose limiting. Otherwise usually well tolerated. Nausea, vomiting, diarrhea, stomatitis, and anorexia are uncommon. Alopecia is generally mild. Elevated liver function findings can occur but are not usually clinically significant. Allergic reactions, hypotension, fatigue, seizures, somnolence, fever, renal insufficiency, and secondary leukemia are all rare.

Indications: FDA-approved for childhood acute lymphoblastic leukemia. Not used commonly for other malignancies but does have activity against small cell lung cancer.

Dosing: 100 mg/m² once or twice weekly or 20 to 60 mg/m² per day for 5 days as a slow intravenous infusion (at least 30 minutes).

THIOGUANINE
(Tabloid, 6-TG, Aminopurine-6-Thiol-Hemihydrate)

Drug class, mechanism of action: Purine analogue antimetabolite, cell cycle dependent.

Form: 40-mg tablets.

Storage: Tablets are stored at room temperature and should be discarded after the label expiration date.

Mixing instructions: None.

Drug interactions: None noted.

Metabolism, pharmacokinetics: Thioguanine has modest but slow oral route absorption. It is almost completely metabolized in the liver and has an elimination half-life of up to 11 hours.

Excretion: Metabolites are excreted in the urine.

Toxicity: Thioguanine is usually well tolerated. Leukopenia and thrombocytopenia are common and dose limiting. Nausea and vomiting, stomatitis, diarrhea, rash, elevated liver function findings, hyperuricemia, and renal insufficiency are uncommon.

Indications: FDA-approved for acute myelogenous leukemia in all phases of treatment. May be useful in other leukemias. An injectable formulation does not yet have FDA approval.

Dosing: The usual dose for leukemias is 2 to 3 mg/kg per day as part of an ongoing multidrug regimen.

THIOTEPA
(TSPA, TESPA, Triethylenethiophosphoramide)

Drug class, mechanism of action: Classical alkylating agent; cell cycle independent.

Form: Available as lyophilized powder in vials containing 15 mg of drug.

Storage: Vials should be stored at 4°C and discarded after expiration date. Reconstituted drug at 10 mg/mL and drug further diluted in normal saline or D_5W are stable for 24 hours at room temperature and 5 days at 4°C.

Mixing instructions: Dissolve the contents of a vial in 1.5 mL of sterile water to yield a 10-mg/mL stock solution; further dilute in D_5W for intravenous infusion.

Drug interactions: None noted.

Metabolism, pharmacokinetics: With poor oral bioavailability, thiotepa is available only by the parenteral route. Extensive metabolism occurs in the liver, and the drug has an elimination half-life of 2 to 3 hours.

Excretion: Metabolites are excreted in the urine.

Toxicity: Myelosuppression, predominantly leukopenia, is expected, dose limiting, and sometimes cumulative. Nausea, vomiting, anorexia, stomatitis, and diarrhea are uncommon. Infertility, fever, angioedema, and urticaria are uncommon. Second malignancies such as acute leukemia are rare. With high-dose therapy and bone marrow rescue, stomatitis and cognitive impairment can be severe. Intravesical administration leads to predominant urinary symptoms, including pain, hematuria, hemorrhagic cystitis, and rare ureteral obstruction.

Indications: FDA-approved for the treatment of breast and ovarian carcinoma, as well as Hodgkin's disease and non-Hodgkin's lymphoma. Used for intravesical therapy of superficial bladder cancer and may also be used for intracavitary and intrathecal administration. Used in the transplant setting for ovarian and breast carcinoma.

Dosing: The usual dose is 12 to 16 mg/m^2 intravenously over 10 minutes every 1 to 4 weeks. In the transplant setting doses up to 900 mg/m^2 have been used. The bladder instillation dose is 30 to 60 mg weekly for 4 weeks. The intrathecal dose is 1 to 10 mg/m^2 once or twice a week.

TOPOTECAN
(Hycamtin, hycamptamine)

Drug class, mechanism of action: Semisynthetic campto-thecin molecule; inhibits topoisomerase I, which is required by cells for both transcription and replication.

Form: 5-mg vials of lyophilized powder.

Storage: Topotecan vials should be stored at 4°C and dis-carded after expiration date. Reconstituted at 20 to 100 μg/mL in normal saline or D$_5$W, it is stable for 48 hours at room tem-perature.

Mixing instructions: Dissolve the contents of each vial in 2 mL sterile water; dilute the desired dose in 100 mL or more of normal saline or D$_5$W for infusion.

Drug interactions: None noted.

Metabolism, pharmacokinetics: No oral form of this drug is available. After intravenous administration, the drug is not ex-tensively metabolized, and it has an elimination half-life of about 3 hours.

Excretion: A significant portion of the drug is excreted un-changed in the urine.

Toxicity: Myelosuppression, especially leukopenia, is ex-pected and dose limiting. Thrombocytopenia and anemia are common but mild. Nausea, vomiting, and diarrhea are common but usually not severe. Headache, fever, fatigue, anorexia, malaise, and elevated liver function findings are also common. Hypertension, tachycardia, urticaria, renal insufficiency, hema-turia, neuropathy, and mucositis are uncommon.

Indications: FDA-approved for the treatment of refractory, relapsed ovarian carcinoma. Also may have activity in lung can-cer and myeloid leukemias.

Dosing: The standard dose for ovarian cancer is 1.5 mg/m^2 per day for 5 days as a 30 minute infusion.

TOREMIFENE
(Fareston)

Drug class, mechanism of action: Nonsteroidal antiestrogen with cytostatic effects on estrogen-dependent and estrogen-independent malignant cells.

Form: 60-mg tablets.

Storage: Tablets are stored at room temperature and should be discarded after expiration date.

Mixing instructions: None.

Drug interactions: None noted.

Metabolism, pharmacokinetics: Toremifene has good oral bioavailability and is extensively bound to plasma proteins. It is metabolized in the liver to active metabolites and has an elimination half-life of about 5 days.

Excretion: Parent drug and metabolites are excreted in the bile.

Toxicity: Toremifene is usually very well tolerated. Hot flashes, nausea, sweating, dizziness, and fatigue are the most common side effects. Vomiting, diarrhea, anorexia, vaginal discharge, vaginal bleeding, and headache are less common. Venous thrombosis and pulmonary embolism are rare.

Indications: FDA-approved for the treatment of post-menopausal or estrogen receptor–positive metastatic breast cancer.

Dosing: 60 mg orally every day.

TRASTUZUMAB (HERCEPTIN [TM])

Drug class, mechanism of action: A genetically engineered humanized mouse monoclonal antibody directed against the HER-2/*neu* growth factor receptor overexpressed on many invasive breast carcinomas. Mechanism of action for clinical activity in breast cancer is unknown but may be complement-mediated cell lysis, antibody-dependent cellular cytotoxicity, or induction of apoptosis.

Form: Vials of 440 mg.

Drug interactions: None noted.

Metabolism, pharmacokinetics: Binding studies show strong binding to cells overexpressing HER-2/*neu* molecules. Very little else is known regarding the distribution and metabolic fate of this molecule. The half-life should be very short with minimal distribution outside the vascular compartment and minimal clearance by kidneys or liver (similar to other monoclonal antibodies and polypeptide agents).

Toxicity: Common toxicities include acute fever, chills, nausea, vomiting, and headache. Trastuzumab seems to worsen leukopenia, anemia, and diarrhea when given with chemotherapy compared to chemotherapy alone. Also, trastuzumab may have uncomon acute cardiotoxicity that may add to the more common anthracycline-induced cardiotoxicity; therefore, the use of trastuzumab with doxorubicin is not indicated by the FDA.

Indications: This product was approved by the FDA on 9/25/98. The package insert is not yet available. It is indicated for HER-2/*neu* overexpressing metastatic or locally advanced breast cancer and has shown clinical benefit as a single agent and in conjunction with paclitaxel-based chemotherapy.

Dosing: Loading dose of 250 mg or 4 mg/kg intravenously, followed by weekly intravenous infusions of 100 mg or 2 mg/kg for up to 10 weeks or longer).

TRETINOIN (VESANOID,
ALL *TRANS* RETINOIC ACID [ATRA])

Drug class, mechanism of action: Naturally occurring retinoid; induces differentiation and apoptosis of malignant promyelocytes in acute promyelocytic leukemia.

Form: 10-mg capsules.

Storage: Capsules should be stored at room temperature protected from light and discarded after expiration date.

Mixing instructions: None.

Drug interactions: None noted.

Metabolism, pharmacokinetics: This drug has good oral bioavailability and a very short elimination half-life, about 40 minutes. It induces its own metabolism in the liver, leading to decreased levels and clinical effect with continued administration.

Excretion: Because of nearly complete metabolism, no appreciable excretion of the parent compound is evident.

Toxicity: Tretinoin is teratogenic, so women of child-bearing age who take this drug must use optimal contraceptive measures. Leukostasis and hemorrhage due to leukocytosis are dose limiting but not usually life threatening if the drug is stopped. Retinoic acid syndrome, although not common, can be dose limiting; it consists of fever, chest pain, dyspnea, hypoxia, pulmonary infiltrates, and pleural and/or pericardial effusions. It can be lethal but improves with cessation of the drug and is treatable with corticosteroids. Dry skin, exfoliation, xerostomia, and cheilitis are common. Elevations in liver function findings and hyperlipidemias are also common. Headache is often seen, but pseudotumor cerebri and other neurologic occurrences are uncommon.

Indications: FDA-approved induction therapy for acute promyelocytic leukemia; also useful in the maintenance phase of this disorder and may have clinical activity in other hematologic malignancies.

Dosing: For induction, the dose is 45 mg/m^2 per day orally for 30 to 90 days, depending on the clinical response.

TRIMETREXATE
(TMQ, TMTX)

Drug class, mechanism of action: Antifolate antimetabolite; chemically similar to methotrexate.

Form: Lyophilized powder in vials containing 25 mg of drug.

Storage: Store unopened vials at room temperature and discard after expiration date. Reconstituted drug (12.5 mg/mL) is stable at room temperature for 7 days; diluted drug (0.1 to 4 mg/mL in D$_5$W) is stable for 24 hours at room temperature.

Mixing instructions: Dissolve the contents of the 25-mg vial with 2 mL sterile water. Further dilute the desired dose in D_5W. Cannot be diluted in saline.

Incompatibilities: incompatible with chloride and other anion-containing solutions.

Drug interactions: None noted.

Metabolism, pharmacokinetics: Good oral bioavailability but not available in pill form. After intravenous administration the drug is extensively protein-bound and is metabolized in the liver. The elimination half-life is 11 to 16 hours, prolonged in patients with hypoalbuminemia.

Excretion: Parent drug and metabolites are excreted primarily by the kidneys.

Toxicity: Leukopenia and mucositis are the two dose-limiting toxicities, and both are expected and can be severe. Leucovorin rescue can diminish these toxicities. Maculopapular rash is common but usually self-limited. Fever is common; nausea, vomiting, anorexia, malaise, and elevations of liver function findings and creatinine are uncommon. Toxicities are more pronounced in patients with significant hypoalbuminemia.

Indications: Orphan drug status with clinical activity demonstrated in squamous cell cancers and non-small cell lung cancer.

Dosing: The usual dose range is 8 to 12 mg/m^2 per day intravenously over 15 minutes or longer for 5 days, repeated every 3 to 4 weeks.

VINBLASTINE
(VLB, Velban, Velsar, Vincaleukoblastine)

Drug class, mechanism of action: Vinca alkaloid; inhibits tubulin polymerization, hence mitosis. G2 phase specific.

Form: Vials in solution (1 mg/mL) or 10 mg lyophilized powder.

Storage: Store at 4°C and discard after expiration date. The solution is stable at room temperature for 14 days. Diluted drug at 0.01 mg/mL is stable for 5 days at room temperature.

Mixing instructions: The vial of solution is ready for dilution; the powder must first be dissolved in 10 mL of normal saline to yield a 1-mg/mL solution; further dilute in normal saline or D_5W.

Incompatibilities: Incompatible in solution with furosemide and heparin.

Drug interactions: None noted.

Metabolism, pharmacokinetics: Poor oral bioavailability. After an intravenous dose, the drug undergoes deacetylation in the liver to an active metabolite, followed by further metabolism. The elimination half-life is about 20 hours.

Excretion: Excretion is predominantly via the bile.

Toxicity: Vinblastine is a soft tissue vesicant, requiring extravasation precautions during administration. Myelosuppression, especially leukopenia, is expected and dose limiting. Anemia and thrombocytopenia are less common. Peripheral and autonomic neuropathy are less common than those observed with vincristine. Nausea and vomiting are uncommon, but constipation is more often seen. Acute reactions during administration, including dyspnea, wheezing, chest pain, tumor pain, and fever are uncommon. Syndrome of inappropriate antidiuretic hormone secretion occurs rarely, as does angina pectoris.

Indications: FDA-approved for multiple hematologic and solid neoplasms. Most often used for Hodgkin's disease, non-Hodgkin's lymphoma, germ cell tumors, and breast cancer.

Dosing: Typical doses are 6 to 10 mg/m^2 by intravenous push every 2 to 4 weeks, combined with other drugs. Can also be given as a continuous infusion over 96 hours at 1.7 to 2 mg/m^2 per day.

VINCRISTINE
(VCR, Oncovin, Vincasar, Leurocristine)

Drug class, mechanism of action: Vinca alkaloid, inhibitor of tubulin polymerization, and thereby mitosis. G2 phase specific.

Form: Solution (1 mg/mL) in 1- to 5-mg vials 1- and 2-mg syringes.

Storage: Store vials or syringes at 4°C and discard after expiration date. Stable for 4 days as a 20 μg/mL solution at room temperature.

Mixing instructions: Intravenous push doses can be given directly; longer infusions require dilution of the desired dose in 50 mL or more of normal saline or D$_5$W.

Drug interactions: L-Asparaginase may decrease hepatic metabolism of vincristine.

Metabolism, pharmacokinetics: Vincristine is bioavailable only by the intravenous route. It is metabolized by the liver. The elimination half-life is variable but usually longer than 10 hours.

Excretion: Parent drug and metabolites are primarily excreted in the bile.

Toxicity: Vincristine is a vesicant and should be administered with extravasation precautions. Neurotoxicity is dose limiting in the form of peripheral neuropathy, which is related to total cumulative dose. Autonomic neuropathy is less common, and central nervous system toxicity is rare. Myelosuppression is mild. Nausea and vomiting are rare, but constipation is fairly common. Acute cardiopulmonary or pain symptoms occurring during administration are uncommon. Transient elevation of liver function findings is sometimes seen.

Indications: FDA-approved for Hodgkin's disease and other lymphomas, acute leukemias, rhabdomyosarcoma, neuroblastoma, and Wilm's tumor. Used for many other neoplasms as well.

Dosing: The usual dose is 0.5 to 1.4 mg/m^2 intravenous push every 1 to 4 weeks. A continuous infusion of 0.5 mg/m^2 per day over 96 hours has also been used.

VINORELBINE
(Navelbine [NVB], 5'-Noranhydrovinblastine)

Drug class, mechanism of action: Semisynthetic vinca alkaloid; inhibits tubulin polymerization, hence mitosis. G2 phase specific.

Form: Vial of 10 mg/mL solution.

Storage: Vials should be stored at 4°C protected from light. Undiluted drug in vials is stable at room temperature for 72 hours. Stability of diluted drug is not provided, so it should be used as soon as possible after dilution.

Mixing instructions: Dilute the desired dose in 100 mL normal saline or D$_5$W for 20-minute intravenous infusion.

Drug interactions: None noted.

Metabolism, pharmacokinetics: This drug has fair oral bioavailability but is available only as an intravenous preparation. It is metabolized by the liver and has an elimination half-life of about 24 hours.

Excretion: Excretion is predominantly in the bile.

Toxicity: Vinorelbine is a mild vesicant requiring extravasation precautions. Myelosuppression, mostly leukopenia, is expected and dose limiting. Significant nausea and vomiting are uncommon. Neurotoxicity in the form of neuropathy is less common and milder than is seen with vincristine. Tumor pain during administration has been reported. Acute reactions such as dyspnea, chest pain, and wheezing have occurred during administration; they may be prevented by premedication with corticosteroids.

Indications: FDA-approved for the treatment of relapsed metastatic breast cancer. Also used for non-small cell lung cancer.

Dosing: The recommended dose is 30 mg/m^2 intravenously over 20 minutes every week with dose adjustments based on leukocyte counts.

BIBLIOGRAPHY

Baltzer, L, Berkery, R, eds. Oncology pocket guide to chemotherapy. 2nd ed. St Louis: Mosby–Year Book, 1995.

Clinical pharmacology online. Version 1.13. Gold Standard Multimedia, October 14, 1997.

Fischer DS, Knobf MF, Durivage HJ, eds. The cancer chemotherapy handbook. 4th ed. St Louis: Mosby–Year Book, 1993.

Micromedex computerized clinical information system. Vol 94. Micromedex, 1997.

Perry MC, ed. The chemotherapy source book. 2nd ed. Baltimore: Williams & Wilkins, 1996.

Physicians' desk reference. 52nd ed. Montvale, NY: Medical Economics, 1998.

Section Three

Symptom Control

6
Gastrointestinal Complaints

Mary Johnson and Michael C. Perry

ANOREXIA

Loss of appetite, or anorexia, is a common problem in the cancer population, and untreated, it leads to weight loss and malnutrition. Although many agents to alleviate this condition have been tried, few have been found successful in controlled trials. Antihistamines and androgens either are ineffective or have significant side effects that prohibit their use. The current standard for both cancer and acquired immunodeficiency syndrome (AIDS) patients is megestrol acetate (Megace), typically started at 160 mg of the oral suspension daily. Corticosteroids and tetrahydrocannabinol are poor second choices.

CONSTIPATION

Constipation is a major concern and a source of discomfort for patients with cancer. Smooth muscles of the gastrointestinal tract can be affected by the neurotoxic effects of antineoplastic agents such as vincristine, vinorelbine, and vinblastine, resulting in constipation. Granisetron and ondansetron, frequently prescribed to control chemotherapy-induced nausea and vomiting, also cause constipation. Other factors contributing to constipation in this population include age, immobility, decreased fluid and fiber intake, concurrent medical problems such as stroke or hypothyroidism, hypercalcemia, hypokalemia, and medications, especially opioid analgesics, cholinergics, iron preparations, and aluminum antacids. Failure to prevent or to treat effectively contributes to nausea, anorexia, and general discomfort and can progress to obstipation or paralytic ileus. Interventions to prevent or control constipation include correction of fluid and electrolyte imbalances, dietary alterations, routine toileting, increased exercise, and the use of laxatives, rectal suppositories, or enemas.

Laxatives are classified as stimulants or irritants, saline derivatives, bulk-forming agents, wetting agents, osmotic agents, and lubricants. Selection of specific treatment choice is affected by severity of constipation, drug availability and cost, and personal preferences of patients. Rectal suppositories and enemas should be avoided in the presence of leukopenia and thrombocytopenia.

Table 6.1 identifies medications and treatments to prevent or control constipation.

DIARRHEA

Diarrhea, with or without abdominal cramping, may indicate hypermotility of the intestinal tract due to cellular damage caused by the administration of antineoplastic agents. Antimetabolites, especially 5-FU, dactinomycin, and irinotecan, are the agents most commonly associated with chemotherapy-induced diarrhea. Uncontrolled diarrhea may result in serious fluid and electrolyte imbalances, even death. It also contributes to patients' nutritional problems and feelings of fatigue, and it causes painful irritation of perianal skin.

Assessment should include the date of administration of last chemotherapy, the amount and number of stools, presence of blood, fluid and food intake, and aggravating and alleviating factors. Other possible causes of diarrhea include *Clostridium difficile* infection, inflammatory fecal disorders of the bowel, lactose deficiency, nutritional supplements, abdominal or pelvic irradiation, impaction, and medications.

Irinotecan can induce both early and late forms of diarrhea, which appear to be caused by different mechanisms. Early diarrhea, occurring within 24 hours of administration of the drug, is a cholinergic reaction that may be preceded by diaphoreses, flushing, and abdominal cramping. Intravenous atropine is the recommended treatment unless clinically contraindicated (Table 6.2). Late-onset diarrhea, which occurs 2 to 14 days after drug administration, is caused by a cytotoxic reaction. Prompt treatment of chemotherapy-induced diarrhea with an agent such as loperamide (Imodium) or diphenoxylate hydrochloride with atropine (Lomotil) is recommended. Diarrhea not responding to these treatments may require a drug such as codeine, paregoric, or octreotide. Octreotide is very effective in controlling 5-FU-associated diarrhea, but its use is limited by its parenteral route of administration and expense, especially in patients with milder symptoms.

Additional therapy includes fluid and electrolyte replacement, dietary alterations to minimize irritation of the gastrointestinal tract, and initiation of skin care measures for the perianal area (Tables 6.3 and 6.4).

NAUSEA AND VOMITING

Nausea and vomiting are two of the most common and feared symptoms associated with chemotherapy. Uncontrolled nausea and vomiting are unpleasant, contribute to anorexia and fatigue, and can result in serious problems such as fluid and electrolyte imbalance or noncompliance with treatment.

Table 6.1. Laxatives

Drug	Onset of Action	Special Considerations
Bulk laxatives: absorb water and expand to increase moisture content and bulk in stool		
Methycellulose (Citrucel)	12–24 hr	Do not administer within 1 hour of other medications (interferes with absorption); follow with an additional 8 oz fluid; most physiological laxative; safest
Psyllium (Metamucil)	Up to 72 hours	Do not administer within 1 hour of other medications (interferes with absorption); mix with 8-oz fluid and follow with an additional 8 oz; most physiological laxative; safest
Lubricants: increase water retention in stool, causing reabsorption of water in stool		
Mineral oil	6–8 hr	Increased effect of oral anticoagulants; decreased absorption of fat-soluble vitamins; avoid aspiration
Wetting agents, softeners: reduce surface tension of liquids in the bowel		
Docusate (Colace, Surfak/Dialose)	24–72 hr	Do not take within 1 hour of antacids, milk, or H_2-blockers
Stimulants: increase peristalsis by direct effect on the intestines		
Bisacodyl (Dulcolax, Correctol, Feen-A-Mint)	6–12 hr	Causes gastric irritation if taken within 1 hour of antacids, milk, H_2-blockers.
Cascara	6–12 hr	Do not take within 1 hour of other drugs.
Senna (Senokot, SenokotXtra)	6–12 hr	Urine may turn pink, red, or black
Saline laxatives: draw water into the intestinal lumen		
Magnesium salts (Milk of Magnesia)	30 min–6 hours	Administer with 8 oz water
Sodium biphosphate, sodium phosphate (Phospho-soda)	30 min–6 hours	Do not take within 1 hour of other medications
Magnesium citrate (Citroma)	30 min–6 hours	Administer with 8 oz fluid Use with caution in the presence of renal disease

continued

Table 6.1. Laxatives *continued*

Drug	Onset of Action	Special Considerations
Osmotics: increase distention and promote peristalsis		
Glycerin suppository or rectal solution	15–30 min	Patient should remain recumbent after administration to prevent headache from cerebral dehydration
Lactulose (Chronulac)	24–48 hr	Mix with juice, water, or milk to counteract sweet taste
Sorbitol	24–48 hr	
Combinations: stool softener plus stimulants		
Docusate sodium, Casanthranol (Peri-Colace, DSS plus)		Do not take within 1 hour of antacids, milk, or H_2-blockers

ANTICONSTIPATION RECIPES

Ingredients	Preparation	Dose
Fruit paste 1 lb pitted prunes 1 lb raisins 1 lb figs 3½–4 oz pkg senna tea 1 cup brown sugar 1 cup lemon juice	Prepare tea: Use about 3½ cups boiling water per pkg of tea Steep 5 minutes Strain tea to remove tea leaves Add only 2 cups tea to large pot Boil tea and fruit 5 minutes Remove from heat; add lemon juice and sugar Cool Use food processor or blender to turn mixture into smooth paste Place in glass or plastic containers; store in freezer. Paste will not freeze but keeps for a long time.	Take 1 or 2 tablespoons daily
Alternative fruit recipe 12 oz each prunes, raisins, dates, figs 2 oz powdered senna	Grind fruits Add powdered senna Mix well Pat into 9 × 13 pan Cut into 1½ × 1½ in. squares Refrigerate or freeze for later use	Usual dose is 1 square

continued

Table 6.1. Laxatives *continued*

ANTICONSTIPATION RECIPES		
Ingredients	Preparation	Dose
Bran recipe 2 cups bran 2 cups applesauce 1 cup prune juice	Mix well	2–3 tablespoons b.i.d.

Table 6.2. Antidiarrheal Agents

Drug	Dose	Comments
Atropine	0.25 mg–1 mg IV	Used for early onset irinotecan-induced diarrhea; OTC
Kaolin, pectin (Kaopectate)	2 caplets or 300 mL; repeat as needed after each loose stool; maximum 12 caplets/24 hr	
Diphenoxylate, atropine (Lomotil)	2 tabs p.o. q.i.d. or 2 tabs initially, then 1 after each additional stool; maximum of 8 tabs/24 hr	Opioid
Codeine	30–60 mg p.o. 4–6 hr	
Loperamide (Imodium)	4 mg p.o. initially, then 2 mg after each loose stool; maximum 16 mg/24 hr	Nonopioid; OTC
Tincture of opium	0.6 mL p.o. q 4–6 hr	Opioid; 6 mg morphine equivalent to 0.6-mL dose
Paregoric	5–10 mL p.o. q.d.–q.i.d.	Opioid; 2 mg morphine equivalent to 5-mL dose
Octreotide	50–200 µg s.q. b.i.d.–t.i.d.	

OTC, over the counter.

The physiology of emesis is better understood than nausea. The vomiting center in the lateral medullary radicular formation of the brain is the final common pathway for stimuli causing vomiting. Central and peripheral neurologic pathways that can stimulate the vomiting center include pharyngeal afferents, vagal afferents, midbrain afferent, chemoreceptor trigger zone, and vestibular system. The vagus nerve is thought to

Table 6.3. Diarrhea: Dietary Alterations and Fluid Replacement

Drink at least 3 L/24 hours fluids containing glucose to induce resorption of sodium and decrease stool volume: Gatorade, bouillon, apple juice, gelatin, grape juice

Eat small, frequent meals, avoiding hot or cold foods

Avoid milk or milk products in presence of lactose intolerance. Buttermilk and yogurt are generally tolerated.

Low-residue diet high in protein and calories

    Rice, spaghetti, and noodles

    Ice cream, sherbet, and gelatin

    Eggs, cheese, and cottage cheese

    Bananas, applesauce

    Cooked fruits and vegetables without seeds or skins

    White, refined wheat, or light rye bread

    Refined cereals such as cream of wheat, cornflakes, puffed rice

    Tender meat, poultry, or fish

Table 6.4. Diarrhea: Perianal Skin Care

Cleanse the perianal area with tepid water and mild soap after each bowel movement; peri-bottle may help reduce irritation of cleansing. Dry skin with a hair dryer on low setting.

Frequent sitz baths.

Allow area to be exposed to air as much as possible. Wear loose-fitting clothing, preferably cotton undergarments.

Use A&D or zinc-containing ointment on irritated areas.

be the most important afferent for chemotherapy-associated emesis. Nausea is completely subjective and does not always result in vomiting.

Three phases of nausea and vomiting have been identified. The acute phase occurs within minutes to hours after the administration of chemotherapy and lasts about 24 hours. Delayed nausea and/or vomiting begins 24 hours after administration and may last for several days. The mechanisms causing delayed nausea and/or vomiting may differ from those of the acute phase; they have not been well defined. Anticipatory nausea or vomiting is a conditioned response to prior chemotherapy administration that caused nausea or vomiting.

Helping the patient prevent or manage nausea and vomiting is more complex with multiple-day drug administration and/or combination chemotherapy. With multiple-day administration the acute phase is repeated daily and the mechanisms associated with delayed nausea or vomiting continue. Combination chemotherapy may increase the severity of the potential for nausea or vomiting, depending on the emetic potential of the individual agents (Table 6.5).

Clinicians can be aided in selecting an antiemetic regimen by considering drug-related factors and patient-related factors. Drug-related factors include the emetogenic potential of each neoplastic agent, expected time of onset, and duration of the symptoms. Important patient-related factors include age, gender, history of chemotherapy (especially if nausea and vomiting were not controlled), coexisting illness, drug allergies or sensitivities, concomitant medications, and alcohol intake. Use of antiemetic drugs from several classifications may be necessary to control nausea and vomiting through the acute and delayed phases (Table 6.6). In selecting these agents the site of action and relative efficacy of the drug or drugs, potential side effects, cost, and patient's preferences should all be considered.

Symptoms of esophageal reflux such as retrosternal burning or water brash may contribute to the patient's discomfort. Patients may even confuse these symptoms with nausea. These patients may benefit from the addition of medications used to treat acid peptic disease (Table 6.7).

MUCOSITIS

Cytotoxic effects of antineoplastic agents on replicating mucosal cells can result in mucositis. Mucositis causes mild to severe discomfort, effects fluid and nutritional intake, interferes with communication, and may require treatment delays and/or chemotherapy dose reductions.

The agents most commonly associated with oral mucositis are 5-FU, doxorubicin, daunorubicin, methotrexate, bleomycin, busulfan, mitomycin, dactinomycin, and cytarabine. Other risk factors include radiation therapy to the head and neck area, smoking, alcohol use, malnutrition, age, steroids, and preexisting dental disease. The onset of oral mucositis or stomatitis is typically 5 to 7 days after the administration of antineoplastic agents, and healing occurs 10 to 14 days after cessation of therapy. Indirect stomatotoxicity secondary to myelosuppression can occur. Indirect effects on the oral mucosa occur 12 to 14 days after chemotherapy administration, during the granulocyte nadir. Patients may be at risk for local bacterial, viral, or fungal infections, which may lead to systemic infection.

Pretreatment dental evaluation is ideal, and good oral hygiene should be reinforced or implemented. Cryotherapy may help decrease the incidence or severity of oral mucositis. To use cryotherapy, patients suck on ice for 5 minutes prior to the

Table 6.5. Emetogenic Potential of Antineoplastic Agents

Incidence	Agent	Onset (hours)	Duration (hours)
High: >90%	Carmustine >200 mg/m^2	2–4	4–24
	Cisplatin ≥50 mg/m^2	1–4	24–120
	Cyclophosphamide >1,000 mg/m^2	2–12	< 24
	Dacarbazine ≥500 mg/m^2	1–3	1–12
	Ifosfamide ≥1.5 g/m^2	2–6	< 24
	Lomustine ≤60 mg/m^2	3–6	< 24
	Mechlorethamine	0.5–3	8–24
	Streptozocin	2–4	< 24
Moderately high: 60–90%	Carmustine <200 mg/m^2		
	Cisplatin <50 mg/m^2		
	Cyclophosphamide		
	Cytarabine >500 mg/m^2	6–12	3–12
	Dacarbazine <500 mg/m^2	1–3	1–12
	Dactinomycin	1–4	4–20
	Daunorubicin >50 mg/m^2	2–6	6–24
	Doxorubicin >60 mg/m^2	4–6	6–24
	Methotrexate >1,000 mg/m^2	4–12	3–12
	Procarbazine	24–27	Varies
Moderate: 30–60%	Altretamine		
	Carboplatin	1–6	4–24
	Cyclophosphamide <600 mg/m^2		
	Daunorubicin <50 mg/m^2		
	Doxorubicin <50 mg/m^2		
	Estramustine		
	Fluorouracil >1,000 mg/m^2	3–6	2–24
	Idarubicin		
	Irinotecan		
	L-Asparaginase		
	Mitomycin	1–4	48–72
	Mitoxantrone	2–6	6–24
	Pentostatin		
	Topotecan		
Moderately low: 10–30%	Bleomycin	3–6	1–4
	Cladribine		
	Cyclophosphamide (oral)		
	Docetaxel		
	Etoposide	3–8	1–4
	Fludara		
	Gemcitabine		
	Melphalan		

continued

Table 6.5. Emetogenic Potential of Antineoplastic Agents *continued*

Incidence	Agent	Onset (hours)	Duration (hours)
	Mercaptopurine		
	Methotrexate <100 mg/m²		
	Paclitaxel	4–8	—
	Teniposide		
	Thioguanine		
	Thiotepa		
Low: <10%	Busulfan		
	Chlorambucil		
	Hydroxyurea		
	Vinblastine		
	Vincristine		
	Vinorelbine		

Adapted with permission from Borison & McCarthy, Ettinger, & Lindley et al.

administration of agents likely to cause oral mucositis during drug administration and for 30 minutes afterward. This intervention is not practical for prolonged or continuous infusions.

The goals of therapy for established oral mucositis are to provide comfort, maintain nutritional status, prevent bleeding, and prevent infection or institute early treatment of it. Nutritional guidelines are listed in Table 6.8. Patients with severe oral mucositis who are unable to maintain adequate fluid intake may require parenteral support.

Topical focal application of anesthetic agents is preferred to avoid the discomfort of generalized oral mucosal anesthesia. However, topical rinses and/or systemic analgesia may be required to control the discomfort of extensive oral mucositis (Table 6.9). Patients at risk for bleeding (platelet count less than 20,000/mm³) should modify oral hygiene regimens to decrease trauma to oral tissue.

The most frequent cause of oral infection is fungus, which appears as superficial white plaques on mucosal surfaces. Herpes simplex virus is the most common viral pathogen affecting the oral cavity. Cultures of suspicious areas are recommended, as these lesions are often difficult to distinguish from other infectious lesions or chemotherapy-induced mucositis. Options for treatment are included in Table 6.9.

The mucosal lining of the esophagus is histologically the same as the oral cavity, and patients with oral mucositis may develop esophagitis as well. The risk is increased if the patient is receiving

Table 6.6. Antiemetic Agents

Drug	Route, Dose	Common Side Effects	Special Considerations
Serotonin antagonists: block serotonin centrally and peripherally			
Dolasetron (Anzemet)	p.o. 100 mg before chemotherapy	Constipation, headache	Antiemetic efficacy increased by adding dexamethasone
Granisetron (Kytril)	p.o. 1–2 mg before chemotherapy; may repeat 1 mg in 12 hr i.v.p. 10 µg/kg 1 mg before chemotherapy Or	Constipation, headache	Antiemetic efficacy increased by adding dexamethasone
Ondansetron (Zofran)	p.o. 4–8 mg q 8 hr i.v.p.b. 15 mg/kg q 2–4 hr × 3 doses Or 24–30 mg loading dose	Headache, constipation	Antiemetic efficacy increased by adding dexamethasone Give larger i.v. doses over 30–45 min to prevent dizziness
Corticosteroids: may inhibit prostaglandin release, enhance effects of the other antiemetic agents			
Dexamethasone (Decadron)	p.o. or IV 10–20 mg before chemotherapy; 10 mg q 6–12 hr on multiple day infusions tapering doses afterward		Rapid IV administration causes perineal burning/itching

Benzodiazepines: block
cortical pathways;
anxiolytic amnesic

Lorazepam (Ativan)   p.o. 0.5–2 mg q 4 hr
SL 0.5–2 mg q 4 hr
i.v. 0.5–2 mg q 4 hr   Sedation, blurred vision,
confusion, postural
hypotension, amnesia,
urinary incontinence   Reduce doses in the elderly; use
with caution in patients with
hepatic, venal, or respiratory
dysfunction; may aggravate
CNS effects of ifosfamide

H-Receptor antagonists:
block histamine response,
may block chemoreceptor
trigger zone, decrease
vestibular stimulation;
primarily treat or prevent
extrapyramidal symptoms

Diphenhydramine
(Benadryl)   p.o. 25–50 mg q 4 hr
i.v. 12.5–50 mg q 4 hr   Dizziness, euphoria, dry
mouth, urinary retention,
sedation, blurred vision   Decrease effect of oral
anticoagulants and heparin;
compatible in solution with
metoclopramide,
dexamethasone

Substituted benzamides:
central and peripheral
blocking of dopamine at
chemoreceptor trigger
zone; high concentrations
block serotonin receptors
in GI tract; stimulate
upper GI tract

continued

Table 6.6.   Antiemetic Agents *continued*

Drug	Route, Dose	Common Side Effects	Special Considerations
Metoclopramide (Reglan)	i.v. 1–3 mg/kg before chemotherapy; then 1–3 mg/kg q 2–3 hr × 3–5 doses p.o. 0.5 mg/kg q.i.d. for delayed nausea and vomiting	Extrapyramidal symptoms, sedation, dry mouth, diarrhea	Compatible in solution with dexamethasone, diphenhydramine; resolve acute extrapyramidal symptoms by administering diphenhydramine 50 mg slow i.v.; may give concomitantly with diphenhydramine to avoid extrapyramidal symptoms
Cisapride (Propulsid)	p.o. 10 mg before meals, at bedtime	Minimal extrapyramidal symptoms	
Butyrophenones: dopamine antagonists in chemoreceptor trigger zone			
Droperidol (Inapsine)	i.v. 0.5–2.5 mg q 4 hr	Extrapyramidal symptoms may be severe; sedation, chills, facial sweating, postural hypotension	Use with other CNS depressants may have additive effect; decreases efforts of anticonvulsants; resolve acute extrapyramidal symptoms by administering diphenhydramine 50 mg slow i.v.

Drug	Mechanism	Dosage	Side effects	Comments
Haloperidol (Haldol)		p.o. 3–5 mg q 4 hr i.v. 1–2 mg q 2–6 hr	Extrapyramidal symptoms, drowsiness	More effective in younger adults; increased CNS toxicity in the elderly
Cannabinoids: depress CNS, indirectly blocking vomiting center Dronabinol (Marinol)		p.o. 5–10 mg q 4 hr	Mood changes, disorientation, drowsiness, increased appetite, impairment of coordination	
Phenothiazines: centrally block dopamine receptors in chemoreceptor trigger zone; peripherally decrease vagal stimulation of vomiting center				
Chlorpromazine (Thorazine)		p.o. 25–50 mg q 4–6 hr i.v. 12.5–50 mg q 4–6 hr	Extrapyramidal symptoms, akathisia, anxiety, dizziness, limb dystonia, oculogyric crisis, torticollis, tremor, trismus, drowsiness	Use with caution in the elderly; causes postural hypotension; resolve acute extrapyramidal symptoms by administering diphenhydramine 50 mg slow i.v.
Prochlorperazine (Compazine)		p.o. tablets 10 mg q 4–6 hr p.o. sustained release 10–15 mg q 8–12 hr i.v. 10–20 mg q 4 hr PR 25 mg q 4–6 hr		Resolve acute extrapyramidal symptoms by administering diphenhydramine 50 mg slow i.v.

continued

Table 6.6. Antiemetic Agents *continued*

Drug	Route, Dose	Common Side Effects	Special Considerations
Thiethylperazine (Torecan)	p.o. 10 mg q 4 hr i.m. 10 mg q 4 hr pr 10 mg q 4 hr	Extrapyramidal symptoms	Resolve acute extrapyramidal symptoms by administering diphenhydramine 50 mg slow i.v.
Promethazine— Phenothiazine derivative (Phenergan)	p.o. 25 mg q 4 hr i.v. 12.5–25 mg q 4 hr pr 12.5–25 mg q 4 hr	Drowsiness	Inadvertent intra-arterial injection can result in gangrene of affected extremity; i.v. rate should not exceed 25 mg/min

Table 6.7. Medications Used to Control Gastroesophageal Reflux Symptoms

Medication	Dose
Histamine receptor antagonists	
Cimetidine (Tagamet)	400 mg b.i.d., Or 800 mg at h.s.
Famotodine (Pepcid)	20 mg b.i.d., Or 40 mg at h.s.
Ranitidine (Zantac)	150 mg b.i.d., Or 300 mg at h.s.
Proton pump inhibitors	
Omeprazole (Prilosec)	20 mg daily

Table 6.8. Dietary Guidelines for Patients with Oral Mucositis

Avoid foods that are irritating to oral mucosa, especially spiced, acidic, or salted foods.

Use blenderized foods if necessary. Avoid extremely hot or cold foods.

Add extra calories to soups, cereals, and milkshakes with dry powdered milk or dietary supplements.

Encourage fluids. Fruit nectars or juices strained from canned fruit may be soothing to oral mucosa and add extra calories.

concurrent radiation therapy that includes the esophagus. Symptoms include dysphagia, odynophagia, and epigastric discomfort. In addition to the interventions listed in the table these patients may benefit from the addition of an H_2-blocker or proton pump inhibitor. Flexible endoscopy with brushings may be indicated to diagnose suspected infections.

XEROSTOMIA

Xerostomia (dry mouth) is a common complication after radiation of the head and neck, whether for primary head and neck cancers or lymphomas. There are numerous proprietary and home-made artificial saliva solutions available to replace the loss of salivary secretions. The latest treatment is the use of oral pilocarpine (Salagen), which is moderately successful. The dose is one 5-mg tablet three times daily, gradually increased to maximum benefit with minimal side effects. Side effects include sweating, nausea, headache, frequent urination, chills, dizziness, runny nose, flushing, and visual changes, especially at night. The ophthalmic solution has also been used orally but is

Table 6.9. Prevention and Management of Oral Mucositis

Agent and Use	Schedule	Comments
Cleansing agents; routine oral cleaning after meals, at bedtime, as needed; avoid commercial mouthwashes containing alcohol		
Normal saline, baking soda 1 tsp each in 1 quart water	After meals, at bedtime, as needed	
Hydrogen peroxide 3% diluted to ¼ strength	After meals, at bedtime	Mix before using; not recommended with ulceration; prevents tissue granulation
Lubricating agents; use only water-soluble agents		
K-Y Jelly	As needed	
Stay Moist Lip Balm	As needed	
Coating agents		
Hurricane	As needed for discomfort	Available as gel, liquid, spray; no systemic absorption
Hydrocortisone acetate (Orabase)	As needed	Apply often; short duration of action
Oral benzocaine (Oratect Gel)	Use up to q.i.d.	Transient stinging when applied; do not remove film
Sucralfate	After meals, at bedtime	No anesthetic action
Zilactin	Use up to q.i.d.	Transient burning sensation on application
Topical anesthetics; apply locally or use as rinse		
Dyclonine hydrochloride 0.5%	15 mL as needed for discomfort; swish and spit	Minimal absorption
Magic mouthwash: equal parts viscous lidocaine, calcium carbonate (Maalox), diphenhydramine syrup	10–15 mL as needed for discomfort; swish, gargle, and spit or may swallow	If swallowed, limit doses; diphenhydramine may cause drowsiness

continued

Table 6.9. Prevention and Management of Oral Mucositis *continued*

Agent and Use	Schedule	Comments
Mu-Coat: nystatin, hydrocortisone sodium succinate (Solu-Cortef), lidocaine 1%, sucralfate, Ora-Plus, Syrpalta	10–15 mL as needed for discomfort; swish, gargle, and spit or may swallow	Anesthetic and coating action
Ulcerease	15 mL; swish and spit q 2 hr as needed for discomfort	
Lidocaine (Xylocaine Viscous) 2%	Swish and spit as needed; do not exceed 120 mL in 24 hr	Systemically absorbed; adding warm water may increase palatability
Antifungal agents		
Clotrimazole	10-mg troche 5×/ day × 14 days	
Fluconazole	200 mg day 1; 100 mg/day × 7–14 days	Decrease dose for impaired renal function
Ketoconazole	200 mg/day × 7–14 days	No antacids for 2 hr after administration
Nystatin	400,000–600,000 U q.i.d. × 7–14 days; must swish 5 min	No food or water for 30 min after use
Antiviral agents		
Acyclovir	200 mg 5×/day × 10 days	
Famciclovir	500 mg t.i.d. × 7 days	
Valacyclovir	1,000 mg b.i.d. × 10 days	

not approved for this use. Pilocarpine ophthalmic solution 4% is used: 4 drops equals 5 mg. Any amount of liquid may be used. Dosing usually starts with 5 mg three times daily titrated to maximum benefit with minimal side effects as mentioned earlier.

BIBLIOGRAPHY

Anorexia

Loprinzi CL, Michalia JC, Schaid DJ, et al. Phase III evaluation of four doses of megestrol acetate as therapy for patients with cancer anorexia and/or cachexia. J Clin Oncol 1993;11:762–767.

Nelson KA, Walsh TD, Sheehan FA. The cancer anorexia-cachexia syndrome. J Clin Oncol 1994;12:213–225.

Puccio M, Nathanson L. The cancer cachexia syndrome. Semin Oncol 1997;24:277–287.

Constipation

Hogue V. Diarrhea and constipation. In: Herfindal E, Gourley D, eds. Textbook of therapeutics: drug and disease management. Baltimore: Williams & Wilkins, 1996;517–531.

Levy MH. Constipation and diarrhea in cancer patients. Cancer Bull 1991;43:412–422.

Wright PE, Thomas S. Constipation and diarrhea: the neglected symptoms. Semin Oncol Nurs 1995;11:289–297.

Diarrhea

Gebbia V, Garseca I, Testa A, et al. Subcutaneous octreotide versus oral loperamide in the treatment of diarrhea following chemotherapy. Anticancer Drugs 1993;4;443–445.

Camptosar. Irinotecan hydrochloride. Kalamazoo, MI: Pharmacia & Upjohn, 1997.

Cascinu S, Fedeli A, Fedeli S, et al. Octreotide versus loperamide in the treatment of fluoroaracil induced diarrhea: a randomized trial. J Clin Oncol 1993;11: 148–151.

Nausea and Vomiting

Andrews P, Davis C. The mechanism of emesis induced by anticancer therapies. In: Andrews P, Sanger E, eds. Emesis in anticancer therapy: mechanisms and treatment. New York: Chapman and Hall Medical, 1993;113–161.

Borison H, McCarthy L. Neuropharmacology of chemotherapy induced emesis. Drugs 1993;25: 8–17.

Ettinger D. Preventing chemotherapy induced nausea and vomiting: an update and review of emesis. Semin Oncol 1995;22(Suppl):6–18.

Gralla R, Rittenberg C, Peralta M, et al. Cisplatin and emesis: aspects of treatment and a new trial for delayed emesis using oral dexamethasone plus ondansetron beginning at 16 hours after cisplatin. Oncology 1996;1:86–91.

Hesketh P, Kris M, Grunberg S., et al. Proposal for classifying the acute emetogenicity of cancer chemotherapy. J Clin Oncol 1997;15:103–109.

Hesketh P, Murphy W, Lester E, et al. GR38032F (GR-507/75): a novel compound effective in the prevention of acute cisplatin-induced emesis. J Clin Oncol 1989;7:700–705.

Italian Group for Antiemetic Research. Persistence of efficacy of three antiemetic regimens and prognostic factors in patients undergoing moderately emetogenic chemotherapy. J Clin Oncol 1995;13:2417–2426.

Lindley C, Bernard S, Fields S. Incidence and duration of chemotherapy induced nausea and vomiting in the outpatient oncology population. J Clin Oncol 1989;7:1142–1149.

Mucositis

Madeya M. Oral complications from cancer therapy: part 2. Nursing implications for assessment and treatment. Oncol Nurs Forum 1996;23:808–819.

Mahood DJ, Dose A, Loprinzi C, et al. Inhibition of fluorouracil-induced stomatitis by oral cryotherapy. J Clin Oncol 1991;9:449–452.

Peterson D. Oral toxicity of chemotherapeutic agents. Semin Oncol 1992;19:478–491.

Sonis S, Clark J. Prevention and management of oral mucositis induced by antineoplastic therapy. Oncology 1991;5:11–18.

Xerostomia

Johnson JT, Ferretti GA, Nethery, et al. Oral pilocarpine for post-irradiation xerostomia in patients with head and neck cancer. N Engl J Med 1993;329:390–395.

LeVeque FG, Montgomery M, Potter D, et al. A multicenter, randomized, double-blind, placebo-controlled, dose-titration study of oral pilocarpine for treatment of radiation-induced xerostomia in head and neck cancer patients. J Clin Oncol 1993;11:1124–1131.

7
Pain Control
Mary Johnson and Michael C. Perry

GENERAL GUIDELINES

Pain is almost certainly the most feared consequence of cancer and its treatment, and there is ample evidence that in spite of general agreement that pain relief is attainable in more than 90% of patients, many patients continue to suffer. Analgesic programs should be tailored to the type and degree of pain. The patient's description of the pain is the first step in determining its origin and causation. The examiner should note the location and character of the pain and any precipitating, aggravating, and relieving influences; delineate the progress or course of the pain; and assess any associated symptoms. This is also the time to estimate the effects of age, gender, and cultural and psychological influences on the patient's pain. We ask the patient to grade the pain on a scale of 1 to 10, with 10 being the worst pain imaginable and 0 no pain at all. This is also helpful to measure success in pain relief.

A routine physical examination and a specific neurologic examination should be performed, and a diagnostic evaluation, which may include routine radiographs, computed tomography, magnetic resonance imaging, radionuclide scans, and so on. It is also useful to assign the patient's pain to one of three categories: musculoskeletal, visceral, or neuritic. This guides the use of specific therapies for specific types of pain. Table 7.1 lists analgesics by class.

Musculoskeletal pain often responds to nonsteroidal anti-inflammatory drugs (NSAIDs), with or without opioids. Painful bony metastases often respond well to radiation therapy, reducing the need for opioids. Samarium and strontium are radioisotopes that concentrate in bone, providing palliation in patients with bone metastases from breast or prostate cancer.

Neuritic pains are often the most difficult to control; Table 7.2 lists some adjuvant analgesic agents that are occasionally effective, even if we do not fully understand their mechanisms of action. Refractory pain may require transcutaneous electrical stimulation (TENS), anesthetics, or neurosurgical intervention.

Several opioid analgesics are available for severe visceral pain, but they are often used in less than optimal fashion, at

Table 7.1. Nonopioid Agents

Class	Agent	Starting Dose, Schedule
NSAIDs		
Acetic acids	Diclofenac	25 mg q 8 hr
	Indomethacin	25 mg q 8 hr
	Ketorolac (long-term use not recommended)	10 mg q 6 hr after 20-mg loading dose
	Sulindac	150 mg q 12 hr
	Tolmetin	200 mg q 8 hr
Propionic acids	Flurbiprofen	100 mg q 12 hr
	Ibuprofen	400 mg q 6 hr
	Ketoprofen	25 mg q 6 hr
	Naproxen	250 mg q 12 hr
Salicylate	Aspirin	650 mg q 4 hr
Antidepressants	Amitriptyline	10–25 mg q.d.
	Desipramine	10–25 mg q.d.
	Doxepin	25–50 mg q.d.
	Imipramine	10–25 mg q.d.
	Nortriptyline	25–50 mg q.d.
	Trazodone	50 mg t.i.d.
Corticosteroid	Decadron	2–20 mg q 12 hr
Para-aminophenol derivative	Acetaminophen	650 mg q 4–6 hr
Anticonvulsants	Carbamazepine	200 mg q 6–8 hr
	Clonazepam	0.5 mg q 12 hr
	Phenytoin	300 mg q.d. at bedtime
	Valproic acid	15 mg/kg q.d.

doses that are too small and at intervals that are too long. The appropriate choice of a drug is directed by the needs of the individual patient and the physician's knowledge of the pharmacologic properties of the analgesic drug. A detailed knowledge of several agents is better than a casual knowledge of many. When switching opioid analgesics, it is important to use equianalgesic doses (Table 7.3).

The oral route of administration is preferred for convenience if possible, but opioids can also be given by parenteral, rectal, or transdermal routes. Oral analgesics take longer to have an effect than parenteral drugs, but the effect is longer lasting. We prefer to give a long-acting opioid such as oxycodone (OxyContin) or morphine sulfate (MS Contin) along with a shorter-acting agent such as oxycodone or MSIR for breakthrough pain. The goal is to provide adequate plasma levels of the drug for satisfactory relief.

Table 7.2. Selected Opioid Agents

Drug	Starting Dose (mg)		Duration of Action (hours)	Comments
	Oral	i.v., i.m.		
Short acting				
Codeine	30	30 i.m.	4–6	Often used in combination
Oxycodone	5	—	3–5	Elixir available
Hydromorphone	4–8	75	2–3	
Meperidine	100	75	3	
Morphine	15–30	10	4–6	Elixir available
Long acting				
Morphine controlled release	15–30	—	8–12	
Oxycodone (OxyContin)	10	—	8–12	
Morphine sustained release	20	—	24	
Fentanyl patch	Starting dose not to exceed 25 mg/hr for opioid-naive patient		72	

Table 7.3. Opioid Agents: Equianalgesic Doses

Drug	i.v., i.m. (mg)	Oral (mg)	Conversion Factor, i.v. to Oral	Duration of Action (hours)
Codeine	130	200	1.5	3–4
Hydrocodone	—	30	—	3–4
Hydromorphone	1.5	7.5	5	2–3
Meperidine	100	300	4	2–3
Methadone	10	20	2	6–8
Morphine	10	30	3	3–4
Oxycodone	—	30	—	3–5
Propoxyphene	—	65–130	—	4–6

Every patient who is taking opioids should also be on a prophylactic bowel program, with high-fluid, high-fiber intake and stool softeners or laxatives as needed. Many patients believe they are "allergic" to codeine and its derivatives because of nausea and vomiting when the drug is ingested. An antiemetic such as prochlorperazine given in advance may make these drugs tolerable.

Patients should be reevaluated daily about the degree and duration of their pain relief and any medication-related side effects. Many patients develop tolerance as a natural consequence of prolonged opioid use. Increased analgesic requirements therefore may not mean progressive disease. These patients simply need more analgesics.

MUSCULOSKELETAL PAIN

There are three major causes of musculoskeletal pain following chemotherapy: paclitaxel administration, steroid withdrawal, and postchemotherapy rheumatism. The introduction of paclitaxel (Taxol) has brought an unusual adverse event, musculoskeletal pain, into notice. More than half of patients receiving it have arthralgias and myalgias that last 2 to 3 days. The symptoms are typically worst in the back and legs. For a small proportion of patients the symptoms are severe enough that if untreated, they lead to noncompliance with treatment. It is not clear whether the syndrome is seen more frequently with shorter infusion times, but prior to treatment patients should be warned of the possibility of developing musculoskeletal pain and encouraged to report it at once if it occurs.

Mild cases of arthralgia–myalgia syndrome can be managed with NSAIDs and moderate cases with corticosteroids. Prednisone 40 mg daily has been used effectively. Severe cases may require opioid analgesics. Some physicians use prophylactic therapy with dexamethasone 4 mg twice a day, starting 2 days after paclitaxel and continuing for 3 days, then 4 mg daily for 3 days.

There are two other important syndromes following chemotherapy: steroid withdrawal and postchemotherapy rheumatism. Many patients, especially older patients, find that their arthritic complaints improve when they are first placed on corticosteroids, only to find that they feel increased pain and discomfort following steroid withdrawal. The solution to this is to taper the corticosteroids slowly, typically by cutting the dose 50% daily.

Postchemotherapy rheumatism has been described in women receiving adjuvant chemotherapy for breast cancer, although it may be seen in other patient populations. Patients developed myalgias and/or arthralgias 1 to 3 months after chemotherapy with cyclophosphamide and 5-FU; resolution occurred over several months. Recognition of the possibility of this syndrome is key, as it appears to be self-limiting.

NEUROPATHIC PAIN

Neuropathic pain is the burning, dysesthetic numbness that occasionally follows a surgical procedure such as mastectomy, thoracotomy, or amputation. Some patients continue to experience this disabling pain for months to years after the procedure, and treatment is often unsuccessful. Current theory holds that substance P, a member of the tachykinin peptide family, is the cutaneous neurotransmitter causing these painful nociceptive impulses. Capsaicin, found in hot chili peppers, depletes substance P in small sensory neurons, both peripherally and centrally. It causes the release of substance P from stores within the sensory neurons and then inhibits both resynthesis and the axonal transport of substance P. In a recent clinical trial comparing capsaicin with placebo, capsaicin, applied to the affected area four times daily, decreased postsurgical neuropathic pain despite more toxicities than the placebo. In our experience it may be helpful for postherpetic neuralgia as well.

BIBLIOGRAPHY

General Guidelines

Foley KM. The treatment of cancer pain. N Engl J Med 1985;313:84–95.

Perry, MC. Pain management. In: Philip S Schein, ed. Decision making in oncology. Philadelphia: BC Decker, 1989;222–225.

Musculoskeletal Pain

Good TA, Benton JW, Kelley VC. Symptomatology resulting from withdrawal of steroid hormone therapy. Arthritis Rheum 1959;2:299–321.

Loprinzi CL, Duffy J, Ingle JN. Postchemotherapy rheumatism. J Clin Oncol 1993;11:768–770.

Palmieri F, Thomas M. Management of arthralgia/myalgia associated with semisynthetic Taxol (paclitaxel) injection administration. Princeton, NJ: Bristol-Myers Squibb, 1997.

Schiller JH, Storer B, Tutsch K, et al. A phase I trial of 3-hour infusions of paclitaxel (Taxol) with or without granulocyte colony-stimulating factor. Semin Oncol 1994;21:9–14.

Neuropathic Pain

Ellison N, Loprinzi CL, Kugler J, et al. Phase III placebo-controlled trial of capsaicin cream in the management of surgical neuropathic pain in cancer patients. J Clin Oncol 1997;15:2974–2980.

8
Other Problems

Mary Johnson and Michael C. Perry

CESSATION OF MENSES

It is fairly common for a premenopausal woman to undergo chemotherapy that carries the risk of thrombocytopenia, which can produce heavier than usual bleeding with the onset of a regular menstrual period. This situation is not usually a problem when the thrombocytopenia is expected to be minimal or brief. However, in the setting of prolonged and severe thrombocytopenia, following the induction of marrow aplasia after antileukemic therapy or high-dose chemotherapy prior to stem cell rescue, for example, this can be a significant bleeding risk. Cessation of menses can be accomplished with the continuous use of birth control pills such as Ortho-Novum 1/35–28 until platelet counts are sufficient. A second option is the administration of methoxyprogesterone (Depo-Provera) 150 mg intramuscularly prior to the onset of chemotherapy. This has the advantage of minimizing the risks of noncompliance. A third option is megestrol (Megace) 40 mg orally daily.

COUGH

Although usually a protective mechanism, a persistent cough can be debilitating. Treatment of sinus drainage may be all that is required, but some patients have a cough that is due to tumor involvement, typically an endobronchial lesion from lung cancer. If the lesion cannot be treated with radiation therapy or chemotherapy, suppression with oxycodone syrup starting at 5 mg every 4 hours may be helpful.

DYSPNEA

Many of the causes of shortness of breath, or dyspnea, can be specifically addressed: draining a pleural effusion or administering transfusions for anemia, for example. Lymphangitic carcinoma, which most commonly results from breast cancer, produces dyspnea, often extreme. Corticosteroids, starting at prednisone 20 to 40 mg daily, may produce symptomatic relief until chemotherapy reduces the intrapulmonary tumor.

FATIGUE

Complaints of fatigue and weakness are very common in an oncology practice and often go without a clear explanation. It is important to consider nonmalignant causes, such as hypothyroidism, adrenal insufficiency, and poorly controlled diabetes, as potential causes. Many patients who have just started to take opioid analgesics have some fatigue. Most patients tolerate some degree of anemia, but virtually all become symptomatic at hemoglobin levels of 7 g or less. Anemia due to hypoproliferative erythropoiesis may be improved with the use of erythropoietin 10,000 U weekly or 150 U/kg three times weekly.

FEVER

Fever accompanied by shaking chills or rigors is fairly common following the administration of either amphotericin B or interferon. Prophylactic meperidine (Demerol) may prevent both chills and fever through an unknown mechanism. Doses of 50 to 100 mg an hour before administration of the causative agent are often successful. Fever from bleomycin administration is fairly common and can often be prevented with acetaminophen 650 mg and diphenhydramine (Benadryl) given beforehand.

FLUID RETENTION

A unique fluid retention syndrome characterized by poorly tolerated peripheral edema, ascites, pleural or pericardial effusions, or anasarca occurs in up to 6% of patients who receive docetaxel chemotherapy, despite the use of a 3-day dexamethasone premedication schedule. It is cumulative in incidence and severity. The cause is unknown; it is not associated with any cardiac, renal, hepatic, or metabolic disorder. It is reversible with the ces-

Table 8.1. Pharmacologic Treatment for Hiccups

Medication	Typical Dose
Chlorpromazine	25–50 mg i.v. over several hours
	25–50 mg i.m. 3–4 times daily
Haloperidol	2–5 mg i.m., then 1–4 mg p.o. t.i.d.
Diphenylhydantoin	200 mg slowly i.v., then 300 mg p.o. q.d.
Valproic acid	15 mg/kg p.o. or PR (short-term therapy only)
Carbamazepine	200 mg q.i.d.
Metoclopramide	10 mg i.v. or i.m., then 10–20 mg q.i.d.
Amitriptyline	25 mg b.i.d
Baclofen	10 mg p.o. q.i.d.

PR, per rectum.

Table 8.2. Overview of Natural Remedies for Menopausal Symptoms

Remedy	Mechanism of Action	Dosage	Possible Side Effects	Cost
Vitamin E	Unknown	800 IU daily	None at this dose	400-IU capsules (100) $5.59
Hesperidin + Vitamin C (Peridin C)	Maintains vascular integrity	2 t.i.d. with meals	Perspiration odor	100 tablets $18
Gamma oryzanol (ferulic acid)	? Enhances pituitary function	300 mg daily	Unknown	—
Angelica (Dong Quai, *Angelica sinensis*)	? Stabilizes blood vessels	Take 3 times a day: Powdered root or tea 1–2 g Or Tincture (1:5): 4 ml OR Fluid extract 1 ml	Unknown	250 mg tablets (30) $7.99
Licorice root (*Glycyrrhiza glabra*)	? Increases estrogen to progesterone ratio	Take 3 times a day: Powdered root or tea 1–2 g Or Fluid extract (1:1) 4 mL Or Solid 250–500 mg	Hypertension (HTN), hypokalemia, sodium retention	250 mg capsules (3) $5.99
Chasteberries (*Vitex agnus-castus*)	? Alters FSH, LH secretion	Take 3 times a day: Powdered root or tea 1–2 g Or Fluid extract (1:1) 4 mL Or Solid 250–500 mg	Unknown	—

continued

Table 8.2. Overview of Natural Remedies for Menopausal Symptoms

Remedy	Mechanism of Action	Dosage	Possible Side Effects	Cost
Black Cohosh (*Cimicifuga racemosa*)	? Decreases LH levels	Take 3 times a day: Powder berries or tea 1–2 g Or Fluid extract (1:1) 4 mL Or Solid 250–500 mg	Unknown	540 mg capsules (100) $7.95
Ginseng (*Eleutherococcus senticosus*)	Unknown	? 410 mg capsules, 2 t.i.d.	Vaginal bleeding, HTN, breast swelling	410 mg capsules (100) $7.95
Evening primrose oil (gamolenic acid)	? Increases FSH, LH levels	? 500–1,000 mg daily	Unknown	500-mg soft capsules (100) $11.99

Reprinted with permission from NSABP.

Table 8.3. Nonhormonal Interventions for Hot Flashes

Drug	Classification	Dose	Mechanism of Action	Side Effects
Vitamin E[a]	Vitamin	800 IU q.d.	Unknown	None at this dose
Vitamin B₆[a]	Vitamin	200 mg q.d.	Unknown	None at this dose
Peridin-C[a]	Bioflavonoid	2 tablets t.i.d.	Enhances capillary tone	Perspiration may have an unpleasant odor
Clonidine (Catapres-TTS)	α-Adrenergic agonist	0.1-mg patch; change weekly	Reduces vascular reactivity; stabilizes thermoregulatory center	Hypotension; dizziness; fatigue
Methyldopa (Aldomet)	α-Adrenergic agonist	250 mg. b.i.d.	Reduces vascular reactivity; stabilizes thermoregulatory center	Dry mouth; fatigue; headache
Bellergal-S (ergotamine tartrate with L–belladonna alkaloids	Autonomic stabilizer	1 p.o. at bedtime; if ineffective, try 1 p.o. b.i.d.	Inhibits adrenergic, cholinergic impulses locally	Dry mouth; dizziness; drowsiness; addictive potential

[a]*Available over the counter.*

sation of docetaxel therapy, but this may take several months or more. Early aggressive diuretic therapy may be helpful once retention has occurred. The incidence may be reduced by the use of lower single doses or by alternative schedules, such as days 1 and 8 of a 21-day schedule.

HICCUPS

Unless they are persistent, hiccups are merely an inconvenience. When persistent they can contribute to insomnia, malnutrition, dehydration, and fatigue. If an underlying cause can be identified and corrected, no further remedy is needed. Patients with chronic hiccups may need pharmacologic treatment (Table 8.1). Mostly anecdotal reports suggest chlorpromazine, haloperidol, diphenylhydantoin, valproic acid, carbamazepine, baclofen, metoclopramide, and amitriptyline as effective.

HOT FLASHES

Regardless of how menopause is induced (naturally, surgically, or by chemotherapy), hot flashes are a common symptom. They can also be a side effect of the antiestrogen tamoxifen, and in some women may be intolerable enough that patients refuse further treatment. The measures that have been tried to eliminate or minimize hot flashes include vitamin E, ginseng, clonidine, ergotamine tartrate with L–belladonna alkaloids (Bellergal-S), and megestrol acetate. Tables 8.2 and 8.3 list these and

Table 8.4. Pharmacologic Agents for Insomnia

Medication (Trade Name)	Usual Dose[a] (mg/day)	Time to Onset (min)	Half-life (hr)
Clonazepam (Klonopin)	0.5–2	20–60	19–60
Clorazepate (Tranxene)	3.75–15	30–60	6–8, 48–96
Estazolam (ProSom)	1–2	15–30	8–24
Lorazepam (Ativan)	1–4	30–60	8–24
Oxazepam (Serax)	15–30	10–15	2.8–5.7
Quazepam (Doral)	7.5–15	20–45	15–40, 39–120
Temazepam (Restoril)	15–30	45–60	3–25
Triazolam (Halcion)	0.125–0.25	15–30	1.5–5
Chloral hydrate (Noctec)	500–2,000	30–60	4–8
Haloperidol (Haldol)	0.5–5	60	20
Trazodone (Desyrel)	50–150	30–60	5–9
Zolpidem (Ambien)	5–10	30	1.5–4.5

Modified with permission from Kupfer DJ, Reynolds CF III. Management of insomnia. N Engl J Med 1997;336:341–346.
[a]*Geriatric doses are usually half of the standard adult dose.*

other options. Interestingly, hot flashes also occur in men post-orchiectomy or when treated with tamoxifen.

INSOMNIA

Inability to sleep on a short-term basis is common and seldom requires therapy except in unusual circumstances, such as hospitalization. Chronic insomnia is vexing and troublesome to both patient and physician. Pharmacologic agents for treating insomnia are listed in Table 8.4. The article by Kupfer and Reynolds lists nonpharmacologic interventions that should be considered first.

BIBLIOGRAPHY

Fatigue

Glaspy J, Bukowski R, Steinberg D, et al. Impact of therapy with epoetin alpha on clinical outcomes in patients with nonmyeloid malignancies during cancer chemotherapy in community oncology practice. J Clin Oncol 1997;15:1218–1234.

Fever

Podrasky DL. Amphotericin B: the nurse' role in controlling adverse reactions. Focus Crit Care 1989;16:194–198.

Fluid Retention

Rowinsky EK, Donehower RC. Microtubule-targeting drugs. In: Perry MC. The chemotherapy source book. 2nd ed. Baltimore: Williams & Wilkins, 1996;387–423.

Hiccups

Rousseau P. Hiccups. South Med J 1995;88:175–181.

Kolodzik PW, Eilers MA. Hiccups (singultus): review and approach to management. Ann Emerg Med 1991;20:565–573.

Hot Flashes

Aikin, JL, Coping with menopausal symptoms caused by cancer therapies. Innovat Breast Cancer Care 1995;1:17–18.

Goldberg RM, Loprinzi CL, O'Fallon JR, et al. Transdermal clonidine for ameliorating tamoxifen-induced hot flashes. J Clin Oncol 1994;12:155–158.

Loprinzi CL, Michalak JC, Quella SK, et al. Megestrol acetate for the prevention of hot flashes. New Engl J Med 1994;331:347–352.

Insomnia

Kupfer DJ, Reynolds CF III. Management of insomnia. N Engl J Med 1997;336:341–346.

Index

Page numbers followed by a "t" denote tables. Acronyms in main entries may refer to multidrug regimens.

ABCM, 344
ABDIC, 331
Abdominal distention, 20
Abdominal mass, 55
Abdominal pain, 11, 23, 381
ABV, 265
ABVD, 44, 327, 329
AC
  breast cancer, 96, 100, 268
  endometrial cancer, 301
  neuroblastoma, 348
ACE, 325
Actinomycin D (see Dactino-
    mycin)
Acute leukemia
  from MDS, 30
  smoldering, 26–31
Acute lymphocytic leukemia
  Burkitt's cell, 4, 9
  in children, 310–311
  CNS prophylaxis, 9, 311,
    314–315
  cytogenetics, 5–6t, 7t
  diagnosis, 4, 7t
  etiology, 3
  risk factors, 3
  salvage therapy, 10
  symptoms, 4
  treatment, 8–9, 310–314
Acute myelogenous leukemia
  CNS prophylaxis, 318
  diagnosis, 12
  elderly patients, 317
  etiology, 11
  gingival infiltration, 11
  orbital involvement, 12
  risk factors, 11
  salvage therapy, 15
  skin infiltration, 11
  symptoms, 11–12
  treatment, 13, 14, 315–319

Acute myeloid leukemia, 389
Acute nonlymphocytic leukemia,
    iatrogenic, 45
Acute promyelocytic leukemia, 14
Addisonian syndrome, 373
Adenopathy (see Lymphadenopa-
    thy)
ADIC, 351
Adrenal insufficiency, 395, 504
Adrenal tumors
  assessment, 156–157
  chemotherapy, 276
  cortical carcinomas, 157–161
  pheochromocytomas, 161–163,
    276
AFP (see α-Fetoprotein)
African Americans
  and ovarian cancer, 215
  and plasma cell dyscrasias, 32
  and testicular cancer, 190
Agricultural chemicals, 20
AI (doxorubicin, ifosfamide),
    227, 352
AIDS
  anal cancer, 263
  cervical cancer, 262–263
  Kaposi's sarcoma, 255–258,
    259t, 265–267
  non-Hodgkin's lymphoma, 47,
    258–261, 262t, 267–268
  patients with, 153, 258–259
Alanine aminotransferase, 383,
    389–390
Alkaline phosphatase, 389–390
  leukocyte, 24
Alkylating agents
  and floxuridine, 381
  risk of subsequent MDS and
    leukemia, 26, 45
ALL (see Acute lymphocytic
    leukemia)
All-*trans* retinoic acid (see
    Tretinoin)
Allergy, 366t
Allopurinol, 342, 382
Alopecia, 362t

Altretamine
    ovarian cancer, 220, 305, 306,
        307
    profile, 407
    toxicity, 399
Amenorrhea, 369t (*see also*
        Menopause)
Amifostine, 399, 407–408
Aminoglutethimide, 99, 395,
        408
AML (*see* Acute myelogenous
        leukemia)
Amputation pain, 501
Amsacrine, 408–409
Amylase levels, 367t
Anagrelide, 409
Anal cancer, 151–155, 277–278
    AIDS-related, 262
Analgesics, 497–500, 498t, 499t
Anasarca, 504–508
Anastrazole, 99, 395, 409–410
Androgens
    ablation, 182–183
    and breast cancer, 99
    and MDS, 28
Anemia (*see also* Fanconi's ane-
        mia; Hemolytic anemia;
        Iron)
    CLL, 17
    CML, 24
    HCL, 20
    multiple myeloma, 34
Anorexia
    and ALL, 4
    and AML, 11
    grading, 359t
    management, 477, 493–494
Antibiotic prophylaxis, 273
Antigens
    cancer, 207
    cell surface, and HCL, 21
Antihistamines, 130
Antiretroviral agents, 263
APL (*see* Acute promyelocytic
        leukemia)
Appendix tumors, 128–130
APUD tumors, 128–130
Ara-C (*see* Cytarabine)
Aromatase inhibitors, 99
Arthralgias, 28, 367t, 500
Ascites (*see* Effusions)

Asians
    and ovarian cancer, 215
    and testicular cancer, 190
Asparaginase (*see* L-asparaginase)
Aspartate amino transferase
        levels, 390
Astrocytomas, 66–67, 68–69
Ataxia-telangiectasia, 3, 11, 47
Atomic radiation, 11, 23
ATRA, 14, 318, 470
Auer rods, 12
Autoimmune diseases, and NHL
        risk, 47
5-azacytidine
    multiple myeloma, 346
    myelodysplastic syndrome, 29
    profile, 411–412
AZT, 260

B-CAVe, 326
B-cell ALL, 3, 10, 314–315
Bacillus Calmette-Guérin
    bladder cancer, 166
    profile, 412–413
BACOP, 333
BCAP, 344
BCD, 348–349
bcl-2, 16
BCNU (*see* Carmustine)
Behavior change, 365t
Bence Jones proteinuria, 36
Benzene, 20, 26
BEP
    CNS tumors, 68–69
    ovarian germ cell tumors, 222,
        304
    testicular cancer, 194, 195, 197,
        298
    unknown primary, 275
Biclutamide, 296, 395, 413
Bile duct cancer, 136–139, 279
Bilirubin
    daunorubicin, 385
    doxorubicin, 386
    and MDS, 28
    methotrexate, 383
    vinblastine, 390
    vincristine, 391
Biochemotherapy, and
        melanoma, 62–63
Biodegradable wafers, 68

Biologic therapy (*see*
  Immunotherapy)
BIP, 300
Bladder cancer, 165t, 166t
  chemotherapy, 291–293
  incontinence, 167
  metastatic, 168, 168t
  radical cystectomy, 167t
  staging, 165t, 166t
Bladder toxicity
  grading, 361t
  ifosfamide, 376–377
Bleeding (*see also* Hemorrhage)
  and ALL, 4
  and AML, 11
  and MDS, 28
  and multiple myeloma, 34
Bleomycin (*see also* ABDIC;
    ABVD; B-CAVe; BEP;
    CBVD; m-BACOD; Stan-
    ford V; VABCD)
  cervical cancer, 204, 300
    AIDS-related, 263
  CNS tumors, 68–69
  esophageal cancer, 284, 285
  gestational trophoblastic tu-
    mors, 212, 304
  melanoma, 61, 343
  non-Hodgkin's lymphoma,
    333, 334, 335, 339
  osteosarcoma, 348–349
  penile cancer, 188, 294
  profile, 413–414
  pulmonary toxicity, 45
  testicular cancer, 194, 195, 197,
    298, 299
  toxicity management, 384–385,
    504
  unknown primary, 252, 275
Blood pressure, 364t (*see also*
    Hypotension)
Bloom's syndrome, 3, 11
BOMP, 300
Bone marrow transplant
  allogeneic
    and ALL, 8–9, 10
    and AML, 15
    and CML, 23, 25
    disadvantages, 9, 36
    and MDS, 30
    and multiple myeloma, 36

autologous
    and Hodgkin's disease, 45
    and multiple myeloma, 36–37
  melanoma, 60
  non-Hodgkin's lymphomas, 55
Bone metastases, 497
Bone pain (*see also* Pain, muscu-
    loskeletal)
  and ALL, 4
  and AML, 11
  and multiple myeloma, 34
Breast cancer
  adjuvant therapy, 94–97
  bone metastases, 497
  cardiac dysfunction, 96
  chemotherapy, 100, 101t,
    268–274
  ductal and lobular in situ carci-
    nomas, 100–102
  estrogen-receptor status, 95
  follow-up monitoring, 100–101,
    102t
  hormone therapy, 98–100
  lobular carcinoma in situ, 102
  monoclonal antibody therapy,
    97
  ovarian ablation, 94–95, 99
  prognosis, 90–93, 91t, 92t, 95
  risk factors, 85t, 86t
  staging, 88–90, 89t, 90t
Breast tumors, post Hodgkin's
    disease, 45
Burkitt's cell ALL, 4, 9
Burkitt's lymphoma, 48, 54, 55,
    339–340, 341–342
  AIDS-related, 259
Buserelin, 414–415
Busulfan
  profile, 415
  toxicity, 373–374
BV, 266
BVCPP, 328

C-MOPP
  Hodgkin's disease, 329
  non-Hodgkin's lymphoma, 334
CA-125, and ovarian cancer,
    216–217, 219
CAF, 96, 100, 268–269
Calcitonin, and thyroid cancer, 83
Calcitriol, 293

Calcium
  and ALL, 4
  and AML, 12
  goserelin, 396
  grading toxicity, 367t, 368t
  and lymphoblastic lymphoma,
    55
  mithramycin, 401–402
  and multiple myeloma, 34
  and non-Hodgkin's
    lymphomas, 48
  tamoxifen, 98, 398
  testolactone, 398
Calvert formula, 355
CaN, 321
Cancer and Leukemia Group B,
    29
Cancer antigen, 107
CAP
  bladder cancer, 168, 291
  lung cancer, 109, 321
  ovarian cancer, 305
CAP-M, 291
Capsaicin, 501
Carbo/VP-16, 348
CarboC, 305
Carboplatin (see also Carbo/VP-
    16; CF; CP)
  dosage adjustment, 374–375,
    374t
  endometrial cancer, 207–208
  head and neck cancer, 309
  lung cancer, 110, 321, 322, 325
  non-Hodgkin's lymphoma, 338
  ovarian cancer, 219, 220, 305
  profile, 415–416
  retinoblastoma, 240
  testicular cancer, 197
  unknown primary, 252, 275, 276
  Wilm's tumor, 246, 248
Carcinoembryonic antigen
  and colorectal cancer, 148
  and thyroid cancer, 83
Carcinoid syndrome, 129
Carcinoid tumors, 128–130,
    287–288
Carcinoma of unknown primary,
    250–254, 275–276
Cardioprotective agents, 386
Cardiotoxicity
  daunorubicin, 385

  doxorubicin, 45, 386
  floxuridine, 381
  grading, 363t
  idarubicin, 13, 387–389
Carmustine
  biodegradable wafers, 68
  CNS tumors, 67, 68, 346
  cutaneous lymphoma, 54
  Hodgkin's disease, 328, 331
  macroglobulinemia, 38
  melanoma, 61, 342
  multiple myeloma, 36, 344, 346
  profile, 416–417
  toxicity and dosage, 375
Castleman's disease, 32
CaT, 322
Cataracts, 98
Caucasians
  and ovarian cancer, 215
  and testicular cancer, 190
CAV, 325
CAV/PE, 326
CAVE, 326
CBVD, 331
CC, 305
CCNU (see Lomustine)
CD-20, 53
CD4 count, 260, 261
2-CdA
  and CLL, 320
  and CML, 321
  and HCL, 22
  and macroglobulinemia, 38
CDE, 261, 267–268
Central nervous system
  and ALL, 4, 9, 311
  and AML, 11
  lymphoma of, 260, 261
  and macroglobulinemia, 38
  and non-Hodgkin's lym-
    phomas, 48, 54, 55
  prophylactic therapy, 267–
    268
  tumors
    adult, 65–69, 346–347
    pediatric, 347–348
CEP, 332
CEPP(B), 333–334
Cerebellar symptoms, 399
Cervical cancer
  AIDS-related, 262–263

chemotherapy, 300–301
premalignant conditions, 199
staging, 200t, 201t, 202t
CEV, 326
CF, 292, 293
CFP, 269
Children
with ALL, 4, 11, 310–311
and MDS, 26
Chili peppers, 501
Chills, 367t, 504
Chlorambucil
cervical cancer, 204
CLL, 18–19, 320
Hodgkin's disease, 328
profile, 417
Chlorodeoxyadenosine
CLL, 320
CML, 321
HCL, 22
macroglobulinemia, 38
profile, 418–419
toxicity, 380
Chloroma
and ALL, 4
and AML, 11
and CML, 23, 25
ChlVPP, 328
CHOP
in AIDS patients, 261
non-Hodgkin's lymphomas, 52,
53, 55, 334
Chromosomal abnormalities
ALL, 4, 5–6t, 7t
AML, 12
CLL, 16
MDS, 26, 27t, 28
Chronic lymphocytic leukemia,
16–19, 17t (see also
Macroglobulinemia)
blast crisis, 24, 25
chemotherapy, 320
and IgM paraprotein, 38
PLL subtype, 17, 18
Chronic myelogenous leukemia,
23–25
Cimetidine, 173, 272, 305
13-cis retinoic acid (see
Isotretinoin)
CISCA, 291
Cisplatin (see also EVAP; FAP; 5-

FU-MMC-RT; M-VAC;
VC)
adrenal tumors, 160, 276
anal cancer, 153, 154, 277
bladder cancer, 167–169, 291,
292, 293
cervical cancer, 203, 204, 300
AIDS-related, 263
CNS tumors, 68–69
dosage adjustments, 375–376
endometrial cancer, 207–208,
302
esophageal cancer, 116, 282,
283, 284, 285, 286
gastric cancer, 286, 287
gestational trophoblastic tumors, 212, 304
head and neck tumors, 74–75,
309, 310
lung cancer, 109, 110, 111,
321–322, 323, 324, 326, 327
melanoma, 61, 62–63, 342, 343
neuroblastoma, 348
neuroendocrine tumors, 253
non-Hodgkin's lymphoma, 337
osteosarcoma, 349
ovarian cancer, 217–218, 219,
220, 305, 306, 307
germ cell tumors, 222, 304
penile cancer, 188, 294
profile, 417–418
prostate cancer, 184
rhabdomyosarcoma, 242, 243,
244t, 351
testicular cancer, 194, 195, 197,
299, 300
thyroid cancer, 277
unknown primary, 252, 253,
275
CIS/TAX, 305
CIS/TAX (PT), 306
CLL (see Chronic lymphocytic
leukemia)
CMF, 94, 96, 100, 269
CMFP, 270
CMFVP, 96, 100
CML (see Chronic myelogenous
leukemia)
CMV, 292
CNF, 270
CNOP, 335

CNS (*see* Central nervous system)
Coagulation toxicity, 368t
COD-BLAM IV, 335
Cold agglutinin disease, 37–38
Colon cancer
 adjuvant therapy, 146, 279–280
 endometrial cancer risk factor, 205
 hepatic metastases, 147
 metastatic disease therapy, 280–282
 postoperative monitoring, 148
 staging, 145t
 vaccine, 147
Coma, 401
COMLA, 336
Congestive heart failure, 99
Conjunctivitis, 369t
Constipation, 365t, 477–478, 479–481t, 493–494
Cooper Regimen, 99, 270
COP
 CLL, 19
 non-Hodgkin's lymphoma, 336
COPP, 336
Coronary artery disease, 45
Corticosteroids (*see also* Hydrocortisone)
 for gastrointestinal toxicity, 477
 and MDS, 28–29
 withdrawal, and pain, 500
Cough, 503
CP, 292
 pulse, 320
CPT-11
 cervical cancer, 204
 lung cancer, 110
Creatinine clearance, 355, 360t (*see also* Renal impairment)
Cryosurgery, prostate cancer, 181
Cryptorchidism, 190
CTCL, 54–55
Cushingoid syndrome, 369t
Cutaneous T-cell lymphoma, 54–55
Cutaneous toxicity (*see* Dermatologic toxicity)
CVD
 melanoma, 61, 342
 pheochromocytoma, 276

CVP
 CLL, 320
 non-Hodgkin's lymphoma, 53, 336
Cyclophosphamide (*see also* AC; BVCPP; C-MOPP; CAF; CDE; CHOP; CMF; CMFP; CNF; Cooper Regimen; CVP; FAC; m-BACOD; M2; PAC; PCVP; TAC)
 ALL, 8, 9, 10, 311–312, 313–314
  B-cell, 314–315
 AML, 15
 and autologous BMT candidates, 36
 bladder cancer, 168, 291
 breast cancer, 94, 96, 268–272
 carcinoid tumors, 130
 CLL, 19, 320
 Ewing's sarcoma, 229, 347
 gestational trophoblastic tumors, 210, 212, 303, 304
 hematologic toxicity, 376
 lung cancer, 109, 321, 325, 326, 327
 multiple myeloma, 35–36, 344, 345, 346
 neuroepithelial tumors, 229
 non-Hodgkin's lymphoma, 333–334, 335, 336, 339, 341
 osteosarcoma, 348–349
 ovarian cancer, 219, 305, 306, 307
  germ cell tumors, 222
 penile cancer, 188
 pheochromocytoma, 163
 profile, 419–420
 prostate cancer, 184, 294, 295
 retinoblastoma, 240
 rhabdomyosarcoma, 242, 243, 244t, 350, 351
 and rheumatism, 500
 soft tissue sarcoma, 352, 354
 Wilm's tumor, 246, 248
Cystitis, 361t
Cytarabine
 ALL, 311, 313–314, 314
 AML, 13, 14, 315–316, 318–319
 in elderly patients, 380
 and hepatic insufficiency, 380
 high-dose
  and ALL, 8, 9, 10

and AML, 13, 14, 15, 319
and non-Hodgkin's lym-
phoma, 337
Hodgkin's disease, 331, 332
intrathecal
and ALL, 311, 315
and AML, 318
and non-Hodgkin's lym-
phoma, 54, 267, 340
and retinoblastoma, 240
and rhabdomyosarcoma,
243
low-dose
and AML, 13
and CML, 25
and MDS, 29–30
myelodysplastic syndrome, 29
non-Hodgkin's lymphoma,
335, 336, 337, 341
profile, 420–421
Cytomegalovirus, 255
Cytosine arabinoside (*see* Cytarabine)
CYVADIC, 227, 352

Dacarbazine (*see also* ABDIC;
ABVD; VABCD)
carcinoid tumors, 130
hematologic toxicity, 376
melanoma, 61, 62, 342, 343
pheochromocytoma, 163
profile, 421–422
rhabdomyosarcoma, 242, 243,
244t
soft tissue sarcoma, 227, 351,
352, 353
Dactinomycin
and diarrhea, 478
Ewing's sarcoma, 229, 347
gestational trophoblastic tumors, 210, 211–212, 303,
304
neuroepithelial tumors, 229
osteosarcoma, 348–349
profile, 422
rhabdomyosarcoma, 242, 244t,
350
soft tissue sarcoma, 227, 354
testicular cancer, 299
Wilm's tumor, 247–248, 248t
Dartmouth regimen, 61, 342

DAT, 318
Daunorubicin
ALL, 8, 312, 313
AML, 13, 14, 315–316, 318–319
Kaposi's sarcoma, 266
profile, 422–423
toxicity, 13, 385
DBV, 266
DCIS in situ, 100–102
2'-deoxycoformycin, 22
Dermatologic toxicity
aminoglutethimide, 395
docetaxel, 390
grading, 366t
liposomal doxorubicin, 386,
387t
pentostatin, 383
perianal skin care, 482t
Dermatosis, acute neutrophilic,
28
DES (*see* Diethylstilbesterol)
Dexa-BEAM, 331
Dexamethasone (*see also* FND;
m-BACOD)
AIDS-related lymphoma, 261
ALL, 314–315
colorectal cancer, 281
for fluid retention, 504
high dose, 261
Hodgkin's disease, 331, 332
intrathecal, 315
multiple myeloma, 36, 344,
345
non-Hodgkin's lymphoma,
335, 337, 338
and paclitaxel, 272, 305
profile, 423–424
Dexamethasone suppression test,
156–157
Dexrazoxone, 424
DHAP, 337
Diarrhea
grading, 359t
and irinotecan, 393t, 478
management, 478, 481t, 482t,
483t
and procarbazine, 379
Diazoxide, 132
DIC (*see* Disseminated intravascular coagulation)
DICE, 337

Diethylstilbesterol
  breast cancer, 97, 99
  profile, 425
  prostate cancer, 183, 295
  toxicity, 395
Diffuse small non-cleaved cell
      lymphoma (*see* Burkitt's
      lymphoma)
Diphenhydramine, 272, 305
Diplopia, 397
Dipyridamole, 290
Disseminated intravascular
      coagulation, 4, 8, 12
Dizziness, 366t
Docetaxel (*see also* TA; TAC)
  breast cancer, 100, 271
  cervical cancer, 204, 300
  dosage adjustments, 389
  fluid retention, 504
  head and neck cancer, 308
  lung cancer, 110, 323, 324
  ovarian cancer, 220, 306
  profile, 425–426
  soft tissue sarcoma, 227
Down's syndrome
  and ALL, 3
  and AML, 11
  and MDS, 26
  and teniposide, 392
DOX/CY, 295
Doxorubicin (*see also* ABDIC;
      ABVD; AC; B-CAVe;
      CAF; CDE; CHOP; DVM;
      EVA; FAC; FAM; FAP;
      Liposomal anthracyclines;
      m-BACOD; M-VAC; Stan-
      ford V; TA; TAC; VABCD;
      VAD; VAM; VATH;
      VBAP; VD)
  adrenal tumors, 161
  ALL, 311–312, 314, 315
  AML, 316
  anal cancer, 154
  bile duct cancer, 137
  bladder cancer, 167–169, 291,
      293
  breast cancer, 96, 99–100,
      268–272
  cardiotoxicity, 45, 386
  cervical cancer, 204
  dosage modifications, 386

endometrial cancer, 207–208,
      301, 302
  esophageal cancer, 284
  Ewing's sarcoma, 229, 347
  gastric cancer, 286, 287
  hepatocellular carcinoma, 136
  Kaposi's sarcoma, 267
  lung cancer, 109, 321, 323, 325,
      326, 327
  multiple myeloma, 344, 345,
      346
  neuroendocrine tumors, 130,
      131, 253
  neuroepithelial tumors, 229
  non-Hodgkin's lymphoma,
      333, 335, 338, 339, 341
  osteosarcoma, 349–350
  ovarian cancer, 220, 305, 306,
      307
    germ cell tumors, 222
  pancreatic islet cell tumors, 290
  profile, 426–427
  prostate cancer, 184, 295
  retinoblastoma, 240
  rhabdomyosarcoma, 242, 243,
      244t, 350, 351
  soft tissue sarcomas, 226, 227,
      351, 352, 353
  thyroid cancer, 83, 277
  unknown primary, 253
  Wilm's tumor, 246, 247–248,
      248t
Drowsiness, 395
DTIC (*see* Dacarbazine)
Ductal carcinoma in situ, 100–102
DVM, 271
Dysgerminomas, 221–222
Dysphagia, 359t, 491
Dyspnea
  busulfan, 374
  and HCL, 20
  management, 503
  and MDS, 28
  and tretinoin, 402

EAP, 286
Early Breast Cancer Trialists' Col-
      laborative Group, 93, 94
Eastern Cooperative Oncology
      Group (ECOG)
  bile duct cancer trial, 137

gallbladder cancer trial, 141
melanoma trial, 60
Edatrexate, 227, 427–428
Edema, 364t, 504–508
Effusions (*see also* Fluid retention)
and methotrexate, 383
and mitoxantrone, 389
ELF, 286
EMA-CE, 212
EMA/CO, 210, 212, 302–303
Embolism
diethylstilbesterol, 99
grading, 364t
medroxyprogesterone, 397
megesterol acetate, 398
tamoxifen, 98
Endocrine toxicity
aminoglutethimide, 395
busulfan, 373–374
grading, 369t
Endocrine tumors (*see* Neuroendocrine tumors)
Endometrial cancer, 205–208, 206t
after tamoxifen, 98
and diethylstilbesterol, 395
EP, 299
Ependymomas, 67, 68
Epidermal growth factor, 91–92
Epidophyllotoxins
and AML, 11
and secondary leukemia risk,
26
Epirubicin, 167, 227
Epstein-Barr virus
and cervical cancer, 3, 40, 47
and Kaposi's sarcoma, 255
Erythema
cutaneous lymphoma, 54
MDS, 28
Erythropoietin
for anemia, 504
and MDS, 29
profile, 428
ESHAP, 337
Esophageal cancer
chemotherapy, 115, 116t,
282–286
staging, 114t
Esophageal reflux, 483, 491t
Esophagitis, 359t, 485–491
Estradiol, 396

Estramustine
and hepatic and renal impairment, 399–400
profile, 428–429
prostate cancer, 184, 295
Estrogens (*see also specific drugs*)
endometrial cancer, 205
prostate cancer, 183
Etidronate, 400–401
Etoposide (*see also* BEP;
Carbo/VP-16; CDE; CEP;
Dexa-BEAM; EVA; EVAP;
Mini-BEAM; Stanford V;
VFP)
adrenal tumors, 160, 276
AML, 15, 316, 319
CNS tumors, 68–69
esophageal cancer, 284, 285
Ewing's sarcoma, 229, 347
gastric cancer, 286
gestational trophoblastic tumors, 210, 212
hematologic toxicity, 391
hepatocellular carcinoma, 136
lung cancer, 111, 325, 326,
327
neuroepithelial tumors, 229
non-Hodgkin's lymphoma,
333–334, 335, 337, 338, 339,
341
ovarian cancer, 220, 307
profile, 429–430
retinoblastoma, 240
rhabdomyosarcoma, 242, 243,
244t, 351
and secondary acute leukemia,
26
testicular cancer, 194, 197, 298,
299, 300
unknown primary, 252, 253,
275
Wilm's tumor, 246, 247
Etoposide phosphate, 392
EVA, 332
EVAP, 332
Ewing's sarcoma, 228–229, 347
Exercise tolerance, and MDS, 28
Eye dryness, 369t (*see also* Ocular
toxicity)

FAC, 96, 100, 271

FAM
  bile duct cancer, 137, 279
  gastric cancer, 287
  pancreatic cancer, 288–290
FAMTX, 287
Fanconi's anemia, 3, 11, 26
FAP
  esophageal cancer, 284
  pancreatic cancer, 288
Fareston, 98
Fatigue
  leukemia, 4, 11, 23
  management, 504, 509
  multiple myeloma, 34
Ferritin, 28
Fertility
  grading toxicity, 369t
  and MOPP, 45
  and RAI, 82
α-Fetoprotein
  ovarian cancer, 216
  testicular cancer, 192
  unknown primary, 253
Fever
  ALL, 4
  AML, 11
  CLL, 16
  CML, 23
  grading toxicity, 366t
  Hodgkin's disease, 41
  management, 504
  MDS, 28
  non-Hodgkin's lymphoma, 48
Fibrinogen, 368t
Filgrastim, 430–431
Finasteride, 176
5-FU (see Fluorouracil)
FLEP, 285
Floxuridine
  and alkylating agents, 381
  colon cancer, 281
  prior radiotherapy, 381
  profile, 431–432
  renal cell cancer, 173, 297
  toxicity, 381
Fludarabine
  CLL, 18, 320
  macroglobulinemia, 38
  non-Hodgkin's lymphoma, 53, 338

  profile, 432
  toxicity, 380–381
Fluid retention, 504–508, 509
Flulike symptoms, 367t
5-Fluorouracil (see also CAF;
    CMF; CMFP; CNF; Cooper
    Regimen; FAC; FAP; 5-FU-
    MMC-RT; Hexa-CAF;
    MFL; NFL)
  and AIDS patients, 153, 262
  anal cancer, 153, 154, 277
  bile duct cancer, 137, 279
  bladder cancer, 167, 292
  breast cancer, 94, 96, 268–272
  carcinoid tumors, 288
  cervical cancer, 203, 204, 262
  colon cancer, 146–147, 279–282
  diarrhea, 478
  dose modifications, 381
  endometrial cancer, 207–208, 302
  esophageal cancer, 116, 282, 283, 285, 286
  gastric cancer, 286, 287
  head and neck tumors, 74, 309, 310
  hepatocellular carcinoma, 136
  infusion, 148, 173, 188
  neuroendocrine tumors, 130, 131, 253
  pancreatic tumors, 125, 288, 289, 290, 291
  penile cancer, 186, 188, 294
  profile, 433
  rectal cancer, 148–149
  renal cell cancer, 173–174, 298
  and rheumatism, 500
Fluoxymesterone, 99, 396, 433–434 (see also VATH)
Flutamide
  hepatic toxicity, 396
  and leuprolide flare reaction, 397
  profile, 434
  prostate cancer, 183, 296
FND, 53, 338
Fotemustine, 61
5-FU-MMC, 282
5-FU-MMC-RT, 278, 289
5-FU-RT, 289
FUCI, 280

FUDR (*see* Floxuridine)

G-CSF (*see* Granulocyte colony-stimulating factor)
Gallbladder cancer, 139–141, 140t, 141t
Gallium nitrate, 293, 401, 434–435
Gamma globulin, 18
Gastric cancer, 120t, 121t, 286–287
Gastrinoma, 132
Gastritis, 359t
Gastrointestinal lymphomas, 47, 54
Gastrointestinal Oncology Study Group, 125, 148
Gastrointestinal toxicity (*see specific conditions*)
Gemcitabine
  bladder cancer, 292
  breast cancer, 271
  clearance, 381
  lung cancer, 110, 323, 324
  ovarian cancer, 220, 306
  pancreatic cancer, 289
  profile, 435–436
  renal cell cancer, 173
  toxicity, 381–382, 382t
Gene therapy, and melanoma, 63
Genes
  and breast cancer, 84–85, 92
  MEN-1, 128
  and pancreatic cancer, 122
  and prostate cancer, 175
  and Wilm's tumor, 246
Genitourinary fistula, 361t
Germ cell tumors (*see* Ovarian germ cell tumors; Testicular cancer)
Germinomas, pineal, 68–69
Gestational trophoblastic tumors, 209–213, 302–304
Gingival infiltration, AML, 11
GITSG trials, 125, 148
Glaucoma, 369t
Gliadel wafers, 68
Glioblastoma multiforme, 66
Gliomas, malignant, 65, 66–67
  brainstem, 68
Glucagonomas, 128, 132
Glucose serum levels, 367t, 383

GM-CSF (*see* Granulocyte macrophage colony-stimulating factor)
GOG trial, 219
Goserelin, 99, 296, 396, 436
Graft versus host disease, 9
Granisetron, 477
Granulocyte colony-stimulating factor
  ALL, 9
  AML, 15
  breast cancer, 272
  head and neck cancer, 309
  lung cancer, 322
  myelodysplastic syndromes, 29
Granulocyte macrophage colony-stimulating factor
  AML, 15
  myelodysplastic syndromes, 29
Granulocytopenia, and MDS, 28
Gynecological Oncology Group trial, 219
Gynecomastia, 369t

Haemophilus influenzae, 18
Hairy cell leukemia, 20–22
Halotestin (*see* Fluoxymesterone)
Hand-foot syndrome, 386
HCG (*see* Human chorionic gonadotropin)
HCL (*see* Hairy cell leukemia)
HCV, 47
Head and neck cancer
  chemotherapy for advanced, 75t, 308–310
  neoadjuvant chemotherapy, 73
  staging, 72t
Hearing change, 365t, 375–376
Helicobacter pylori, 47, 54
Hematologic toxicity
  in AIDS patients, 263
  aminoglutethimide, 395
  busulfan, 374
  carboplatin, 374, 374t
  carmustine, 375
  cyclophosphamide, 376
  dacarbazine, 376
  docetaxel, 389
  dosage adjustments, 372t
  doxorubicin, 386, 388t
  etoposide, 391

Hematologic toxicity—*Continued*
  fludarabine, 380
  fluorouracil, 401
  gemcitabine, 381–382, 382t
  grading, 358t
  hexamethylmelamine, 399
  hydroxyurea, 382
  idarubicin, 388–389
  ifosfamide, 376
  interferon-α, 398
  irinotecan, 392, 393t
  levamisole, 401
  lomustine, 377, 377t
  mechlorethamine, 377
  mithramycin, 401
  mitomycin, 378, 378t
  paclitaxel, 390
  pentostatin, 383
  procarbazine, 379
  streptozocin, 379
  teniposide, 392
  6-thioguanine, 384
  thiotepa, 379
  vinblastine, 390
  vinorelbine, 391
Hemolytic anemia, 28
Hemolytic uremic syndrome, 378
Hemorrhage, 358t (*see also*
  Bleeding)
Hepatic dysfunction
  chlorodeoxyadenosine, 380
  cytarabine, 380
  daunorubicin, 385
  diethylstilbesterol, 395
  docetaxel, 389–390
  doxorubicin, 386
  estramustine, 399
  etoposide, 391
  gemcitabine, 382
  idarubicin, 389
  letrozole, 397
  medroxyprogesterone, 397
  methotrexate, 383
  mithramycin, 401
  mitoxantrone, 389
  paclitaxel, 390
  streptozocin, 379
  teniposide, 392
  thioguanine, 384
  thiotepa, 379
  vinblastine, 390

  vincristine, 391
  vinorelbine, 391
Hepatic metastases, colon cancer,
  147
Hepatic toxicity
  busulfan, 374
  floxuridine, 381
  fluoxymesterone, 396
  flutamide, 396
  grading, 373t
  interferon α, 398–399
  ketoconazole, 397
  L-asparaginase, 394
  thioguanine, 384
Hepatitis B, 255
Hepatocellular carcinoma, 133–136
Hepatomegaly, 20, 28
Hepatosplenomegaly, 4, 11, 16, 38
Hepatotoxicity
  fluoxymesterone, 99
Herbicides, 47
Herceptin, 97, 469
Herpes simplex virus, 198
Herpesvirus
  and Kaposi's sarcoma, 255–256
  and plasma cell dyscrasias, 32
Hexa-CAF, 306–307
Hexamethylmelamine (*see* Altretamine)
Hiccups, 504t, 508, 509
HIV
  and cervical cancer, 198
  and Hodgkin's disease, 40
Hodgkin's disease
  AIDS-related, 258–259
  classification, 41t
  extranodal, 41
  lung tumors after, 45
  risk factors, 40
  staging, 42–43, 42t
  toxicity of therapy, 45
  treatment, 43–45, 44t, 327–333
HOP, 338
Hormone ablation, 182
Hormone receptors, 91, 95, 96, 98
Hormone therapy
  breast cancer, 98–100
  dosage modifications, 395–398
  endometrial cancer, 207, 208
  and ovarian cancer risk, 215
  prostate cancer, 182, 183, 295–297

Hot flashes, 369t, 507t, 508, 509
HTLV, 3, 47, 54
Human chorionic gonadotropin
  molar pregnancy, 210
  ovarian cancer, 216
  testicular cancer, 192
  unknown primary, 253
Human immunodeficiency virus
  and cervical cancer, 198
  and Hodgkin's disease, 40
Human papilloma virus, 198, 255
Human t cell lymphoma-
  leukemia virus, 3, 47, 54
Hurthle cell carcinoma, 82
Hydrea, 321
Hydrocortisone (*see also* Cortico-
  steroids)
Hodgkin's disease, 329
  intrathecal
    and ALL, 311
    and non-Hodgkin's lym-
      phoma, 54
  retinoblastoma, 240
  rhabdomyosarcoma, 243
Hydroxyurea
  ALL, 8
  AML, 319
  cervical cancer, 203, 301
  CML, 25
  dosage modification, 382
  melanoma, 61
  profile, 436–437
Hyperleukocytosis, 8, 12, 13, 25
Hypertension, 364t
Hyperthermia, 97
Hyperuricemia, 4, 12
Hyperviscosity syndrome, 34,
  37–38
Hypogammaglobulinemia, 18
Hypophosphatemia, 4, 12
Hypotension, 364t
  orthostatic, 395
Hypothyroidism, 504

Iatrogenic disorders
  acute nonlymphocytic
    leukemia, 45
  MDS, 26–27
ICE
  and non-Hodgkin's lym-
    phoma, 338

unknown primary carcinoma,
  275
Idarubicin
  AML, 13, 317
  dosage modifications, 387–389
  profile, 437–438
Ifosfamide (*see also* VIG)
  ALL, B-cell, 314
  cervical cancer, 204, 300
  CNS tumors, 68
  Ewing's sarcoma, 229, 347
  hematologic toxicity, 376
  neuroepithelial tumors, 229
  non-Hodgkin's lymphoma,
    337, 338–339, 341
  ovarian cancer, 220, 307
  profile, 438–439
  retinoblastoma, 240
  rhabdomyosarcoma, 242, 243,
    244t, 351
  soft tissue sarcomas, 227, 352,
    353
  testicular cancer, 299, 300
  unknown primary, 275
IgM paraprotein, 38
Immunocompromised patients,
  261, 263
Immunophenotyping, HCL, 21
Immunosuppression,
    chlorodeoxyadenosine-
    induced, 380
Immunotherapy (*see also*
    Vaccines; *specific agents*)
  melanoma, 60, 62, 342, 343
  renal cell cancer, 173–174
Impotence
  and bladder cancer, 167
  grading toxicity, 369t
  and prostate cancer, 181
IMVP-16, 338–339
Incontinence
  and cystectomy, 167
  grading, 361
  and prostate cancer surgery,
    181
Indolent myeloma, 32
Infants, dosage, 246
Infections
  and CLL, 18
  grading toxicity, 358t
  and multiple myeloma, 34

Insecticides, 26, 47
Insomnia, 366t, 508t, 509
Insulinomas, 132
Interferon α
  carcinoid tumors, 287
  CLL, 19, 22
  CML, 25, 321
  diabetes patients, 398
  heart failure patients, 398
  high dose, 58, 62, 398–399
  Kaposi's sarcoma, 257–258, 266
  lung disease patients, 398
  and macroglobulinemia, 38
  and melanoma, 58, 60, 62, 342, 343
  and multiple myeloma, 37
  myelodysplastic syndromes, 29
  non-Hodgkin's lymphoma, 53
  pancreatic islet cell tumors, 290
  profile, 439–440
  renal cell cancer, 173–174, 297, 298
  toxicity management, 398–399, 504
Interferon-γ, 29, 53, 440
Interleukin 2
  and CLL, 19
  for melanoma, 58, 62, 343
  profile, 440–441
  and renal cell cancer, 173–174, 297, 298
  withholding, 399, 400t
Interleukin 12, 63
Interleukin 15, 63
Intestinal fistula, 359t
Intestinal obstruction, 359t
Intestinal tumors (see Colon cancer; Small intestine)
Intra-arterial therapy, 236
Intralesional administration, 257
Ireland regimen, 283
Irinotecan
  cervical cancer, 204
  colorectal cancer, 147–148, 281
  diarrhea, 393t, 478
  dosage modifications, 392, 393t
  profile, 442
Iron, 28 (see also Anemia)
IRS-IV pilot, rhabdomyosarcoma, 351
Isotretinoin, 29, 443

Kaposi's sarcoma, 255–258, 259t, 265–267
Kaposi's sarcoma-associated herpes virus (KSHV), 47
Karnofsky performance scale, 354
Keratitis, 369t
Ketoconazole, 339
Klinefelter's syndrome, 190

L-asparaginase
  ALL, 4, 8, 310, 312, 313
  AML, 412
  profile, 410–411
  toxicity, 394
Lactate dehydrogenase, 24, 28, 192
Lactic acid dehydrogenase, 49
Lactic acidosis, 4, 12
Lactose dehydrogenase, 229
LAP score, 24
Large cell lymphoma, 18
Larson regimen, 313–314
Larynx preservation, 309
Laxatives, 477, 479t
LDH (see Lactic dehydrogenase; Lactose dehydrogenase)
Lethargy, and CML, 23
Letrozole, 99, 397
Leucovorin
  with 5FU, 146–147, 279, 280, 281 (see also ELF; FLEP; NFL)
  and gestational trophoblastic tumors (see EMA/CO)
  head and neck cancer, 310
  MTX rescue, 314–315, 339–340, 348–349, 349–350 (see also COD-BLAM IV; COMLA; EMA/CO; Linker regimen; MFL; ProMACE-CytaBOM; Stanford Regimen, non-Hodgkin's lymphoma)
  profile, 443–444
  with trimetrexate, 384
Leukapheresis, in CML, 25
Leukemia (see specific leukemia type)
Leukocyte alkaline phosphatase, 24
Leukopenia (see also Hematologic toxicity)
  and HCL, 20

Leuprolide
  breast cancer, 99
  profile, 444–445
  prostate cancer, 183, 296, 397
Levamisole
  with 5FU, 146–147, 279, 401
  profile, 445–446
Li-Fraumeni syndrome, 85
Libido, 99, 369t
Linker regimen, 312–313
Liposomal anthracyclines, 258
  daunorubicin, 266
  doxorubicin, 267, 271, 306, 386, 387t, 388t
Listeria, 18
Lobular carcinoma in situ, 102
Lomustine
  and CNS tumors, 68, 347
  hematologic toxicity, 377, 377t
  and Hodgkin's disease, 328, 331, 332, 333
  and melanoma, 61
  profile, 446
Lung cancer
  adjuvant chemotherapy, 109
  cranial metastases, 110, 111
  non-small cell, 104, 107–111, 321–325
  occult or in situ, 108
  small cell, 104–105, 111, 325–327
  staging, 105, 106t, 107t
Lung metastases, colorectal primary, 148
Lung tumors, after Hodgkin's disease, 45
Luteinizing hormone-releasing hormone, 99
Lymphadenopathy
  ALL, 4
  AML, 11
  CLL, 16
  Hodgkin's disease, 41
  macroglobulinemia, 37–38
  non-Hodgkin's lymphoma, 48
Lymphoblastic lymphoma, 48, 54, 55
Lymphocytosis, and CLL, 16

Lymphoma (*see also specific types*)
  large cell, 18
  primary central nervous system, 260, 261
  splenic villous, 21

M-VAC
  and bladder cancer, 167–169, 293
  breast cancer, 272
  and endometrial cancer, 301
MAC III, 304
MACOP-B, 339
Macroglobulinemia, 32, 37–38
Magnesium, 368t
Magrath protocol, 339–340
MAID, 227, 353
Malaise
  ALL, 4
  AML, 11
  CML, 23
  grading, 367t
Malignant melanoma (*see Melanoma*)
Malignant meningiomas, 68
MALT lymphomas, 47, 54
Mantle cell lymphoma, 55
Marrow
  and CML, 24
  and melphalan, 35
Mastectomy pain, 500–501
Mayo Clinic regimen, 147
M-BACOD, 340
m-BACOD
  in non-Hodgkin's lymphoma, 340
  AIDS-related, 261, 267
MBC, 285
MCA, 301
MDS (*see* Myelodysplastic syndromes)
Mechlorethamine
  cutaneous lymphoma, 54
  hematologic toxicity, 377
  Hodgkin's disease, 329, 330
  profile, 447
Mediastinal mass, 55
Mediastinal radiation, 45
Medroxyprogesterone, 397, 447–448
Medulloblastoma, 68

Megestrol acetate
  for anorexia, 477
  breast cancer, 98–99
  endometrial cancer, 301
  for hot flashes, 98
  menses cessation, 503
  profile, 447–448
  renal cell cancer, 173
  thromboembolism, 398
Melanoma
  adjuvant therapy, 60–61,
    342–343
  after Hodgkin's diseases, 45
  clinical types, 58
  disseminated, 61–62, 253
  staging, 58, 59t, 60t
  vaccine, 63
Melphalan
  autologous marrow transplant,
    36
  bioavailability, 377
  dosage adjustments and toxic-
    ity, 35, 378
  Hodgkin's disease, 331
  macroglobulinemia, 38
  multiple myeloma, 35–36, 344,
    345, 346
  profile, 449
Memory loss, 401
MEN (multiple endocrine neoplasia), 83, 128, 163
Meningiomas, malignant, 68
Menopause (*see also* Amenorrhea)
  induction, 503
  symptom management,
    505–506t, 507t, 508
Mercaptopurine
  ALL, 311, 313–314
  and allopurinol, 382–383
  profile, 450
Mesna
  for bladder protection, 377
  cervical cancer, 300
  and Ewing's sarcoma, 347
  non-Hodgkin's lymphoma,
    337, 338, 341
  profile, 450–451
  soft tissue sarcoma, 227, 352,
    353
  unknown primary, 275
  Wilm's tumor, 246, 247–248

Metabolic abnormalities
  ALL, 4
  AML, 12
Metabolic toxicity, 367t–368t
Methotrexate (*see also* CMF;
    CMFP; Cooper Regimen;
    Hexa-CAF; m-BACOD;
    MFL; MVAC)
  ALL, 311–312, 313–314
    B-cell, 314–315
  bladder cancer, 167–169, 291,
    292, 293
  breast cancer, 94, 100
  and effusions, 383
  esophageal cancer, 284, 285
  gestational trophoblastic tu-
    mors, 210, 211–212,
    302–303, 304
  head and neck cancer, 308
  high dose
    and ALL, 8, 9
    and non-Hodgkin's lym-
      phoma, 339–340, 341
    and osteosarcoma, 349–350
  intrathecal
    and ALL, 311, 312, 313, 315
    and gestational trophoblastic
      tumors, 303
    and non-Hodgkin's lym-
      phoma, 54, 340, 341
    and retinoblastoma, 240
  non-Hodgkin's lymphoma,
    335, 336, 339, 341
    AIDS-related, 267–268
    Burkitt's lymphoma, 55,
      339–340, 341–342
  osteosarcoma, 348–349
  penile cancer, 188, 294
  pretreatment for, 287
  profile, 451–452
  soft tissue sarcoma, 227
Methoxyprogesterone, 98–99, 503
Metyrosine, 163
MF, 294
MFL, 282
MGUS, 32, 38–39
Michigan Regimen, 283
Microangiopathic hemolytic ane-
  mia, 378
Migraine, 397
MIME, 341

Mini-BEAM, 331
Mithramycin, 401–402
  and ALL, 319
  profile, 459–460
Mitomycin C (*see also* BOMP;
      DVM; MF; VAM)
  anal cancer, 153, 154
  bile duct cancer, 137
  breast cancer, 274
  esophageal cancer, 116, 282, 286
  gastric cancer, 286
  lung cancer, 324
  pancreatic cancer, 288, 290
  profile, 452–453
  toxicity and dosage, 378, 378t
Mitotane
  adrenal tumors, 160, 276
  dosage, 402
  profile, 453–454
  toxicity, 160
Mitoxantrone (*see also* CNF; FND;
      NFL)
  AML, 15, 317, 319
  breast cancer, 96
  and hepatobiliary system, 389
  hepatocellular carcinoma, 136
  non-Hodgkin's lymphoma,
    335, 338, 341
  and pleural effusion, 389
  profile, 454
  prostate cancer, 184, 295
MOF, 146
Molar pregnancy, 209–210
Monoamine oxidase inhibitors,
  130
Monoclonal antibodies
  and colon cancer, 147
  for non-Hodgkin's lymphoma,
    53
Monoclonal antibody therapy for
    breast cancer, 97
Monoclonal gammopathy, 32,
  38–39
Mood change, 365t, 399
MOPP
  and fertility, 45
  for Hodgkin's disease, 43–44,
    329
  subsequent MDS and leukemia
    risk, 26
MOPP/ABVD, 329

MP
  and multiple myeloma, 36
  and prostate cancer, 295
M2
  and macroglobulinemia, 38
  and multiple myeloma, 36,
    344–345
Mucosa-associated lymphoid
    tissue lymphoma, 47, 54
Mucosal toxicity
  doxorubicin, liposomal, 388t
  floxuridine, 379
  grading, 360t
  management, 483–491, 494–495
  methotrexate, 383
  procarbazine, 379
  teniposide, 392
Multiple endocrine neoplasia, 83,
  128, 163
Multiple myeloma
  and African Americans, 32
  as CLL transformation, 18
  diagnostic criteria, 33t
  indolent, 32
  staging, 33t
  treatment, 34–37, 344–346
MVP, 324
MVPP, 330
MVVPP, 330
Myalgias, 367t, 500
-*myc* oncogene, 16
Mycosis fungoides, 54–55
Myelodysplastic syndromes,
  26–31
  dysplastic changes, 27–28,
    27t
  iatrogenic, 26–27, 45
  morphological classification,
    27t
  treatment, 28–30, 346
Myocardial ischemia, 381

N-*myc* amplification, 231, 232
National Surgical Adjuvant
    Breast Project, 91, 93, 98
  colon cancer trial, 146
Nausea
  altretamine, 399
  grading, 358t
  management, 478–483,
    494

NCCTG trials, 146, 148
Neoadjuvant chemotherapy
  bladder cancer, 167
  head and neck cancer, 73–74
  neuroblastoma, 233
  osteosarcoma, 236
  pancreatic cancer, 289
  penile cancer, 188
Nephrotoxicity
  cisplatin, 376
  dosage adjustments,
    372t
  etidronate, 400–401
  gallium nitrate, 401
  grading, 360t–361t
  L-asparaginase, 394
  mitomycin, 378
Neuroblastoma, 230–234, 232t,
    233t, 348
Neuroendocrine tumors, 128–132,
    253
Neuroepithelial tumors, 228–229
Neurologic toxicity
  altretamine, 399
  cytarabine, 380
  docetaxel, 390
  fludarabine, 380
  fluorouracil, 401
  grading, 364t–366t
  ifosfamide, 376
  levamisole, 401
  paclitaxel, 390
  procarbazine, 379
  vincristine, 391
Neuropathies
  and hyperviscosity syndrome,
    38
  and multiple myeloma, 34
  and non-Hodgkin's lym-
    phomas, 48
Neutropenia (see also Hemato-
    logic toxicity)
  ALL, 4, 8
  AML, 11, 13
  CLL, 17
Neutrophilia, and MDS, 28
NFL, 272
NHL (see Non-Hodgkin's
    lymphoma)
Night sweats, 16, 41, 48
Nilutamide, 297

Non-Hodgkin's lymphoma (see
    also Macroglobulinemia)
  after Hodgkin's disease, 45
  AIDS-related, 258–261, 262t,
    267–268
  classification, 48–49, 48t, 50t,
    51t
  CNS involvement, 54, 55
  extranodal, 48, 49, 55
  and IgM paraprotein, 38
  indolent versus aggressive,
    49–54
  risk factors, 47, 49
  staging, 49, 51t, 52
  treatment, 52–54, 333–342
North Central Cancer Treatment
    Group trials, 146, 148
NSABP trial, 91, 93, 98
  colon cancer trial, 146
Nutrition, total parenteral, 8

Obesity, 381, 382, 385
Octreotide
  carcinoid tumors, 288
  and 5FU-induced diarrhea, 478
  neuroendocrine tumors, 130,
    131
  pancreatic islet cell tumors, 290
  pituitary tumors, 277
  profile, 454–455
Ocular toxicity, 369t, 397
Oligodendrogliomas, 66–67
Omeprazole, 132
Oncogenes, 91–92
Oncogenicity, of Hodgkin's dis-
    ease therapy, 45
Ondansetron, 477
Opioids, 497–500, 499t
Oprelvekin, 455–456
Osteolytic lesions, multiple
    myeloma, 34
Osteosarcoma, 235–237, 348–349
Ototoxicity, 375–376
Ovarian cancer
  borderline tumors, 220
  cellular classification, 214–215
  chemotherapy, 305–308
  staging and treatment, 217–220,
    218t
Ovarian germ cell tumors,
    221–222, 304

PA, 302
PAC, 302
PAC-I, 307
PACE, 327
Paclitaxel
    bladder cancer, 292, 293
    breast cancer, 100, 272
    cervical cancer, 204, 301
    endometrial cancer, 212
    esophageal cancer, 285, 286
    gestational trophoblastic tu-
        mors, 304
    head and neck cancer, 309
    lung cancer, 110, 322–323, 324,
        325
    musculoskeletal pain, 500
    ovarian cancer, 217, 219, 220,
        305, 306, 308
    premedication, 272, 305, 306
    profile, 456–457
    toxicity and dosage adjust-
        ments, 390
    unknown primary, 252, 275,
        276
Pain
    abdominal, 11, 23, 381
    musculoskeletal, 497, 498t, 500,
        501 (see also Bone pain)
    neuropathic, 500–501
        neuritic, 497, 499t
    visceral, 497–498, 499t
Pallor, 20, 23, 28
Pamidronate, 402, 457–458
Pancreatic cancer, 122–127, 124t,
        126t, 288–290
    islet cell tumors, 130–132, 131t,
        290–291
Pancreatic toxicity, 394
Pancytopenia, 4, 11 (see also
        Hematologic toxicity)
Papilledema, 397
Paroxysmal nocturnal hemoglo-
        binuria, 3, 11, 28
PCE, 275
PCV, 68, 347
PCVP, 333
Pegaspargase, 394, 411
Penile cancer, 186–189, 187t, 294
Pentostatin, 383–384, 458–459
Performance scales, 354–355
Peritoneal carcinomatosis, 252

Petechiae, 4, 11
Petroleum products, 32
PF, 285, 310
PFL, 310
Phenacetin, 170
Pheochromocytomas, 161–163
Philadelphia chromosome, 4, 23,
        24
Philadelphia-positive ALL, 9–10
Phlebitis, 364t
    chemical, 329
Phosphate, 4
Pineal germinomas, 68–69
Piritrexim, 293
Pituitary adenoma, 277
Pituitary insufficiency, 28
Plasma cell dyscrasias, 32–39
Plasmacytoma, 37
Plasmapheresis, 8, 13
Platelets, in CML, 24 (see also
        Thrombocytopenia)
PLL (see Prolymphocytic
        leukemia)
Pneumocystis carinii, 18
Pneumonitis, 45
Potassium, 4, 12, 157, 368t
Prednimustine
    and Hodgkin's disease, 332
    profile, 460
Prednisone (see also ABDIC;
        BVCPP; ChlVPP; CHOP;
        CMFP; Cooper Regimen;
        CVP; MOPP; M2; MVPP;
        MVVPP; PCVP)
    ALL, 8, 310, 311, 312, 313–314
        B-cell, 314–315
    CLL, 19, 320
    multiple myeloma, 35–36, 344,
        345
    for musculoskeletal pain, 500
    non-Hodgkin's lymphoma,
        333, 334, 335, 336, 337, 338,
        339, 341
    profile, 460–461
    prostate cancer, 184, 295
Preleukemia, 3, 11, 26–31
Preoperative chemotherapy (see
        Neoadjuvant chemother-
        apy)
Primitive neuroepithelial tumors,
        228–229

Procarbazine (*see also* MOPP)
  CNS tumors, 68, 347
  Hodgkin's disease, 328, 330, 333
  non-Hodgkin's lymphoma, 334, 335, 336
  profile, 461–462
  toxicity, 379
Progestational agents, 98–99
Prolymphocytic leukemia, 17, 18
ProMACE-CytaBOM, 341
Proptosis, 397
Prostate cancer
  advanced, 182–183
  bone metastases, 497
    bone pain, 184
  chemoprevention, 176
  chemotherapy, 184, 294–295
  cryosurgery, 181
  hormone therapy, 295–297
  localized, 176–182
  staging, 177t, 178t
Prostate specific antigen (PSA test), 175, 181
Prothrombin time, 368t
Psoralen with ultraviolet light, 54
Pulmonary toxicity
  bleomycin, 45, 384–385
  busulfan, 374
  grading, 362t–363t
Purine analogs, 22
PUVA, and cutaneous lymphoma, 54
PVB
  dysgerminoma, 222
  gestational trophoblastic tumors, 212, 304
  testicular cancer, 195, 299

Radiation, atomic, 11, 23
Radiation history
  and leukemia, 3, 11, 20
  and lung cancer, 107, 111
  and myelodysplastic syndromes, 26
  and plasma cell dyscrasias, 32
Radioactive iodine, 81, 82
Radioisotopes, 217, 497
Radionuclides, 184
Radiotherapy
  adrenal tumors, 160, 163
  anal cancer, 153, 278
    AIDS-related, 263
  bladder cancer, 167
  bone metastases, 497
  breast cancer, 93–94, 96
  central nervous system
    involvement, in ALL, 312
    prophylaxis, 268, 313, 315, 318
    tumors, 67
  cervical cancer, 200, 202, 203, 204
  chronic leukemias, 18, 25
  colon cancer, 146, 147, 280
  concurrent with chemotherapy, 116–117, 117t, 153, 289
  doxorubicin, 386
  endometrial cancer, 206, 207
  esophageal cancer, 115, 116–117, 117t, 282, 283
  gastric cancer, 119
  head and neck tumors, 74, 309, 310
  Hodgkin's disease, 43, 45
    and interferon a, 398
  Kaposi's sarcoma, 257
  lung cancer, 108, 109, 110
  non-Hodgkin's lymphoma, 52, 53, 54
  osteosarcoma, 236
  ovarian cancer, 217
    germ cell tumors, 222
  pancreatic cancer, 125, 137, 289
  penile cancer, 186, 188
  prostate cancer, 181, 182, 183
  rectal cancer, 148, 149, 280
  retinoblastoma, 240
  rhabdomyosarcoma, 241, 242, 351
  soft tissue sarcomas, 226
  testicular cancer, 193
  unknown primary, 253
  and vinblastine, 390
  Wilm's tumor, 246, 248–249
Ranitidine, 272, 305
Rectal cancer (*see also* Anal cancer)
  adjuvant therapy, 146, 279–280
  metastatic disease therapy, 147, 280–282
  postoperative monitoring, 148
  staging, 145t

Rectal carcinoid tumors, 128–130
Reed-Sternberg cells, 40, 41
Regimen 38, 351
Renal cell cancer
  chemotherapy, 173–174,
    297–298
  hereditary papillary carcinoma,
    170
  staging, 171t, 172t
  types, 171
Renal failure, and multiple
    myeloma, 34
Renal impairment (*see also*
    Nephrotoxicity)
  bleomycin, 385
  carboplatin, 374–375
  cladribine, 380
  daunorubicin, 385
  dosage reductions for, 372t
  estramustine, 400
  etoposide, 391, 392
  fludarabine, 380–381
  gallium nitrate, 401
  gemcitabine, 382
  hydroxyurea, 382
  idarubicin, 389
  ifosfamide, 377
  melphalan, 35, 378
  6-mercaptopurine, 383
  methotrexate, 383
  pamidronate, 402
  pentostatin, 383–384
  streptozotocin, 379
  teniposide, 392
  thioguanine, 384
  thiotepa, 379
  topotecan, 393
Retinoblastoma, 238–240
Retinoic acid syndrome, 14, 402
Retinoid agents, 176
Rhabdomyosarcoma, 241–245,
    350–351
Rheumatism, postchemotherapy,
    500
Richter's syndrome, 18
Rituximab, 53, 462
Roswell Park regimen, 147

Samarium, 184
Sarcomas, soft tissue, 223–227,
    225t, 351–354

Sargramostim, 463
Seminoma, 192, 193–194
Small intestine
  toxicity grading, 359t
  tumors, 128–130
SMF, 290
Sodium, 368t
Solvents, 20, 47
Somatostatin, 132
Somatostatinomas, 128
Southwestern Ocology Group
    NHL trial, 52
Speech disturbances, 401
Splenectomy, and acute
    leukemia, 45
Splenomegaly, 20, 23, 28, 48
Stanford V, and Hodgkin's dis-
    ease, 44, 330
Stanford Regimen, and non-
    Hodgkin's lymphoma, 341
Stem cell rescue, 55
Steroid withdrawal, 500
Stomatitis, 359t, 483–491, 491t,
    492–493t
Streptococcus pneumoniae, 18
Streptozotocin
  carcinoid tumors, 288
  neuroendocrine tumors, 130,
    131, 253
  pancreatic tumors, 290, 291
  pheochromocytoma, 163
  profile, 463–464
  toxicity, 379
  unknown primary, 253
Strontium, 184
Subacute leukemia, 26–31
Substance P, 501
Suramin, 161, 184, 464–465
Sweats, 367t
Sweeteners, artificial, 164
Sweet's syndrome, 28

T-cell lymphoma (*see* Lym-
    phoblastic lymphoma)
TA, 273
TAC, 273
Tamoxifen
  breast cancer, 94, 95, 97–98
  endometrial cancer risk, 205
  and hypercalcemia, 398
  melanoma, 61, 342

ovarian cancer, 220
profile, 465
renal cell cancer, 173
side effects, 98
Tartrate-resistant acid phosphatase, 20, 21
Taste change, 366t
Taxanes (*see also specific taxanes*)
breast cancer, 97, 100
head and neck tumors, 75
lung cancer, 110
melanoma, 61
TCF, 286
Temozolamide, 61–62
Teniposide
and acute leukemia risk, 26
ALL, 313, 314
and Down's syndrome patients, 392
neuroblastoma, 348
profile, 465–466
Teratocarcinoma, 192
Testicular cancer
histologic types, 193
metastatic, 195–197, 196t
nonseminoma, 194–195
salvage therapy, 197
seminoma, 193–194
staging, 191t, 192t
tumor markers, 192
Testolactone, 398
Tetrahydrocannabinol, 477
Thioguanine
ALL, 314
AML, 316, 318–319
hematologic toxicity, 384
profile, 466–467
Thiotepa
breast cancer, 273
profile, 467–468
toxicity, 379
Thoracotomy pain, 501
Thorotrast, 170
Thrombocytopenia
leukemias, 4, 11, 17, 20, 24
and mitomycin, 378
myelodysplastic syndromes, 28
Thromboplastin time, 368t
Thrombosis
diethylstilbesterol, 99
grading, 364t

medroxyprogesterone, 397
megesterol acetate, 398
multiple myeloma, 34
tamoxifen, 98
Thyroid dysfunction, 504
Thyroid tumors
after Hodgkin's disease, 45
anaplastic, 79–80
chemotherapy, 277
follicular, 82
Hurthle cell, 82
medullary, 83
papillary, 80–82
postsurgical monitoring, 81
staging, 80t
undifferentiated, 82–83
Tirapazamine, 61–62
TIT, 314–315
TMP/SMX, 339, 341
Tobacco, 3, 11
Topoisomerase-I inhibitors, 147
Topotecan
lung cancer, 110, 327
ovarian cancer, 220, 308
profile, 468
and renal impairment, 383
Toremifene, 98, 468–469
Total parenteral nutrition, 8
Toxicity
grading, 357–369
management bibliography, 493–495
Transcobalamin, 24
Transferrin, 28
TRAP, 20, 21
Trastuzumab, 97, 469
Tretinoin, 14, 318, 402, 470
Trimetrexate
dosage, 384
profile, 470
and prostate cancer, 184
T-10, 348–349
Tumor markers, 192

UCLA regimen, 290
Unknown primary, 250–254, 275–276
Uracil mustard, 379
Uremia, 378
Uric acid serum level, 24, 28

Urinary tract toxicity (*see also* Nephrotoxicity)
  grading, 360t–361t
  ifosfamide, 376–377

VABCD, 333
VABG, 197
VAB-6, 299
VAC
  ovarian germ cell tumors, 222
  rhabdomyosarcoma, 243
  soft tissue sarcoma, 354
Vaccines (*see also* Bacillus Calmette-Guérin)
  colon cancer, 147
  melanoma, 63
VAD, 36, 345
VAdCA+I/E, 347
Vaginal bleeding, 395
VAM, 273
VATH, 273
VBAP, 36, 346
VBD, 343
VBM, 294
VBMCP, 36, 344–345
VC, 274
VCAP, 345
VD, 274
VeIP, 197, 299
VFP, 302
VIG, 293
Vinblastine (*see also* ABVD; B-CAVe; BVCPP; CBVD; ChlVPP; CMV; EVAP; M-VAC; MVPP; MVVPP; PCVP; PVB; Stanford V; VABCD; VAM; VATH; VIG)
  breast cancer, 274
  and cachexic patients, 390
  and elderly patients, 390
  esophageal cancer, 283
  gestational trophoblastic tumors, 212
  Kaposi's sarcoma, 257
  melanoma, 61, 342, 343
  profile, 471–472
  prostate cancer, 184, 295
  renal cell cancer, 173
  and skin ulceration, 390
  testicular cancer, 195, 298, 299

Vincristine (*see also* CHOP; Cooper Regimen; CVP; DVM; EVA; m-BACOD; MOPP; M2; MVVPP; Stanford V; VAD; VBAP; VBMCP; VMCP)
  ALL, 8, 310, 311, 312, 313–314
    B-cell, 314–315
  anal cancer, 154
  bladder cancer, 167–168
  cervical cancer, 300
    in AIDS patients, 263
  CLL, 19, 320
  CNS tumors, 68, 347
  in elderly patients, 391
  Ewing's sarcoma, 229, 347
  gestational trophoblastic tumors, 210, 212, 303
  lung cancer, 325, 326
  multiple myeloma, 344, 345, 346
  neuroepithelial tumors, 229
  neurologic toxicity, 391
  non-Hodgkin's lymphoma, 333, 335, 336, 338, 339, 341
  osteosarcoma, 349
  penile cancer, 188, 294
  pheochromocytoma, 163
  profile, 472–473
  retinoblastoma, 240
  rhabdomyosarcoma, 242, 243, 244t, 350, 351
  soft tissue sarcoma, 227, 352, 354
  Wilm's tumor, 246, 247–248, 248t
Vindesine
  Hodgkin's disease, 332
  lung cancer, 110
Vinorelbine
  breast cancer, 274
  dosage modifications, 391
  and head and neck cancer, 310
  lung cancer, 110, 321, 324
  profile, 473
VIP, 197, 300
VIP-omas, 128, 132
Vision change, 365t, 397
Vitamin B_{12}, 24
Vitamin D_3, 29
Vitamin K, 4, 12

VM-26 (*see* Teniposide)
VMCP, 36, 345, 346
Vomiting
    and altretamine, 399
    emetogenic potential, 484–485t
    grading, 359t
    management, 478–483,
        486–490t, 494
Von Hippel-Lindau disease, 170
VP, and ALL, 310–312
VP-16 (*see* Etoposide)

Waldenstrom's macroglobuline-
    mia, 32, 37–38
Wayne State University
    anal cancer, 153
    esophageal cancer regimen, 283
    head and neck cancer regimen,
        310
Weight change
    and Hodgkin's disease, 41

    and leukemias, 4, 11, 16, 20, 23
    and non-Hodgkin's lym-
        phoma, 48
    toxicity grading, 367t
White blood count, 23, 24–25 (*see
    also* Hematologic toxicity)
Wilm's tumor, 246–249
Wiskott-Aldrich syndrome, 3, 11,
    47
Wood dust, 20

X-linked lymphoproliferative dis-
    ease, 47
Xerostomia, 491–493, 495

Yolk sac tumor, 192

Zidovudine, 260
Zollinger-Ellison syndrome,
    132
Zubrod performance scale, 355